# HORMONE-SECRETING
# PITUITARY TUMORS

Annual symposia on gynecologic endocrinology
held at the University of Tennessee and
published by Year Book Medical Publishers, Inc.


Volume 1
GYNECOLOGIC ENDOCRINOLOGY (1977)


Volume 2
ENDOCRINE CAUSES OF MENSTRUAL
DISORDERS (1978)


Volume 3
THE INFERTILE FEMALE (1979)


Volume 4
CLINICAL USE OF SEX STEROIDS (1980)


Volume 5
ENDOCRINOLOGY OF PREGNANCY (1981)

# HORMONE-SECRETING PITUITARY TUMORS

EDITOR
JAMES R. GIVENS, M.D.

ASSOCIATE EDITORS
ABBAS E. KITABCHI, M.D., Ph.D.
JAMES T. ROBERTSON, M.D.

Based on the proceedings of the Sixth Annual
Symposium on Gynecologic Endocrinology
held March 5–7, 1981 at the University of
Tennessee, Memphis, Tennessee

YEAR BOOK MEDICAL PUBLISHERS, INC.
CHICAGO • LONDON

# Dedication

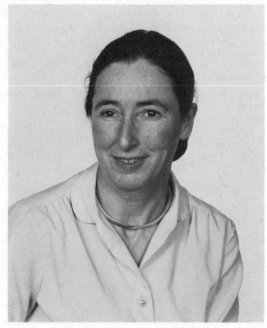

ANNE PAPPENHEIMER FORBES, M.D.

THIS VOLUME is dedicated to Dr. Anne Pappenheimer Forbes for her outstanding contributions to the science of endocrinology. After obtaining A.B. and M.D. degrees from Radcliffe College and the Columbia University College of Physicians and Surgeons, respectively, Dr. Forbes became a pediatric house officer in the Johns Hopkins Hospital. A succession of appointments in the Massachusetts General Hospital and in the Harvard Medical School followed, culminating in her promotion to the rank of Clinical Professor of Medicine.

In the Massachusetts General Hospital, Dr. Forbes first became associated with Dr. Fuller Albright and, as his health worsened, she became not only useful but indispensable to him. It was she who su-

v

pervised the workup of the endocrine cases he attracted from all over the world, and who translated the resulting therapeutic recommendations to his patients. At the same time Dr. Forbes, who with her husband was rearing a family of five children, permitted herself only the briefest of absences from her work. In the course of this arduous but rich apprenticeship, she achieved the refinement of clinical skill that distinguished her ever afterward.

To energy and clinical ability was added a capacity for rigorous thinking. The latter quality, so brilliantly exemplified by Dr. Albright, was systematically inculcated in his trainees. The marshalling of clinical evidence in a manner that permits the systematic testing of hypotheses is discernible in all of Dr. Forbes' work and is well illustrated by the deduction that prolactin (a then uncharacterized human hormone) must be hypersecreted in the syndrome of galactorrhea, amenorrhea and low urinary FSH. She published this remarkable finding in the memorable monograph, "Syndrome characterized by galactorrhea, amenorrhea and low urinary FSH: Comparison with acromegaly and normal lactation" (Forbes A.P., Henneman P.H., Griswold G.C., Albright F.: *J. Clin. Endocrinol. Metab.* 14:265, 1954).

While Dr. Forbes' scholarly contributions to endocrinology reflect her long association with Dr. Albright, they are by no means limited to it. Following his enforced retirement and subsequent death, she remarked that she had ingested "enough calcium for a lifetime." With characteristic imaginativeness, she struck out in new directions. Among the findings that resulted were a demonstration of the frequency of autoimmune disease in patients with gonadal dysgenesis, the existence of ovarian autoantibodies in certain patients with secondary amenorrhea, and the presence of anti-kidney antibodies in the serum of patients with primary tumors of the liver or kidney.

Schooled to abhor shoddy thinking, Dr. Forbes brought discipline as well as integrity to experimentation, colored by such qualities as wit, humaneness, and unfailing kindness to patients. Her students, fellows and colleagues savor her distinction, recognizing the improbability of encountering her like again.

JANET W. McARTHUR, M.D.

# Preface

THIS VOLUME represents the proceedings of the "Functioning Pituitary Tumors: Diagnosis and Treatment" symposium, which was sponsored by the Baptist Memorial Hospital, Memphis, Tennessee, in cooperation with the Pituitary Foundation of America, Inc., and the University of Tennessee College of Medicine. The symposium was held March 5–7, 1981, in the Frank S. Groner Education Center of the Baptist Memorial Hospital in Memphis. The speakers submitted prepared manuscripts of their presentations for publication. The panel discussions are edited transcriptions.

The first section of the book deals with the basic physiology of pituitary function, including neuroendocrine control of pituitary function, modulation of hypothalamic function by opioid and other peptides, and metabolic effects of neuroendocrine peptides. The second section describes the pretreatment hormonal evaluation of the patient. Also discussed in this section are the histopathology of pituitary tumors, as well as their radiologic therapy. The next several sessions of symposium (reproduced in sequential order in this volume) dealt with the diagnosis and management of Cushing's disease, acromegaly and prolactin-secreting tumors.

A particularly enlightening aspect of the program was the definition and clinical features of the amenorrhea-galactorrhea syndrome provided by Dr. Anne Forbes, to whom this volume is dedicated.

Considerable interest was generated by "The Great Debate," which examined the pros and cons of medical vs. surgical treatment of prolactin-secreting tumors. Proposing the medical therapeutic approach was Gordon M. Besser, M.D., and speaking in favor of the surgical treatment was George Tindall, M.D.

The last sections of the book concern the posttreatment evaluation of the pituitary patient and the complications and failures attending surgical management. Also included in this section is a discussion of the treatment of children with pituitary tumors and a review of pituitary tumor epidemiology.

vii

The cooperation and support of the Postgraduate Education Department of the Baptist Memorial Hospital under the able direction of Dr. Kenneth Burch, with the efficient assistance of Ms. Anne Wallace are gratefully acknowledged. The skillful assistance of Gabriela Radulescu and the staff at Year Book Medical Publishers was again essential to the success of this publication. The expert secretarial assistance of Jeanette Austin is gratefully appreciated.

JAMES R. GIVENS, M.D.

# Contributors

CHARLES F. ABBOUD, M.D.
Mayo Medical School, Mayo Clinic, Rochester, Minnesota

JAMES ACKER, M.D.
Department of Neuroradiology, Baptist Memorial Hospital, Memphis, Tennessee

JOHN F. ANNEGERS, PH.D.
Department of Epidemiology, The University of Texas School of Public Health, Houston, Texas

RICHARD M. BERGLAND, M.D.
Department of Neurosurgery, Beth Israel Hospital, Boston, Massachusetts

G. M. BESSER, M.D.
Department of Endocrinology, St. Bartholomew's Hospital, London, England

E. A. COWDEN, M.D.
Department of Physiology, University of Manitoba, Winnipeg, Manitoba, Canada

CAROLYN B. COULAM, M.D.
Department of Obstetrics and Gynecology, Mayo Clinic, Rochester, Minnesota

LOIS DAVIDSON, M.B.A.
President, Pituitary Foundation of America, Inc., Memphis, Tennessee

WILLIAM H. DAUGHADAY, M.D.
Metabolism Division, Washington University School of Medicine, St. Louis, Missouri

MIGUEL A. FARIA, JR., M.D.
Division of Neurosurgery, Department of Surgery, Emory University School of Medicine, Atlanta, Georgia

ix

PAUL A. FITZGERALD, M.D.
Departments of Neurological Surgery and Medicine, and the Metabolic Research Unit, University of California, San Francisco, California

ANNE P. FORBES, M.D.
Endocrine Unit, Massachusetts General Hospital, Boston, Massachusetts

PETER H. FORSHAM, M.D.
Departments of Neurological Surgery and Medicine, and the Metabolic Research Unit, University of California, San Francisco, California

H. G. FREISEN, M.D.
Department of Physiology, University of Manitoba, Winnipeg, Manitoba, Canada

JAMES R. GIVENS, M.D.
Department of Obstetrics and Gynecology, University of Tennessee Center for the Health Sciences, Memphis, Tennessee

EVA HORVATH, M.D.
Department of Pathology, St. Michael's Hospital, University of Toronto, Toronto, Ontario, Canada

RICHARD JORDAN, M.D.
Department of Medicine, University of Arkansas for Medical Sciences, Little Rock, Arkansas

ABBAS E. KITABCHI, M.D., PH.D.
Departments of Medicine and Biochemistry, The University of Tennessee College of Medicine, Memphis, Tennessee

PETER O. KOHLER, M.D.
Department of Medicine, University of Arkansas for Medical Sciences, Little Rock, Arkansas

KALMAN T. KOVACS, M.D., PH.D., F.R.C.P.
Department of Pathology, St. Michael's Hospital, University of Toronto, Toronto, Ontario, Canada

DOROTHY T. KRIEGER, M.D.
Department of Medicine, Division of Endocrinology, Mount Sinai Medical Center, New York, New York

I. LANCRAJAN, M.D.
Department of Physiology, University of Manitoba, Winnipeg, Manitoba, Canada

EDWARD R. LAWS, JR., M.D.
Department of Neurologic Surgery, Mayo Medical School, Mayo Clinic, Rochester, Minnesota

RAYMOND V. RANDALL, M.D.
Division of Endocrinology/Metabolism and Internal Medicine, Mayo Medical School, Mayo Clinic, Rochester, Minnesota

SEYMOUR REICHLIN, M.D., PH.D.
Division of Endocrinology, New England Medical Center Hospital, Boston, Massachusetts

JAMES T. ROBERTSON, M.D.
Department of Neurosurgery, University of Tennessee Center for the Health Sciences, Memphis, Tennessee

ALAN D. ROGOL, M.D.
Departments of Pediatrics and Pharmacology, The University of Virginia School of Medicine, Charlottesville, Virginia

GLENN E. SHELINE, M.D., PH.D.
Department of Radiation Oncology, University of California, San Francisco, California

L. CASS TERRY, M.D., PH.D.
Department of Neuroendocrinology, Veterans Administration Hospital, Memphis, Tennessee

GEORGE T. TINDALL, M.D.
Division of Neurosurgery, Emory University School of Medicine, Atlanta, Georgia

J. BLAKE TYRRELL, M.D.
Departments of Neurological Surgery and Medicine, and the Metabolic Research Unit, University of California, San Francisco, California

CHARLES B. WILSON, M.D.
Department of Neurosurgery, University of California, San Francisco, California

# Contents

# Neuroendocrinology of Pituitary Regulation

SEYMOUR REICHLIN, M.D., PH.D.

*Professor of Medicine, Tufts University School of Medicine; Chief, Endocrine Division, New England Medical Center Hospital*

THE FACT THAT ALL ANTERIOR PITUITARY SECRETIONS are under the control of the hypothalamus has important implications for understanding of the pathogenesis and manifestations of adenoma of the pituitary. New findings that reveal the high incidence of clinically silent adenomas, and the embarrassing inaccuracy of current radiologic techniques for the diagnosis of prolactinoma, the most common pituitary adenoma, have further emphasized the importance of physiologic studies for the identification of pituitary disorder. This chapter reviews current concepts of the nature of the hypothalamic-pituitary control mechanism, and the physiologic basis of neuroendocrine strategies for the clinical evaluation of pituitary adenomas. These topical areas have been recently summarized in comprehensive monographs and reviews.[1-13]

## The Concept of Neurosecretion

Central to the understanding of neural control of the pituitary is the concept of neurosecretion.[14-18] As currently defined, neurosecretion refers to the synthesis and release of chemical substances by neurons (Fig 1). When so defined, it is apparent that virtually all neurons are neurosecretory. Some, like cholinergic neurons, synthesize

---

Laboratory studies referred to in this review were supported by research grants: USPHS—AM 16684, Clinical Study Unit RR0054, and Endocrinology Training Grant AM 07039.

1

SUPRAOPTICOHYPOPHYSIAL HYPOPHYSIOTROPHIC NEUROMODULATORS

RELEASES VASOPRESSIN (ADH) AND OXYTOCIN INTO THE PERIPHERAL CIRCULATION.

RELEASES HYPOPHYSIOTROPHIC HORMONES INTO INTERSTITIAL SPACE OF MEDIAN EMINENCE OF HYPOTHALAMUS, THENCE THE RELEASING FACTORS REACH THE PITUITARY VIA THE HYPOPHYSIAL-PORTAL VESSELS.

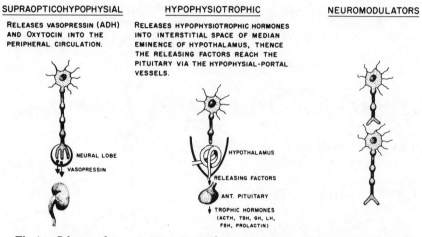

NEURAL LOBE
VASOPRESSIN

HYPOTHALAMUS
RELEASING FACTORS
ANT. PITUITARY
TROPHIC HORMONES (ACTH, TSH, GH, LH, FSH, PROLACTIN)

Fig 1.—Schema of neurosecretory, peptidergic neurons involved in pituitary regulation and neuromodulation. (From Reichlin S., in Williams R.H. (ed): *Textbook of Endocrinology*. Philadelphia: W.B. Saunders Co. In press. Used by permission.)

acetylcholine by enzymatic processes and release their product at presynaptic nerve endings that may terminate on other nerve cells, glandular cells, or muscle cells. Other kinds of neurons may synthesize and release into synapses neurotransmitters, such as norepinephrine, glutamic acid, and γ-aminobutyric acid. Other kinds of neurosecretory neurons may release their product into the blood. Such neurosecretions can be referred to as neurohormones because they satisfy the classic description of a hormone as a substance arising in one structure to influence the activity of another structure at a more remote site. Most of the neurons involved in pituitary regulation are neurohormone-secretory because they release their secretory products (vasopressin and oxytocin, the secretions of the neurohypophysis) directly into the general bloodstream or into the specialized (hypophysial-portal) blood supply that links the hypothalamus and anterior pituitary.

The bulk of neurons involved directly in pituitary gland regulation secrete polypeptides, and for this reason they are called peptidergic neurons. But at least one bioamine, dopamine, is involved in anterior pituitary regulation. All cells giving rise to neurosecretions that ultimately impinge upon the pituitary are themselves influenced by other neurons—some aminergic, some peptidergic. To understand how these interactions are brought about it is necessary to consider the physical structure of the hypothalamus and pituitary.

## Anatomy of the Hypothalamic-Pituitary Unit

The pituitary gland is divided into a glandular portion (adenohypophysis, anterior lobe, pars distalis), intermediate lobe (pars intermedia), and a neural lobe (posterior pituitary, infundibular process) that is a direct downgrowth of tissue from the base of the hypothalamus (Fig 2). The intermediate lobe is rudimentary in man, making up less than 0.8% of total weight. A significant number of intermediate-lobe cells are diffusely distributed in the adenohypophysis and neural lobe of man. The neurohypophysis consists of specialized tissue at the base of the hypothalamus, together with the neural stalk and lobe. The neurohypophysial portion of the hypothalamus forms the base of the third ventricle. Viewed grossly, this region resembles a funnel, and was given the name infundibulum (Latin for funnel) by early anatomists. Indeed, a funnel function was assigned to this re-

**Fig 2.**—Sagittal view of the human hypothalamic-pituitary unit illustrating the anatomical relationships between optic chiasm and pituitary stalk. (From Post K.D., et al. (eds): *The Pituitary Adenoma.* New York: Plenum Medical Book Co., 1980. Used by permission.)

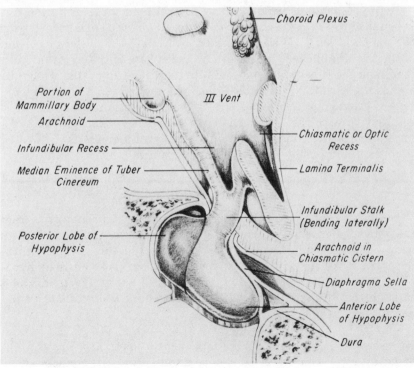

gion by Vesalius, who believed that cerebrospinal fluid drained through this structure into the nose to form mucous. The pituitary gains its name from this fanciful origin of mucus ("pituita"). The central portion of the infundibulum is enveloped from below by the pars tuberalis portion of the anterior pituitary gland and is penetrated by numerous capillary loops of the primary portal plexus of the hypophysial-portal circulation (Fig 3). This neurovascular complex forms a small but conspicuous structure at the base of the hypothalamus that is termed the median eminence of the tuber cinereum. Neurons arising in the hypothalamus in regions adjacent to the pars tuberalis and terminating in the infundibulum are designated tuberoinfundibular (TI) neurons. For the most part, these are regulatory to the pituitary (hypophysis) and are also called hypophysiotropic.

Although the median eminence is anatomically classified as part of the neurohypophysis and is traversed by fibers of the supraoptic and paraventricular neurons, this structure is primarily related to control of the anterior pituitary. In the median eminence, transfer of neurosecretions of hypophysiotropic neurons of the hypothalamus to the pituitary *blood* supply takes place.

The hypothalamus is outlined by several landmarks. Anteriorly, it is bounded by the optic chiasm and laterally by the sulci formed with the temporal lobes. The mammillary bodies are the posterior portion of the hypothalamus. The smooth, rounded base of the hypothalamus is termed the tuber cinereum, and its central region, from which descends the pituitary stalk, is termed the median eminence. The extent of the median eminence can be easily determined because it is coextensive with the distribution of the primary plexus of the hypophysial-portal circulation. Dorsally, the hypothalamus is delineated from the thalamus by the hypothalamic sulcus.

## The Neurohypophysis

The neural lobe develops embryologically as a downgrowth from the ventral diencephalon and retains its neural connections and its neural character in adult life. The dominant features of the neurohypophysis are the supraopticohypophysial and paraventriculohypophysial nerve tracts. These unmyelinated nerve tracts descend through the infundibulum and the neural stalk to terminate in the neural lobe[19] (see Fig 3).

Most cells that originate in these tracts are strikingly large (and hence are called magnocellular) and for the most part are consolidated into well-characterized groups situated in paired nuclei above

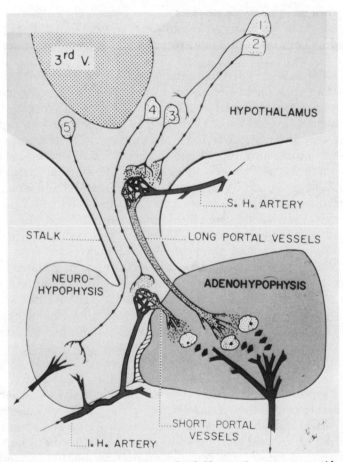

**Fig 3.**—Neural control of the pituitary gland. Neuron 5 represents peptidergic neurons of supraopticohypophysial and paraventricular-hypophysial tracts, with hormone-producing cell bodies in hypothalamus and nerve terminals in neural lobe. Neurons 3 and 4 represent tuberoinfundibular neurons, which secrete hypophysiotropic hormones. Most are peptides (hence the nerves are peptidergic), and at least one group is dopamine secretors (hence dopaminergic). Neurons 1 and 2 represent nerves that regulate hypophysiotropic hormone secretion, either by synapses on soma of hypophysiotropic neurons *(1)*, or ending in the substance of the median eminence *(2)*. These act by releasing neurotransmitter in relation to nerve endings of tuberoinfundibular neurons. (From Gay V.L.: *Fertil. Steril.* 23: 50, 1972. Used by permission.)

the optic tract (supraoptic) and on each side of the ventricle (paraventricular). A few small cells of this system are also distributed between the two nuclei. The other nerve cells of the hypothalamus are relatively small (paravicellular) and do not have any obvious distinguishing characteristics by conventional microscopy. Because of the prominence of the neurohypophysial cell bodies, they have been the subject of study for many years, and have been shown to be richly endowed by capillaries the fenestrated endothelia of which are characteristic of endocrine glands generally.

Specific antiserums directed singly against vasopressin, oxytocin, and the two chief classes of neurophysin (the neurohypophysial carrier protein) have confirmed earlier morphological studies that show that principal projections of the two nuclei terminate in the neural lobe. New specific methods have shown an additional pathway of neurophysin-containing nerve endings within the median eminence in apposition to the primary plexus of the hypophysial-portal circulation. Thus, the neurohypophysial neurons may have a role in anterior pituitary regulation as well as in neural lobe regulation. Direct assays of blood in the portal circulation show high concentrations of neurophysin, vasopressin, and oxytocin, a fact that confirms the anatomical observations, although more recent work suggests that they may also arise by reflux from the pituitary. Most of the cell bodies in the supraoptic nucleus contain vasopressin, but some contain oxytocin. A somewhat smaller percentage (but still the majority of stainable cells) in the paraventricular nucleus contain vasopressin. Most cells contain either one or the other peptide, but studies by Defendini and Zimmerman suggest that a given cell may contain both. Not all authors agree on this point. Because vasopressin and oxytocin release can be dissociated physiologically, the two different types of cells must be regulated individually. Neurophysin-vasopressin-containing neurons arising in the paraventricular nuclei also project to the dorsal hypothalamus, brain stem, and spinal cord. These findings suggest that the neurohypophysial peptides may have a more general function in brain regulation in addition to neurohypophysial secretion. Recently, somatostatin has also been identified in the supraoptic nuclei with projections to the neural lobe.

Neurons of the neurohypophysis are the classic example of neurosecretory cells and are the model of the tuberoinfundibular neurons that regulate anterior pituitary function by way of the hypothalamic hypophysiotropic factors (releasing hormones).

Vasopressin and oxytocin are synthesized mainly in the cell bodies of the supraoptic and paraventricular neurons. Like all neurosecretions, these hormones are transported in small vesicles enclosed by a membrane. Secretory vesicles containing the hormones flow down the axons to the neural lobe, where they are stored and later released when stimulated by a propagated action potentional originating in the neuronal cell body. Neurosecretory cells and cells of this type are called neuroendocrine transducers. They convert (transduce) neural information to hormone information.

The function of neurohypophysial neurons is in turn directly controlled by cholinergic and noradrenergic neurotransmitters; several neuropeptides may also be important regulators of secretion. Release of vasopressin and oxytocin is stimulated by cholinergic impulses. Adrenergic influences, in contrast, are inhibitory to both hormone secretion and electric activity.

The secretion of vasopressin is also stimulated by angiotensin II. This peptide can be synthesized entirely within the brain as well as by the peripheral renin-angiotensin system. Neurohypophysial neurons are also stimulated by endogenous opiates (endorphins). The well-known antidiuretic action of morphine is due to release of vasopressin, an effect that can be duplicated by the administration of β-endorphin.

Plasma osmolarity is the most important determinant of vasopressin secretion, an effect mediated through neural mechanisms. This neuronal activation—and the accompanying release of vasopressin— is functional proof that some type of "osmoreceptor" exists within the perfusion area of the internal carotid artery. Whether the osmoreceptor neuron is distinct from the vasopressin neurosecretory neuron has not been established, but it has been shown by direct electric recording that some neurons that project to the neural lobe are immediately activated following exposure to hypertonic saline. Changes in osmolarity most likely alter the electric properties of the membranes of the osmoreceptor cell, thereby changing its firing rate.

The neurohypophysial neurons also respond to blood-volume receptors located in the left atrium and in other vascular areas. In addition, the secretion of vasopressin is affected by various parts of the "visceral brain" and the reticular activation system—regions involved in the maintenance of consciousness and in emotional expression.

When the supraopticohypophysial system is deprived of neural input from other parts of the brain, neurons in this region are electrically more active than normal and vasopressin secretion is enhanced. Denervation hyperfunction of the neurohypophysis may explain the syndrome of "inappropriate ADH (antidiuretic hormone) secretion," which occurs in certain kinds and locations of brain damage.

Damage to the neurohypophysis or to its central controlling input leads to diabetes insipidus. Excessive secretion by the neurohypophysis can also occur due to an abnormality of the neural regulating system.

## The Median Eminence and Tuberoinfundibular Neurons

Harris and Fink[20] were the first to recognize fully the functional significance of the fact that nearly all the blood that reaches the anterior pituitary has first traversed capillary plexuses located in the median eminence and adjoining neural stalk. Their postulate, originally termed the portal vessel-chemotransmitter hypothesis, was that these vessels formed part of a neurovascular link by which the hypothalamus, through the mediation of neurohumoral substances, regulated the secretion of the anterior pituitary tropic hormones. This hypothesis has been amply proved.

The median eminence consists of a neural component (nerve fibers of the neurohypophysis, nerve endings of the tuberoinfundibular neurons), a vascular component (the hypophysial-portal capillaries and veins), and an epithelial component (the pars tuberalis of the adenohypophysis). Electron microscopic studies show that the infundibulum is composed mainly of densely packed nerve endings, capillaries with conspicuous perivascular spaces, supporting cells that resemble neurohypophysial pituicytes, and specialized ependymal cells (tanycytes) that traverse the median eminence from the lumen of the third ventricle to the outer mantle plexus.

Two classes of tuberohypophysial neurons project to the median eminence. Some are peptidergic (for example, thyrotropin-releasing hormone (TRH), luteinizing-hormone-releasing hormone (LH-RH), and somatostatin) (Fig 4). Others are bioaminergic, the most important of which are dopaminergic.

The large perivascular space contact area and the peculiar vessels in this region, which have fenestrations typical of those seen in ordinary endocrine glands, account for the observation that unlike most of the brain, the neurohypophysis, including the median eminence, is particularly permeable to molecules such as thyroxine, trypan blue, and growth hormone (GH).

The median eminence contains ten or more biologically active substances, including several hypothalamic peptides, neurotransmitters (dopamine, norepinephrine, serotonin, acetylcholine, γ-aminobutyric acid, histamine), and a variety of other active substances. Most workers believe that there are no morphologically demonstrable synapses in the median eminence. As Joseph and Knigge[21] point out: "The extracellular and perivascular space of the median eminence would appear to be a medium of remarkable composition. Although some regional topography is emerging, the phenomenon of diffusion occurring after release alone would suggest that large pools of nerve

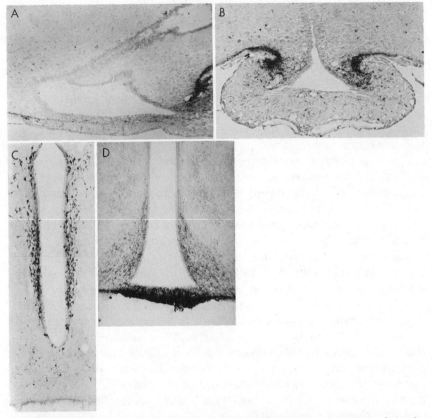

**Fig 4.**—Peptidergic neuronal pathways in the hypophysiotropic system. **A,** sagittal section of rat hypothalamus stained with anti-LHRH antibody by Sternberger sandwich technique. **B,** frontal section of rat hypothalamus shows median eminence stained by using anti-LHRH. **C,** periventricular somatostatinergic neuron cell bodies. **D,** median eminence somatostatinergic nerve endings. (**A** and **B,** courtesy of Dr. Lesley Colton Alpert. **C** and **D,** courtesy of Dr. Ronald Lechan.)

terminals and nonneural elements are bathed in an interstitial fluid containing a multitude of hormones, and excitatory and inhibitory neurotransmitters."

Although classic studies have demonstrated that the direction of blood flow in the long portal vessels is from the hypothalamus to the pituitary, more recent work indicates that flow of blood from pituitary to median eminence also occurs.[22, 23] One consequence of this circular flow is that the hypothalamus is exposed to exceedingly high concentrations of the secretions of both anterior and posterior pituitary lobes.

The epithelial component of the median eminence, the pars tuberalis, is in the form of a thin glandular sheath around the infundibulum and pituitary stalk. In some animals, the epithelial component may make up as much as 10% of the total glandular tissue of the pituitary; several pituitary tropic hormones have been extracted from this region. Moreover, nerve fibers can be traced to the pars tuberalis. Yet the bulk of studies indicates that the pars tuberalis does not have an important physiologic function, but serves merely as the region through which arteries and veins of the hypophysial-portal circulation are conducted.

The hypophysial portal-chemotransmitter hypothesis of pituitary control was introduced as an explanation of how the anterior pituitary gland, which is devoid of secretomotor nerve fibers, could be influenced by the nervous system. According to this hypothesis, which initially was based on purely morphological considerations, neurohumoral substances released from nerve endings in the median eminence enter capillaries of the primary plexus of the hypophysial-portal circulation and are carried by the portal veins of the hypophysial stalk into the sinusoids of the pituitary.

Definitive proof of this hypothesis came when TRH and LH-RH were chemically identified and shown to be present in hypophysial-portal blood. These findings together with the demonstration of neurosecretory tuberohypophysial neurons permit the conclusion that the portal-vessel chemotransmitter hypothesis has been fully validated. For their work on the elucidation of the chemistry of the hypophysiotropic hormones, Roger Guillemin[24] and Andrew Schally[25] were awarded Nobel Prizes in 1977.

The search for hypothalamic neurohumors with anterior-pituitary regulating properties focused on extracts of stalk median eminence (SME) and hypothalmus. Hypophysiotropic materials that stimulate the release of pituitary hormones have been called releasing factors, after the first description of corticotropin-releasing factor (CRF). At present the term releasing factor is still applied to substances of unknown chemical nature, while those with established chemical identity, such as TRH and LH-RH, have been called releasing hormones. Use of the term hypophysiotropic or releasing factor to describe hypothalamic secretions regulating adenohypophysial function is too restrictive. One such regulator is somatostatin, which inhibits GH and TSH secretion. Another hypothalamic secretion that inhibits pituitary secretion is dopamine. The chemical structures of the three peptide pituitary regulating hormones identified thus far are shown in

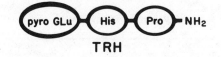

**TRH**

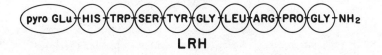

**LRH**

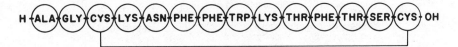

## SOMATOSTATIN

H-Ser-Gln-Glu-Pro-Pro-Ile-Ser-Leu-Asp-Leu-
Thr-Phe-His-Leu-Leu-Arg-Glu-Val-Leu-Glu-Met-
Thr-Lys-Ala-Asp-Gln-Leu-Ala-Gln-Gln-Ala-His-
Ser-Asn-Arg-Lys-Leu-Leu-Asp-Ile-Ala-NH$_2$

**Fig 5.**—Structures of the known peptide hypothalamic pituitary regulating hormones. The structure sequence of ovine CRF is shown at bottom.

Figure 5. Dopamine can also be included in the list of hypothalamic secretions that act directly on the pituitary, since it is present in portal-vessel blood in sufficient concentration to duplicate all its known effects on the pituitary gland. Biologic activities in hypothalamic extracts as yet uncharacterized chemically are shown in Table 1.

Certain hypothalamic factors exert significant inhibitory actions on anterior pituitary function. Inhibitory factors interact with the respective releasing factor to exert dual control of secretion of prolactin, GH, TSH, and to a lesser extent the gonadotropins.

The action of each of the hypophysiotropic hormones is not limited strictly to a single pituitary hormone. For example, TRH is a potent releaser of prolactin, and under some circumstances releases ACTH and GH. LH-RH releases both LH and FSH. Somatostatin inhibits secretion of GH, TSH, and a wide variety of other nonpituitary hormones. The principal inhibitor of prolactin secretion is dopamine, but this potent bioamine acting directly on the pituitary is also inhibitory to TSH and gonadotropin secretion, and under some circumstances is also inhibitory to GH secretion.

TABLE 1.—Hypophysiotropic Hormones of
Established Function but Unknown Structure

| NAME | FUNCTION |
|------|----------|
| Growth-hormone-releasing factor (GRF), somatotropin-releasing factor (SRF) | Releases GH† |
| Prolactin-releasing factor (PRF) | Releases prolactin,‡ not TSH |
| Prolactin-inhibitory factor (PIF) | Inhibits prolactin release§ |

†A number of amino acids and peptides will stimulate release of GH under certain conditions in vivo or in vitro. These include glucagon, MSH, β-endorphin, neurotensin, substance P, TRH, LH-RH, and a decapeptide isolated from porcine hypothalamic extracts that is chemically identical with the alpha chain of porcine hemoglobin. None is now believed to be an authentic GRF because of inconsistencies of effects in various test systems, and because the GH-release system is relatively easily affected by nonspecific factors.

‡TRH, a peptide of established structure, is a potent prolactin-releasing factor and has a role in maintenance of normal prolactin secretion, but is not the most potent releaser of prolactin found in hypothalamic extracts. VIP may be an important PRF.

§Hypothalamic extracts contain several factors that inhibit prolactin release: dopamine, GABA, and His-Pro-diketopiperazine; dopamine is the most important of these.

## Thyrotropin-Releasing Hormone

The chemical structure of TRH was elucidated by investigators working in association with Drs. Roger Guillemin and Andrew Schally. Their work, which was the culmination of more than a decade of effort to identify the nature of the thyrotropin-releasing activity of crude hypothalamic extracts, made neuroendocrinology credible to the general scientific and clinical community. It also made possible the introduction of TRH into clinical medicine, vastly widened the scope of understanding of TRH in other biologic systems, and gave a powerful incentive to efforts to identify other biologic activities in hypothalamic extract.

TRH is a relatively simple substance, a tripeptide amide, (pyro)Glu-His-Pro-NH$_2$. TRH is chemically stable, but is rapidly degraded in plasma by enzymatic action. Following injection in man or in the rat, blood TSH levels rise rapidly and dramatically, a change detected within three minutes; peak values are attained between ten and 20 minutes after injection in normal individuals, somewhat later in patients with pituitary or hypothalamic hypothyroidism (Fig 6). The standard clinical dose commonly administered as a bolus is 500 μg. Transient mild nausea, a sense of urinary urgency, and mild de-

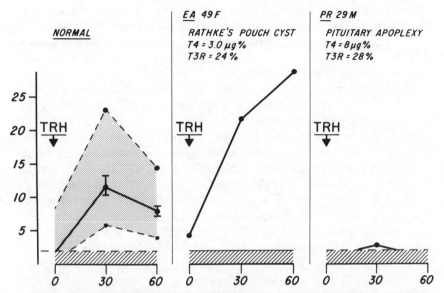

**Fig 6.**—Classical TSH responses to TRH. In normals *(left panel)* 500 μg of TRH is shown to bring about the release of TSH, peaking at 30 minutes. *Middle panel* shows response in a patient with hypothalamic hypothyroidism due to Rathke's pouch cyst. The response is greater than normal, and prolonged. This effect may be due to the hypothyroid state together with low GH levels. *Right panel* shows no response in a patient whose pituitary has been largely destroyed by pituitary apoplexy. Unfortunately, all responses do not fit into these categories. Some patients with TSH deficiency due to hypothalamic deficiency fail to respond to TRH, while some patients with TSH deficiency due to pituitary damage may respond normally.

creases or increases in blood pressure occur as side effects of injection in an appreciable number of patients, but no serious or life-threatening complications have been reported. The surge of TSH release induced by TRH injection leads to a readily detected rise in plasma triiodothyronine and an increase in thyroxine release that may not be large enough to produce significant increase in plasma levels of this hormone.

One of the most important aspects of TRH action on the pituitary is that its effects are blocked by prior treatment with thyroid hormone. The interaction of the negative-feedback action of thyroxine on the pituitary with the stimulating effects of TRH is the basis of the integrated neuroendocrine control system of TSH secretion. Somatostatin also plays a role in regulating TSH release. TRH cannot be used as a diagnostic agent in patients receiving thyroid hormone replacement.

In addition to bringing about TSH release, TRH is also a potent prolactin-releasing factor. The time course of response of blood prolactin levels to TRH, dose-response characteristics, and suppressibility by thyroid hormone pretreatment (all of which parallel changes in TSH secretion) make it seem likely that TRH is involved in the regulation of prolactin secretion.

Despite these striking overlapping effects, the evidence suggests that TRH plays no more than a modulator role in prolactin regulation under normal circumstances.

TRH has no influence on pituitary hormones other than TSH and prolactin in normal individuals. However, under special circumstances, it exerts a number of other effects on pituitary secretion, including the release of ACTH in some patients who have Cushing's syndrome and of GH in some acromegalics. These responses are thought to be due to the presence on pituitary cell membranes of TRH receptors ordinarily obscured by the normal regulatory processes of the pituitary or appearing as a consequence of "derepression" of the adenoma to a more primitive cell resembling an ancestral pituitary stem cell. TRH also releases GH in some patients with anorexia nervosa, in children with hypothyroidism, and in patients with psychotic depression. TRH also inhibits sleep-induced GH release through a central nervous system mechanism and has other central nervous system effects.

## Extrahypothalamic Distribution and Function of TRH

TRH was the first of the hypothalamic hypophysiotropic hormones to be found outside the hypothalamus. This observation was among the findings that led to current interest in peptides as neuroregulators. It has been found by immunoassay or immunohistochemistry in virtually all parts of the brain, including the cerebral cortex and spinal cord, nerve endings abutting on the ventral horn motor cells, the circumventricular structures, the neurohypophysis, and the pineal (for reviews see Jackson and Reichlin[27] and Jackson[28]). TRH has also been found in pancreatic islet cells and in various parts of the gastrointestinal tract. Although present in low concentrations in these areas, the aggregate in extrahypothalamic tissues exceeds the total amount in the hypothalamus. As the phylogenetic scale is descended, the concentration of TRH found in neural tissues outside the hypothalamus increases, so that in the frog, for example, the concentration in all extrahypothalamic brain is fully half that in the hypothalamus.[28, 29] In some species of frogs, TRH is found in the skin in concentrations higher than those found in the hypothalamus, an association presumed to be related to the embryologic origin of skin cells in neuroectoderm. TRH has been detected in the most primitive vertebrate, the larval form of the lamprey; in the amphioxus, a provertebrate; and in snail nerve ganglia. Since the lamprey probably does not synthesize TSH, and amphioxus and snails lack a pituitary gland, it appears that the TRH molecule appeared in evolutionary development as a primitive neurosecretion prior to the development of TSH, and that the pituitary has "co-opted" TRH as its regulatory hormone (for a review, see Jackson[28, 29]). The same might be said for dopamine, which first appears in the nervous nets of the sponge, a primitive invertebrate.

The extensive extrahypothalamic distribution of TRH, its localization in nerve endings, and the presence of TRH receptors in brain tissue strongly suggest that it serves as a neurotransmitter or neuromodulator outside the hypothalamus.

## Gonadotropic-Hormone-Releasing Hormone (GnRH), LH-RH

It has been known for more than 20 years from the work of McCann and of Harris and their respective collaborators that extracts of hypothalamic tissue contain one or more biologically active substances capable of stimulating the release of gonadotropic hormones from the pituitary. This material was isolated in almost pure form from the hypothalami of stockyard animals by Guillemin and by Schally and their collaborators, and the structure was finally elucidated by Schally's group in 1971.

Following intravenous injection, the naturally occurring LH-RH or its synthetic form brings about a prompt dose-related release of LH and FSH in man (Fig 7). The onset of effect on FSH release after a single bolus injection is somewhat delayed as compared with effects on LH secretion; the values peak at ten to 30 minutes after injection. The response to LH-RH is markedly influenced by the prior LH-RH secretory state, the steroid milieu of the patient, the time course of LH-RH injection (i.e., single dose, multiple pulses, or constant infusion), and perhaps by the patient's sex. LH-RH is less effective in patients who have had no prior exposure to the peptide such as those with hypogonadotropic hypogonadism. Repeated injections restore normal sensitivity. Sustained high doses transiently stimulate and then suppress gonadotropin secretion. This is the basis for its proposed use as an ovulation blocker. In women, estrogen administration sensitizes the pituitary to effects of LH-RH. These and other aspects

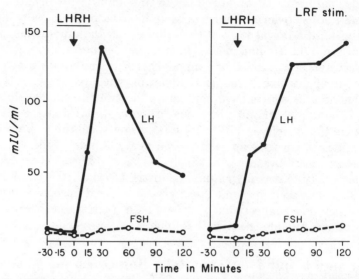

Fig 7.—Gonadotropin secretory response to intravenous injection of LH-RH, 100 μg in a normal woman during the follicular phase of the menstrual cycle. Administration of diethylstilbestrol, 2 mg per day for 7 days, sensitized the pituitary to a second test dose of LH-RH. This sensitization response to female hormone is part of the normal mechanisms that underlie the midcycle ovulatory surge.

of LH-RH effect have limited its use as a diagnostic agent in evaluation of hypogonadism.

Through secondary effects of pituitary activation, and under appropriately defined conditions, LH-RH can induce spermatogenesis and testosterone production in men with hypothalamic hypogonadotropic hypogonadism and ovulation in women with hypothalamic amenorrhea (for a recent review see Casper[30] and Beling[31])

Most reproductive neuroendocrinologists now believe that the LH-RH decapeptide is the only hypothalamic gonadotropin regulator and that observed dissociations of secretion are due to the interacting effects of prior hormone status, steroid pretreatment, and history of exposure to LH-RH, but some observations still cannot be explained by this unitary hypothesis.

## Extrahypothalamic Distribution and Function of GnRH

Unlike TRH and somatostatin, almost all the GnRH in the brain is restricted to the hypothalamus and related neural structures. Small amounts are found in the circumventricular organs, including the pineal gland. LH-RH (as in the case for TRH) has also been found in milk, a discovery that suggests that the breast, a dermal-derived structure with embryologic origins analogous to the primitive neuroectoderm, which is the source of neuroendocrine cells generally, may have LH-RH synthesizing capacity. The possibility that the breast concentrates LH-RH from the blood also has to be considered. LH-RH is also present in the placenta of man, and is the principal neurotransmitter in frog sympathetic ganglia. On direct application to individual nerve cells, LH-RH can enhance or depress certain populations of cells. Even though this peptide is found in a very restricted area, responding cells are localized in many other areas of the brain. The most important neural effects of LH-RH in mammals appear to be those involved in regulation of mating behavior. Direct injection of LH-RH into the hypothalamus has been reported to enhance female sexual responsivity even in animals without a pituitary and hence incapable of responding with gonadotropin-ovarian activation. The effects on sexual function in man are being investigated. There is evidence that LH-RH can stimulate sexual function in man unrelated to activation of pituitary function.

## Somatostatin

During the course of their efforts to isolate GRF from hypothalamic extracts, Krulich and McCann discovered a fraction that inhibited GH release from pituitary incubates in vitro. They named the factor growth-hormone-release-inhibitory factor (GIF), and postulated that GH secretion was regulated by a dual control system, one stimulatory, the other inhibitory. Relatively little attention was paid to GIF when it was first discovered because it was thought by most workers to be a relatively nonspecific effect. Several years later, in 1972, Brazeau and a number of collaborators attempting to isolate GRF in Guillemin's laboratory again identified the inhibitory factor, and with the background in methodology gained from earlier studies of TRH and LH-RH, were able in a relatively short time to isolate and identify a potent peptide from hypothalamic extracts that inhibited GH release in every assay system in which it was studied (for reviews see Guillemin[32] and Reichlin[33]). The material, to which the name somatostatin was applied, is a 14-amino-acid peptide that lacks the amide and pyroglutamic acid termini characteristic of LH-RH and TRH but which contains an S-S cyclic bridge similar to that of vasopressin and oxytocin (see Fig 6). That somatostatin is important as a physiologic regulator of GH release is shown by studies in which the somatostatinergic pathways are damaged or endogenous somatostatin is neutralized by treatment with antisomatostatin antibody.

Shortly after chemically synthesized somatostatin became available for study, it was found to inhibit the secretion of TSH, glucagon, and insulin. Subsequently, somatostatin has been shown to inhibit the secretion of many other secretory structures in the body (including virtually all the glands of the gastrointestinal tract) (Table 2). Contemporary studies of somatostatin content of body tissues, carried out by radioimmunoassay and immunohistochemistry, showed that most tissues that respond to somatostatin contain this peptide in specialized neurosecretory cells. Thus, somatostatin, originally isolated from the hypothalamus, has been shown to be a widely distributed tissue component that in some settings acts as a paracrine secretion ("control of one cell by secretions of an adjacent tissue") and in others as a neuroendocrine secretion (as in the tuberohypophysial neurons of the hypothalamus). It even acts as an autocrine secretion in the pancreas and thyroid parafollicular cells and perhaps elsewhere.

Of the hypophysiotropic hormones thus far isolated, somatostatin has the highest extrahypothalamic concentration, both in other parts of the central nervous system and in extraneural structures, especially the gastrointestinal tract.

## Corticotropin-Releasing Factor

Although corticotropin-releasing factor (CRF) was the first of the releasing factors to be recognized and named by Saffran and Schally, but its chemical nature was not disclosed until 1981 when Vale and

TABLE 2.—GLANDULAR SECRETIONS INHIBITED
BY SOMATOSTATIN

| GLAND | SECRETION |
|---|---|
| Pituitary | GH |
| | TSH |
| Pancreas | Glucagon |
| | Insulin |
| | Vasoactive intestinal peptide (VIP) |
| Gastrointestinal tract | Gastrin |
| | Gastric acid |
| | VIP |
| | Cholecystokinin-pancreazymin |
| | Bombesin |
| | Motilin |
| | Secretin |
| Kidney | Renin |
| Thyroid | Calcitonin |
| | Thyroxine |

colleagues[34] reported that a 42-residue peptide isolated from sheep hypothalamic tissue had all the activity predicted. The material acts only on ACTH release. Although it releases ACTH from all species tested, it is not immunologically cross-reactive with most species. Whether there is another CRF as well is unknown.

## Prolactin-Regulatory Factors

In keeping with the observation that the hypothalamus exerts an *inhibitory* effect on prolactin secretion is the observation that hypothalamic extracts contain one or more substances inhibitory in prolactin release. This activity was termed prolactin-inhibitory factor (PIF) by Meites and collaborators. PIF has been identified in portal-vessel blood by Kamberi, Porter, and their collaborators, an accomplishment that again satisfies the critical requirement of evidence for physiologic significance of a hypophysiotropic hormone.

Dopamine is the most important PIF. This biogenic amine, the secretory product of the tuberohypophysial dopaminergic pathways, has recently been shown to be present in hypophysial-portal vessel blood in sufficient concentration to inhibit prolactin release. γ-Aminobutyric acid (GABA), a constituent of hypothalamic extracts, is also an active PIF, but its presence in portal-vessel blood in appropriate concentrations has not yet been established. Several groups have also claimed that there is at least one additional PIF activity, one distinct from the two that have already been mentioned. One candidate is His-Pro-diketopiperazine, a metabolic breakdown product of TRH.[35] Dopamine alone can explain all the known prolactin-inhibitory functions of the hypothalamus, but not all the PIF activity of hypothalamic extracts.

Although the stalk section and transplantation experiments indicate that the predominant effect of the hypothalamus on prolactin secretion is inhibitory, the acute release of prolactin seen after suckling and acute stress have raised the possibility that there is a prolactin-releasing factor. Crude and partially purified extracts of hypothalamic tissue bring about the release of prolactin. Several well-characterized hypothalamic peptides also release prolactin on systemic injection. These include vasopressin, TRH, neurotensin, VIP, substance P, and β-endorphin. The effects of crude extracts have been shown to be independent of their content of ADH and TRH, but the other factors have not been excluded as the active substance. VIP added directly to pituitary cells is a potent PRF.[36]

## Regulation of Secretion of the Tuberohypophysial Neurons: Neuropharmacology of Hypothalamic Regulation

As outlined in previous sections, the tuberohypophysial neurons form the "final common pathway" of neural control of the anterior pituitary and thereby serve as the ultimate neuroendocrine transducer. This group of neurons is acted on by the feedback effects of hormones secreted by target glands, such as the sex steroids, thyroid hormone, and cortisol, by pituitary peptide hormones (short-loop feedback control), by classic neurotransmitters (through which communication from the rest of the brain is mediated), and by neuropeptide modulators. This complex set of controls is integrated at the neuronal level for the regulation of anterior pituitary secretion.

## Neurotransmitter Regulation of Hypophysiotropic Neurons

The function of central bioaminergic neurotransmitters is of enormous importance for the understanding of psychiatric disease, of behavior, and of effect as well as control of the pituitary[37-41] (Fig 8).

The structures of the important hypothalamic neurotransmitters are reviewed in the chapter by Dr. Terry in this volume.

## Dopaminergic Pathways

An important group of bioaminergic neurons involved in anterior pituitary regulation arise mainly in the arcuate nucleus of the hypothalamus and are distributed to the median eminence. This grouping, termed the dopaminergic tuberohypophysial system, is important mainly for its function in direct control of anterior pituitary secretion. Three other relatively independent dopaminergic systems have also been identified. The best known, and the earliest to be recognized by neurologists, is that involved in extrapyramidal control, namely, the nigrostriatal pathways, which arise in the substantia nigra in the hindbrain, and are distributed to the caudate nucleus and other structures in the forebrain. Parkinson's disease is due to defects in this system. A third dopaminergic system arises in cells adjacent to the hypothalamus and projects to several hypothalamic regulatory areas, and the fourth (mesolimbic) projects to the visceral brain. Dopaminergic neurotransmitters may be of importance by producing either

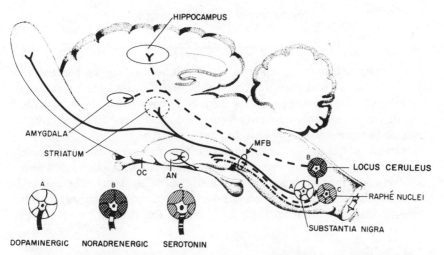

Fig 8.—Ascending monoaminergic pathways in mammalian brain. The principal localization of the neurons containing norepinephrine, dopamine, and serotonin is in the mesencephalon and pons. Axons of these cells are distributed to widespread areas of cortex, limbic system, and striatum. The dopaminergic system of the arcuate is an exception to this general scheme of distribution. *MFB,* medial forebrain bundle; *AN,* arcuate nucleus; *OC,* optic chiasm. (From Martin J.B., et al., in *Clinical Neuroendocrinology,* Philadelphia: F.A. Davis, 1977. Used by permission.)

direct effects on the pituitary or indirect effects on other tuberoinfundibular neurons (or both). This complexity of input underlines the problem of using dopamine agonists and antagonists for analyzing the neuropharmacologic coding of anterior pituitary regulation.

## Noradrenergic Pathways

All the cell bodies of origin of the noradrenergic pathways arise outside the hypothalamus in several nuclear groups in the hindbrain, the most conspicuous of which is the locus ceruleus, a cell group found in the floor of the fourth ventricle. From the locus ceruleus, noradrenergic fibers ascend to the hypothalamus and other midbrain and forebrain structures and descend into the spinal cord. The bulk of noradrenergic fibers involved in neuroendocrine control arise from areas adjacent to the locus ceruleus and also from cells anatomically close to the nucleus of the vagus nerve. These ascend in defined anatomical pathways and terminate on cell bodies of tuberohypophysial neurons, neurohypophysial neurons, and with the median eminence itself.

## Serotonergic Pathways

Most of the serotonergic neurons project to the hypothalamus from cell bodies located in the brainstem (raphe nuclei). They are extensively distributed to neurons, and to a lesser extent to the median eminence, and to ependymal cells. Serotonin-containing nerve endings ramify over the ventricular surface of the brain. There is probably an intrinsic serotonin pathway within the hypothalamus analogous to the tuberohypophysial dopamine pathway.

Dopamine, serotonin, and noradrenaline pathways are the principal control systems, but recent work has demonstrated the presence of adrenergic and histaminergic neural control systems. The cell bodies arise for the most part in hindbrain regions, but there are also smaller intrinsic bioaminergic systems self-contained in the hypothalamus.

## Cholinergic Control

Tuberoinfundibular control is also exerted by cholinergic neurons. Choline acetyltransferase, an enzyme marker of acetylcholine synthesis, is distributed in all defined nuclei in the hypothalamus, including the arcuate, and in the median eminence, two regions especially related to anterior pituitary control. Because only small changes have been noted in medial basal hypothalamic concentration of choline acetyltransferase after surgical isolation of this region of the brain, it has been proposed that there is ". . . a cholinergic tuberoinfundibular pathway similar to the dopaminergic one, which may be responsible for the neuroendocrine effects of cholinergic agents."

GABA has also been demonstrated in fairly high concentration in the hypothalamus and median eminence, and the presence of GABA-sensitive neurons has been demonstrated by microiontophoresis in the hypothalamic ventromedial nucleus as well as other sites in the "endocrine hypothalamus."

Neuropeptides with hypothalamic distribution of nerve endings are substance P, met-enkephalin (an endorphin), angiotensin II, neurotensin, gastrin, and cholecystokinin. The findings of met-enkephalin-containing cell bodies in the hypothalamus and a median eminence distribution support the presence of an intrinsic control system for this peptide as well as a system with projections from other parts of the brain.

When called on to explain neural control of anterior pituitary secretion, the contemporary neuroendocrinologist suffers from an em-

TABLE 3.—NEUROTRANSMITTERS AND
ANTERIOR PITUITARY SECRETION*

| ANTERIOR PITUITARY SECRETION | NEUROTRANSMITTERS† | | | | | |
|---|---|---|---|---|---|---|
| | NE | DA | 5-HT | ACh | H | GABA |
| ACTH | ↓→ | ↓→ | ↑ | ↑ | ↑ | ↓ |
| TSH | ↑ | ↓ | ↓ | → | — | — |
| LH/FSH | ↑ | ↕ | ↓→ | ↑ | ↑ | ↑ |
| GH | ↑ | ↑ | ↑ | → | → | →↓ |
| PRL | ↕ | ↓ | ↑ | ↕↕ | ↑ | ↕↕ |

*Adapted from Muller et al.[42] and Weiner and Ganong.[43] Symbols: (↑), increase; (↓), decrease; (→), no change; (—), not known. The effects of various neurotransmitters is inferred from neuropharmacologic studies using agonists, antagonists, and precursors. It must be emphasized that there are many inconsistencies and contradictions in the literature. These are due in part to species differences, prior functional status, lack of specificity of some drugs, and direct pituitary effects differing from hypothalamic effects.

†NE, norepinephrine (noradrenaline); DA, dopamine; 5-HT, 5-hydroxytryptamine (serotonin); ACh, acetylcholine; H, histamine; GABA, γ-aminobutyric acid.

barrassment of riches with regard to potential neurohumoral mediators. Summarized in Table 3 are the overall effects of the various classes of neurotransmitters and other hypothalamic regulators on anterior pituitary regulation. It should be borne in mind that a given effect of an agonist or antagonist may be due to direct or indirect effects on other regulatory systems and that many of the findings are not uniform in all studies in all animals and under all conditions.

## Endocrine Significance of Neuropeptides

In addition to the enkephalins and the hypophysiotropic peptides, a number of other peptides have been demonstrated to occur in neurons distributed in the hypothalamus and other brain regions.[17] Almost all are represented in characteristic glandular cells of the gastrointestinal tract, believed to arise in embryologic life from the primitive neuroectoderm. Most have effects on anterior pituitary function.[44] Their physiologic role in pituitary regulation remains to be elucidated.

REFERENCES

1. Martin J.B., Reichlin S., Brown G.M.: *Clinical Neuroendocrinology*. Philadelphia: F.A. Davis Co., 1977.
2. Martini L., Besser G.M. (eds): *Clinical Neuroendocrinology*. New York: Academic Press, 1977.
3. Reichlin S., Baldessarini R.J., Martin J.B. (eds): *The Hypothalamus*. New York: Raven Press, 1978.
4. Everett J.W.: The mammalian hypothalamo-hypophysial system, in Jeffcoate S.L., et al. (eds): *The Endocrine Hypothalamus*. New York: Academic Press, 1978.
5. Fuxe K., Hökfelt T., Luft R. (eds): *Central Regulation of the Endocrine System*. New York: Plenum Press, 1978.
6. Jeffcoate S.L., Hutchinson J.S. (eds): *The Endocrine Hypothalamus*. London: Academic Press, 1978.
7. Tolis G., Labrie F., Martin J.B., et al. (eds): *Clinical Neuroendoendocrinology*. New York: Raven Press, 1979.
8. Gotto A.M. Jr., Peck E.J. Jr., Boyd A.E. III (eds): *Brain Peptides: A New Endocrinology*. New York: Elsevier/North-Holland, 1979.
9. Reichlin S.: The control of anterior pituitary secretion, in Beeson P.B., et al. (eds): *Cecil Textbook of Medicine*. Philadelphia: W.B. Saunders Co., 1979.
10. Gauger G.E.: Anatomy of the pituitary and hypothalamus, in Linfoot J.A. (ed): *Recent Advances in the Diagnosis and Treatment of Pituitary Tumors*. New York: Raven Press, 1979.
11. Reichlin S.: Anatomical and physiological basis of hypothalamic-pituitary regulation, in Post K.D., et al. (eds): *The Pituitary Adenoma*. New York: Plenum Medical Book Co., 1980.
12. Krieger D.T., Hughes J.C.: *Neuroendocrinology*. Sunderland, Mass.: Sinauer Associates, 1980.
13. Reichlin S.: Neuroendocrinology, in Williams R.H. (ed.): *Textbook of Endocrinology*. Philadelphia: W.B. Saunders Co. In press.
14. Sawyer C.H.: Neuroendocrine regulation: The peptidergic neuron: introduction and historical background, in Fuxe K., et al. (eds): *Central Regulation of the Endocrine System*. New York: Plenum Press, 1978.
15. Pickering B.T.: The neurosecretory neuron: A model system for the study of secretion. *Essays Biochem.* 14:45, 1978.
16. Klee W.A.: Peptides of the central nervous system. *Adv. Protein Chem.* 33:243, 1979.
17. Hökfelt T., Johansson O., Ljungdahl A., et al.: Peptidergic neurons. *Nature* 284:515, 1980.
18. Martin J.B., Reichlin S., Bick K.L. (eds.): *Neurosecretion and Brain Peptides*. New York: Raven Press, 1981.
19. Zimmerman E.A.: The organization of oxytocin and vasopressin pathways, in Martin J.B., et al. (eds): *Neurosecretion and Brain Peptides*. New York: Raven Press, 1981.
20. Fink G.: The development of the releasing factor concept. *Clin. Endocrinol.* 5(Suppl. 2):45s, 1976.
21. Joseph S.A., Knigge K.M.: The endocrine hypothalamus: Recent anatomical studies, in Reichlin S., et al. (eds): *The Hypothalamus*. New York: Raven Press, 1978.

22. Oliver C., Mical R.S., Porter J.C.: Hypothalamic-pituitary vasculature: Evidence for retrograde blood flow in the pituitary stalk. *Endocrinology* 101:598, 1977.
23. Bergland R.M., Page R.B.: Pituitary-brain vascular relations: A new paradigm. *Science* 204:18, 1979.
24. Guillemin R.: Peptides in the brain: The new endocrinology of the neuron. *Science* 202:390, 1978.
25. Schally A.V.: Aspects of hypothalamic regulation of the pituitary gland: Its implications for the control of reproductive processes. *Science* 202:18, 1978.
26. Sandow J., Konig W.: Chemistry of the hypothalamic hormones, in Jeffcoate S.L., et al. (eds): *The Endocrine Hypothalamus.* New York: Academic Press, 1978.
27. Jackson I.M.D., Reichlin S.: Distribution and biosynthesis of TRH in the nervous system, in Collu R., et al. (eds): *Central Nervous System Effects of Hypothalamic Hormones and Other Peptides.* New York: Raven Press, 1979.
28. Jackson I.M.D.: Distribution and evolutionary significance of the hypophysiotropic hormones of the hypothalamus. *Front. Hormone Res.* 6:35, 1980.
29. Jackson I.M.D.: The releasing factors of the hypothalamus, in Barrington E.J.W. (ed): *Hormones and Evolution.* London: Academic Press, 1979.
30. Casper R.F., Yen S.S.C.: Recent advances in hypothalamic "hormones" and their clinical implications, in Linfoot J.A. (ed): *Recent Advances in the Diagnosis and Treatment of Pituitary Tumors.* New York, Raven Press, 1980.
31. Beling C.G., Wentz A.C. (eds): *The LH-Releasing Hormone.* New York: Masson Publishing, USA, 1980.
32. Guillemin R.: Hypothalamic hormones: Releasing and inhibiting factors, in Krieger D.T., et al. (eds): *Neuroendocrinology.* Sunderland, Mass.: Sinauer Associates, 1980.
33. Reichlin S.: Systems for the study of regulation of neuropeptide secretion, in Martin J.B., et al. (eds): *Neurosecretion and Brain Peptides.* New York, Raven Press, 1981, pp. 573–597.
34. Vale, W., Speiss J., Rivier C., Rivier J.: Characterization of a 41-residue ovine hypothalamic peptide that stimulates secretion of corticotropin and β-endorphin. *Science* 213:1394, 1981.
35. Bauer K., Graf K.J., Faivre-Bauman A., et al.: Inhibition of prolactin secretion by histidyl-proline-diketopiperazine. *Nature* 274:174, 1978.
36. Shaar C.J., Clemens J.A., Dininger N.B.: Effect of vasoactive intestinal polypeptide on prolactin release in vitro. *Life Sci.* 25:2071, 1979.
37. Hökfelt T., Elde R., Fuxe K., et al.: Aminergic and peptidergic pathways in the nervous system with special reference to the hypothalamus, in Reichlin S., et al. (eds): *The Hypothalamus.* New York: Raven Press, 1978.
38. del Pozo E., Lancranjan I.: Clinical use of drugs modifying the release of anterior pituitary hormones, in Ganong W.F., et al. (eds): *Frontiers in Neuroendocrinology.* New York: Raven Press, 1978, vol 5.
39. Kordon C.: Role and regulation of neuropeptide neurons, in Fuxe K., et al. (eds): *Central Regulation of the Endocrine System.* New York: Plenum Press, 1979.

40. Krulich L.: Central neurotransmitters and the secretion of prolactin, GH, LH and TSH. *Ann. Rev. Physiol.* 41:603, 1979.
41. Frohman L.A.: Neurotransmitters as regulators of endocrine function, in Krieger D.T., et al. (eds): *Neuroendocrinology.* Sunderland, Mass.: Sinauer Associates, 1980.
42. Müler E.E., Nistico G., Scapagnini V.: Neurotransmitters and anterior pituitary function. Academic Press, Inc., 1977.
43. Weiner, R.I. and Ganong, W.F.: Role of brain monoamines and histamine in regulation of anterior pituitary secretion. Physiol. Rev. 58:905–976, 1978.
44. Imura H., Kato Y., Katakami H., et al.: Effect of CNS peptides on hypothalamic regulation of pituitary secretion, in Martin J.B., et al. (eds): *Neurosecretion and Brain Peptides.* New York: Raven Press, 1981.

# Neuropharmacologic Regulation of Anterior Pituitary Hormone Secretion in Man

L. CASS TERRY, M.D., PH.D.

*Associate Professor of Neurology*
*University of Michigan and VA Medical Center*
*Ann Arbor, Michigan*

## Introduction

THE REGULATION OF ANTERIOR PITUITARY HORMONE SECRETION by neurotransmitters and neuropeptides has been the subject of extensive research in recent years. Advances in this field were made possible by the development of sensitive radioimmunoassays and radioenzymatic assays for pituitary and hypothalamic hormones and biogenic amines, by development of neuropharmacologic agents that interfered with various aspects of neurotransmitter actions in the brain, by anatomical mapping of peptidergic and monoaminergic systems within the brain using immunohistochemical techniques, and by the study of enzymes involved in the biosynthesis of biogenic amines. From these studies it now appears that hypothalamic peptidergic neurons regulate the secretion of anterior pituitary hormones by direct effects on pituitary cells. Peptidergic neurons are regulated, in turn, by biogenic aminergic neurons that stimulate or inhibit the release of releasing or inhibiting hormones. Prolactin (PRL) may be an exception to this concept, since dopamine has a direct inhibitory action on PRL-secreting pituitary cells.

The abundance of monoamines in the hypothalamus and surrounding regions has been documented,[1-4] and there is convincing evidence to implicate the catecholamines—norepinephrine, dopamine, and the

27

0-8151-3530-0/82/0006-27-44-$03.75

indolamine, serotonin—in the regulation of anterior pituitary hormone secretion (Fig 1).[5-11] Histamine, acetylcholine, and γ-aminobutyric acid (see Fig 1) also influence the secretion of some pituitary hormones,[5-11] but available evidence is less complete and their role in pituitary regulation is not clearly established.

The finding that L-dopa, a biosynthetic precursor of dopamine, and bromocriptine, a dopamine-receptor agonist, inhibit the secretion of PRL from the pituitary gland has provided new insights into the pharmacologic control of neurosecretory mechanisms. Moreover, the suppressive effect of bromocriptine on PRL-secreting adenomas, and GH in acromegaly, has led to medical treatments for these disorders.[12]

The purpose of this chapter is to review recent knowledge concerning the pharmacology and clinical use of biogenic aminergic and peptidergic neurotransmitters that influence the secretion of anterior pituitary hormones in man. The discussion is limited to GH, PRL, and adrenocorticotropin, since they are products of the most common types of hypersecreting pituitary tumors.

## Synthesis and Metabolism of Neurotransmitters

Knowledge of the synthesis and metabolism of neurotransmitters is necessary in order to understand the mechanisms by which neuropharmacologic agents influence neurosecretion. This section focuses on norepinephrine, dopamine, and serotonin because they are biogenic amines that have been studied most extensively in regard to

Fig 1.—Structures of putative neurotransmitters involved in anterior pituitary hormone regulation.

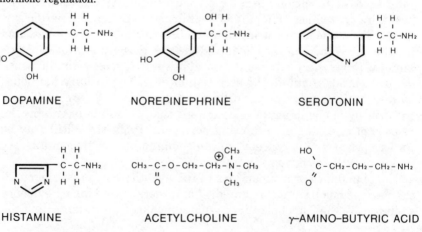

their synthesis, metabolism, and role in neuroendocrine regulation. However, it is important to bear in mind that other neurotransmitters, such as acetylcholine, γ-aminobutryic acid, and histamine, as well as others not yet discovered, may function as regulators of neuroendocrine function. Furthermore, several of the neuropeptides, such as opioids, substance P, and neurotensin, may also be important in the regulation of hypothalamic releasing and inhibiting factors.[5-11] The description that follows is an overview of the subject; the reader is referred to a recent review by Cooper et al.[13] for a more detailed presentation.

## CENTRAL CATECHOLAMINERGIC NEURONS

Tyrosine, an essential amino acid, is transported actively into the brain. L-Dopa is also taken up actively by catecholaminergic neurons. After its entry into cells, tyrosine is hydroxylated by tyrosine hydroxylase to L-dopa. L-Dopa is then decarboxylated by a nonspecific enzyme, L-amino acid decarboxylase, to dopamine, which, in turn, is hydroxylated by the enzyme dopamine-β-hydroxylase to norepinephrine. Norepinephrine can be methylated to form epinephrine by phenylethanolamine-N-methyltransferase.

After their synthesis, dopamine, norepinephrine, and epinephrine are stored in cytoplasmic granules within nerve terminals. In response to neuronal depolarization, granules are extruded from the nerve endings into the synaptic cleft. It is assumed that specific postsynaptic binding sites (receptors) are present on hypothalamic peptidergic neurons. Analogous to the peripheral autonomic nervous system, it is postulated that there are two classes of norepinephrine receptors on hypothalamic neurons, one corresponding to α-receptors and the other to β-receptors. Dopamine receptors are also believed to exist on certain hypothalamic neurons. It appears likely that some hypothalamic neurons may have more than one type of receptor. Agents that mimic the effects of biogenic amines are called agonists or receptor-agonists and agents that block their effects are called antagonists or receptor-blockers.

After catecholamines are released, free neurotransmitter in the synaptic cleft that is not bound to the receptor can be taken up into the presynaptic nerve ending and reincorporated back into storage granules. Postsynaptically bound or free catecholamines are vulnerable to destruction by the enzymes monoamine oxidase (MAO) or catechol-O-methyltransferase (COMT).

## CENTRAL SEROTONERGIC NEURONS

The neuropharmacology of serotonin (5-hydroxytryptamine) has not been characterized as well as that of the catecholamines. However, a hypothetical model has been constructed that explains most of the available information. The function of serotonergic neurons is described as similar to that of the catecholamines.

Tryptophan, the precursor of serotonin, is taken up actively by neurons. It is converted to 5-hydroxytryptophan by tryptophan hydroxylase, and subsequently decarboxylated by L-amino acid decarboxylase to serotonin. In certain brain tissues, such as the pineal gland and retina, serotonin is converted to melatonin. Melatonin may also function as a neurotransmitter, although the evidence is not conclusive at present.

Serotonin is stored in cytoplasmic granules in nerve endings. The storage mechanism for serotonin is similar to that of catecholamines, since it is abolished by the same drugs that cause a depletion of catecholamines. The control of the release process for serotonin has not been completely established. Serotonin is thought to interact with specific postsynaptic receptors. As is the case with catecholamines, the action of serotonin is terminated by re-uptake into the presynaptic nerve endings or enzymatic degradation by monoamine oxidase.

## Sites of Action of Neurotransmitters

The concentration of catecholamines and serotonin is greater in the hypothalamus than in most other regions of the brain,[1-4] and these agents are thought to be the primary central monoaminergic neurotransmitters that regulate neuroendocrine function.[5-11] The monoamines are concentrated in the hypophysiotropic area of the hypothalamus, where the cell bodies of many of the peptidergic neurons that produce hypothalamic peptides are located.[4] In addition, axons from monoaminergic neurons extend into the external lamina of the median eminence, where they are in close contact with peptidergic axons and the hypothalamic-pituitary portal system, which transports releasing factors and neurotransmitters to the pituitary gland.

There are several potential loci at which anterior pituitary hormone secretion could be influenced by neurotransmitters.[5] One possibility is direct axoaxonic synapses between monoaminergic nerve terminals, which liberate a given neurotransmitter, and peptidergic terminals, which contain releasing or inhibiting factors. Secondly, direct axodendritic or axosomatic contacts between neuronal elements, or multisynaptic connections through monoaminergic neurons distant to the peptidergic neuron, are also possible. Thirdly, neurotransmitter release into the portal circulation could directly stimulate or inhibit pituitary hormone release or alter pituitary sensitivity to releasing/inhibiting factors. This appears to be the case with dopamine and PRL. Alternatively, monoamines in the peripheral circulation might affect anterior pituitary function through a direct effect on the pituitary, or indirectly by affecting peripheral nerve pathways communicating with the central nervous system. Finally, neurons may contain both monoamines and peptides, with the former affecting secretion of the latter.

With the exception of prolactin, there is general agreement that the effects of neurotransmitters on anterior pituitary hormones are mediated by releasing and/or inhibiting factors.[5-11] However, recent data suggest that neurotransmitters may have a direct pituitary action. Acetylcholine receptor sites on rat and sheep anterior pituitary glands have been reported.[14-17] Also, $\alpha_2$-adrenergic receptors in cultures of bovine anterior pituitary cells showed close correlation with secretion of adrenocorticotropin.[18] Furthermore, γ-aminobutyric acid was reported to inhibit directly PRL release from isolated rat pituitary glands in doses as low as 0.1 μg/ml,[19] suggesting that γ-aminobutyric acid, in addition to dopamine, may have PRL-inhibiting factor ability.[20-21] Whether these effects are meaningful physiologically still remains to be determined.

## Growth Hormone

Plasma levels of GH, measured at frequent intervals throughout the day and night, show striking variations in man.[5, 22] Individual surges of GH secretion may reach levels of 20 to 60 ng/ml, the largest bursts occurring during the first two hours of sleep.[23] The number and magnitude of spontaneous GH bursts in man are age-dependent, increasing during the growth spurt of adolescence and declining thereafter. Sleep-associated GH release is commonly absent in persons over 50 years of age.

The basis of these physiologic variations in GH has been the subject of extensive research.[5, 22] Factors such as sleep, exercise, and stress, both physical and psychological, account for some of these fluctuations, but many GH surges are spontaneous. Abrupt changes in plasma GH levels are not caused by variations in glucose, amino acids or free fatty acids.

The profile of the secretory bursts of GH and their nonsuppressibility by potential metabolic regulators of GH secretion suggest that the surges are the result of a primary activation of GH secretion induced by neural mechanisms. Numerous studies in laboratory animals indicate that the physiologic GH secretory pattern is regulated by an intrinsic central nervous rhythm that is dependent on neural structures located in the medial-basal hypothalamus. Furthermore, reflex GH secretion, associated with stress or related to sleep, may require neural input from higher centers such as the limbic system.

## NEUROTRANSMITTERS AND GH REGULATION

Growth hormone is believed to be regulated by the release of both inhibitory (somatostatin) and excitatory (GH-releasing factor) hormones.[22] Release of these hypothalamic hormones is, in turn, thought to be regulated by neurotransmitter neurons.[5-11, 22, 24, 25] In general, the effects of neurotransmitters on GH secretion are thought to be mediated at brain sites because direct application of biogenic amines to pituitary cells in vitro is without effect.[22] The finding that several pharmacologic stimuli affect GH secretion in man has led to extensive investigation of the role of neurotransmitters, particularly norepinephrine, dopamine, and serotonin, in normal and abnormal GH secretory states.

The catecholamines, norepinephrine and dopamine, have a stimulatory effect on GH secretion in man.[5, 22, 24, 25] Oral administration of L-dopa, the precursor of dopamine, norepinephrine, and epinephrine, causes release of GH. Evidence that the L-dopa effect is mediated through its conversion to norepinephrine, or possibly epinephrine, is derived from experiments demonstrating that L-dopa-induced GH release is blocked by the α-adrenergic receptor blocker, phentolamine. Additional evidence of α-adrenergic receptors in control of GH is the finding that acute administration of clonidine, a centrally active α-receptor agonist, stimulates release of GH in man.[25]

An additional independent dopaminergic control mechanism for GH probably exists[5, 22, 24, 25] because administration of the dopamine receptor agonists, apomorphine and bromocriptine, also releases GH, and this effect is inhibited by dopamine receptor blockers. Furthermore, pharmacologic blockade of GH release by drugs such as chlorpromazine and haloperidol is probably due to competitive blockade of dopaminergic receptor sites.

In general, most of the stimuli that cause release of GH in man appear to be mediated by central α-adrenergic receptors.[5, 6, 22, 24, 25] GH release induced by insulin-hypoglycemia, arginine, vasopressin, L-dopa, exercise, or certain types of stress is prevented by α-adrenergic blockade (Fig 2). In contrast, propranolol, a β-adrenergic receptor blocker, enhances GH release induced by glucagon, vasopressin, and L-dopa, and β-adrenergic activation with isoproterenol inhibits GH release under certain conditions. These studies indicate that secretion of GH is enhanced by dopaminergic and α-adrenergic-receptor stimulation and inhibited by β-adrenergic receptor activation.[5, 6, 22, 24, 25]

There is increasing evidence of serotoninergic control of GH secre-

**Fig 2.**—Schematic representation of GH regulation by biogenic aminergic and peptidergic neuronal systems. *SRIF,* somatostatin; *GRF,* GH-releasing factor.

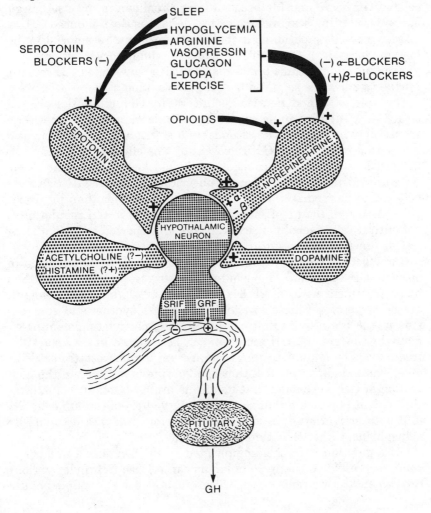

tion.[5, 9–10, 22, 24, 25] Oral administration of the serotonin precursors, L-tryptophan or 5-hydroxytryptophan, causes release of GH in man. Cyproheptadine and methysergide, serotonin antagonists, block insulin-induced GH secretion. Also, cyproheptadine is reported to inhibit nocturnal GH release.

Sleep-associated GH release may be mediated by other mechanisms. Neither α- nor β-adrenergic receptor blockade has an effect on this phenomenon.[6] Methysergide, a serotonin receptor blocker, has been reported to cause an increase in GH release during sleep, whereas other reports have shown either the opposite or no effects.[6, 22] The cholinergic system appears to play some role in sleep-related GH secretion. Methscopolamine bromide, an anticholinergic agent with antimuscarinic properties, decreases sleep-induced GH release,[27] whereas piperidine, a cholinergic nicotinic receptor stimulator, enhances it.[28] These effects suggest stimulatory roles for both muscarinic and nicotinic mechanisms in sleep-associated GH release. Further studies are required to resolve this issue.

The role of other neurotransmitters in GH regulation is not clear.[5–11, 22, 24, 25] Histamine can elicit GH release in man, but the response may be nonspecific, secondary to stress. γ-Aminobutyric acid is reported to stimulate GH release, but this effect is believed to be mediated by dopamine because it can be blocked by dopamine receptor antagonists. However, γ-aminobutyric acid-induced GH release is believed to be mediated at the hypothalamic, rather than pituitary, level. Although the involvement of acetylcholine in GH regulation is not entirely clear, cholinergic pathways are reported to have a facilitative function in insulin-induced GH secretion.[28]

Our laboratory has attempted to define the role of epinephrine in episodic GH secretion. The spontaneous surges of GH are abolished by pretreatment with SK&F 64139 (25 and 50 mg/kg of body weight, given intraperitoneally), an agent that blocks synthesis of epinephrine in the brain by inhibiting the enzyme, phenylethanolamine-N-methyl transferase.[29] GH secretion can be restored in SK&F 64139-treated rats by administration of antiserum to somatostatin or clonidine. These findings suggest that epinephrine is involved in the generation of GH pulses and that its effects are mediated by somatostatin. Also, it is possible that the stimulatory effect of clonidine on GH is due to activation of α-adrenergic receptors that are occupied by epinephrine, rather than norepinephrine.

GH regulation is further complicated by the fact that a number of peptides present in the hypothalamus can release GH under various experimental conditions.[5, 22, 24, 30] These peptides are met-enkephalin, β-endorphin, substance P, neurotensin, thyrotropin-releasing hormone (TRH), luteinizing hormone-releasing hormone, α-melanocyte-stimulating hormone, glucagon, bombesin, vasoactive intestinal peptide, gastrin, myelin basic protein, and cholera endotoxin. However, none of these substances appears to qualify as the physiologic GH-releasing hormone.

### CLINICAL APPLICATION OF NEUROTRANSMITTERS

There is evidence to suggest that there is excessive noradrenergic stimulation of a GH-releasing factor cell in acromegalics, which raises the possibility that drugs that alter catecholamine neurotransmission might be therapeutically useful.[12, 31] Paradoxically, L-dopa, which causes a rise in GH levels in normal people, depresses GH levels in acromegalics.[6, 12, 31] This effect may be due to the presence of altered dopaminergic receptors on the neoplastic GH-secreting pituitary tumor cells. These findings have led to the partially successful use of bromocriptine, a dopamine-receptor agonist, in reducing GH levels in some patients.[12, 31] The efficacy of bromocriptine in acromegaly seems clear, and it may actually reduce tumor size (see Dr. Besser's chapter, "Medical Management of Prolactinomas," in this volume).

Phentolamine and isoproterenol have been reported to decrease GH secretion in acromegaly.[12] However, the therapeutic value of this finding has not been established. Although long-term data on the usefulness of serotonin antagonists (e.g., cyproheptadine and methysergide) are not yet available, this group of pharmacologic agents may be another promising approach to the medical therapy of acromegaly. Thus, the hypersecreting pituitary adenoma appears to retain, to a degree, its dependence on normal GH secretory regulatory hormones.

Somatostatin is also capable of inhibiting GH secretion in acromegaly.[6, 12, 31] Because of its suppressive effects on thyrotropic stimulatory hormone and other nonpituitary hormones and because of the very short biologic half-life of injected somatostatin, various analogues have been synthesized to provide specificity and longer duration of action. Although some success has been demonstrated, the use of somatostatin in the treatment of acromegaly is still investigative.

## Prolactin

PRL is secreted episodically during sleep with peak elevations[6-8, 23] occurring during the later part (usually 2:00 A.M. to 8:00 A.M.). This late nocturnal rise in plasma PRL levels is followed by a decline immediately after awakening. In addition to the nocturnal rise, PRL, like other pituitary hormones, is secreted in a pulsatile manner. PRL secretion is also influenced by a multiplicity of stimuli: suckling, physical and emotional stress, arginine, hypoglycemia, and estrogens all stimulate PRL release. Thus, PRL secretion resembles GH and adrenocorticotropin in its lability to environmental and pharmacologic stimuli.[5, 9–10]

The control of PRL secretion by the hypothalamus is predominantly inhibitory; disruption of hypothalamic-pituitary connections by stalk section, pituitary transplantation, or placement of hypothalamic lesions results in an increase in PRL secretion.[6–8, 11] The finding that the hypothalamus inhibits PRL secretion led to the isolation of PRL-inhibitory factors from hypothalamic extracts and in pituitary-portal vessel blood. The chemical nature of PRL inhibitory factor is unknown. However, because dopamine has a direct inhibitory effect on PRL release in vitro in physiologic concentrations, it is thought that it may act as the primary PRL inhibitory factor. Dopamine is also present in portal vessel plasma. Furthermore, dopaminergic nerve terminals end on median eminence capillaries and could therefore release dopamine into the portal system. Current findings suggest that PRL inhibitory factor activity in hypothalamic tissue is accounted for largely by dopamine because pharmacologically induced reductions in catecholamines also abolish PRL inhibitory factor activity. In addition, dopamine receptors are present on the pituitary gland, but not in the basal hypothalamus, suggesting that dopaminergic effects on pituitary PRL are direct rather than mediated by release of a separate PRL-inhibiting factor from the hypothalamus (Fig 3).

Hypothalamic extracts contain at least two factors that release PRL.[6–8, 11] One of the PRL-releasing factors is TRH, but the other is unknown. These observations indicate that PRL, like GH, is under a complex dual regulatory system that involves both specific inhibitory PRL-inhibiting factor) and stimulatory (PRL-releasing factor) hormones and neurotransmitters.[9–11]

## NEUROTRANSMITTER REGULATION OF PROLACTIN

The monoamines dopamine and serotonin are involved in the control of PRL secretion in man.[9, 10, 12, 31, 32] Dopamine agonists inhibit, and serotonin agonists stimulate, PRL secretion. Administration of L-dopa causes an acute lowering of PRL in man, and is effective in blocking TRH-induced PRL release, suggesting an effect on the pitu-

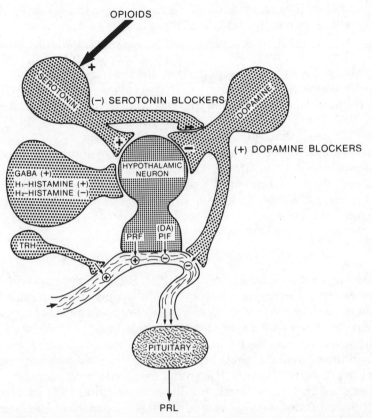

**Fig 3.**—Schematic representation of prolactin *(PRL)* regulation by biogenic aminergic and peptidergic neuronal systems. *PRF*, PRL-releasing factor; *PIF*, PRL-inhibiting factor; *DA*, dopamine; *TRH*, thyrotropin-releasing factor; *GABA*, γ-aminobutyric acid.

itary. Bromocriptine and apomorphine, dopamine receptor agonists, also block PRL release. Thus, dopamine may have both a central nervous system action and a direct pituitary effect. In contrast, several agents that block dopamine receptors, or alter dopamine turnover, elevate PRL levels. Some of these agents are tricyclic neuroleptics, reserpine, chlorpromazine, sulpiride, and metoclopropamide.

Norepinephrine does not appear to have a major function in PRL regulation.[5-11] Clonidine does not significantly modify basal PRL secretion. Moreover, β-adrenergic receptor blockade with pindolol does not affect PRL.

Serotonin precursors cause PRL elevation in humans, whereas serotonin antagonists are reported to decrease PRL levels.[9, 10] However, the inhibitory effects of serotonin antagonists may be due to some nonspecific dopaminergic effects of these drugs.

The role of other neurotransmitters in PRL regulation in humans is not clear.[5-12, 32] Anticholinergic drugs appear to inhibit PRL, and γ-aminobutyric acid may be stimulatory. Evidence from experiments on animals suggests that histamine $(H_1)$-receptors may be involved in the stimulation, and histamine $(H_2)$-receptors in the inhibition of PRL secretion. Acute intravenous administration of cimetidine, an $H_2$-receptor blocker, stimulates PRL release in humans.[33]

Bombesin, neurotensin, substance P, vasoactive intestinal peptide, alytensin, ranatensin, litorin, and arginine vasotocin, all stimulate PRL release in experimental animals. Except for vasoactive intestinal peptide, they do not have a direct effect on the pituitary gland. Their physiologic significance is unknown.[5-11, 30, 32]

## CLINICAL USE OF NEUROTRANSMITTER AGENTS

It is known that L-dopa suppresses PRL levels in patients with hypersecreting pituitary adenomas.[12, 31] More recently, bromocriptine has been used in the treatment of PRL-secreting adenomas because it is more effective and longer lasting than L-dopa.[12, 31, 34] Very recent studies (see the chapters by Drs. Besser, Cowden et al., and Forbes in this volume) indicate that bromocriptine decreases tumor size.[35] Other ergot derivatives (methergoline, lergotrile, and pergolide) are being tested in Europe for their efficacy in treating PRL adenomas. The controversy of medical versus surgical treatment of PRL-secreting adenomas continues.

# Adrenocorticotropin

Adrenocorticotropin (ACTH) is secreted in bursts throughout the day; an average of eight to nine major secretory episodes occur in a 24-hour period.[6-8] Cortisol secretion occurs within five to ten minutes after the ACTH rise. ACTH and cortisol secretory bursts occur predominantly during the latter half of the sleep cycle, but are not related to rapid eye movement (REM) episodes.[23] Also, the rise in ACTH and cortisol occurs even when people are sleep-deprived. The hypothalamic-pituitary-adrenal axis is activated by a wide variety of stressful stimuli, including psychologic ones, such as apprehension or fear; physical ones, such as severe cold exposure, hemorrhage, and electroshock therapy; and insulin-hypoglycemia.[6-8]

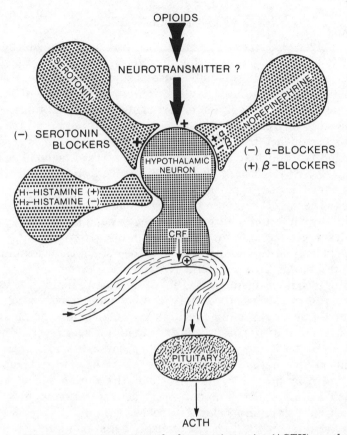

**Fig 4.**—Schematic representation of adrenocorticotropin *(ACTH)* regulation by biogenic aminergic and peptidergic neuronal systems. *CRF,* corticotropin-releasing factor.

The secretion of ACTH is believed to be under the control of a hypothalamic corticotropin-releasing factor, the structure of which is now known.[36] Corticotropin-releasing factor activity, measured in the hypothalamus, shows diurnal variation, and increases in response to stress. The hypothalamic region controlling ACTH secretion involves the basal hypothalamus. In addition to this excitatory factor, there may be an inhibitory area in the posterior hypothalamus. The neural pathways involved in the stress responses and diurnal rhythm appear to be separate. Furthermore, a number of structures outside the hypothalamus are involved in ACTH regulation (Fig 4).

### NEUROTRANSMITTER REGULATION

The control of ACTH secretion by central neurotransmitters has proven to be the most complex of all anterior pituitary hormone systems to analyze.[5-12, 31] This is because various pharmacologic agents appear to have both stimulatory and inhibitory effects on ACTH that are dependent on the specific experimental conditions under which they are tested.

In man, evidence concerning the role of catecholamines in ACTH regulation is inconclusive. Acute administration of L-dopa has no effect on ACTH release in most studies. α-Adrenergic stimulating agents cause a rise in plasma ACTH, while β-Adrenergic blockade enhances the ACTH response to hypoglycemia. These studies suggest a stimulatory effect of α-adrenergic receptors and an inhibitory effect of β-adrenergic receptors in ACTH regulation. However, since there is a large body of conflicting evidence, the role of catecholamines in the control of ACTH in man still remains unresolved.

Serotonin has been implicated in ACTH regulation.[6-12] A variety of studies report activation of the pituitary-adrenal system following administration of serotonin precursors to man and animals. Other studies report an opposite effect. Insulin-hypoglycemia-induced ACTH secretion is inhibited by cyproheptadine, a serotonin antagonist, but not by methysergide. The ACTH response to metyrapone is also blunted by pretreatment with the antiserotonin agent, methergoline. Thus, these drugs do not alter basal secretion of ACTH, but do interfere with pharmacologic responses.

Acetylcholine in the hypothalamus is believed to be involved in stress-induced ACTH release in laboratory animals.[37] In addition, intraventricular administration of histamine stimulates ACTH in dogs. This effect is inhibited by $H_1$-receptor blockers, but not $H_2$-receptor blockers. Moreover, $H_2$-receptor stimulation decreases plasma ACTH. Thus, the effect of histamine on ACTH seems to be due predominantly to an $H_1$-receptor stimulatory effect.

### CLINICAL USE OF NEUROTRANSMITTERS

In adrenal cortical hyperplasia there is often elevated secretion of ACTH from a functioning adenoma of the pituitary, and suggestive evidence for hypersecretion of specific releasing factors is present.[6-8] Thus, it is reasonable to anticipate that pharmacologic agents could be used to suppress corticotropin-releasing factor and/or ACTH secretion. Unfortunately, there has been limited success in the pharmacologic treatment of Cushing's disease or Nelson's syndrome.[9-12, 31]

Cyproheptadine, a serotonin antagonist with antihistamine and antidopamine properties, was reported to be effective in treating Cushing's disease, and in a few cases, Nelson's syndrome. However, other investigators have had very limited success with this drug, or none. Bromocriptine has also been reported to cause a fall in ACTH in Cushing's disease and Nelson's syndrome,[12, 31, 37] but its efficacy remains to be determined. Drugs with both antiserotonin and antidopamine properties, such as lysuride, may prove to be more effective.

## Hormonal Effects of Opioids in Man

The results of studies reporting the acute effects of opioids on anterior pituitary hormone levels are summarized in Figure 5. This subject is reviewed comprehensively in recent reports.[39, 40] Administration of enkephalin analogues increases plasma levels of GH and PRL, and lowers ACTH. However, administration of the specific opiate receptor blocker, naloxone, does not lower GH or PRL. In addition, naloxone does not suppress the sleep-induced GH and PRL rise.

Opiate agonists alter GH responses to arginine and, inconsistently, to hypoglycemia. Methadone potentiates the stimulatory effect of arginine on PRL release. Moreover, L-dopa and apomorphine inhibit the methadone-induced PRL rise. FK-33–824, a stable analogue of met-enkephalin, suppresses ACTH and cortisol release induced by lysine-vasopressin.[41]

**Fig 5.**—Effects of neurotransmitters and opioids on anterior pituitary hormone secretion in man.

| | GROWTH HORMONE | PROLACTIN | ADRENOCORTICOTROPIN |
|---|:---:|:---:|:---:|
| NOREPINEPHRINE α | ↑ | (↑) | (↑) |
| NOREPINEPHRINE β | ↓ | ? | (↓) |
| DOPAMINE | ↑ | ↓ | ? |
| SEROTONIN | ↑ | ↑ | ↑ |
| HISTAMINE H₁ | (↑) | ↑ | ↑ |
| HISTAMINE H₂ | ? | ↓ | ↓ |
| GABA | ↑ | (↑) | ? |
| ACETYLCHOLINE | ↓ | ? | ? |
| OPIOIDS | ↑ | ↑ | ↓ |

↑ STIMULATES    ↓ INHIBITS    ( ) SUGGESTIVE    ? NOT KNOWN

Naloxone diminishes the GH response to arginine and augments the PRL response to TRH. Furthermore, naloxone has no effect on the GH and PRL reponses to L-dopa. Pretreatment with naloxone enhances the cortisol response to stress without affecting GH or PRL responses.

Although naloxone stimulates both ACTH and cortisol secretion in normals, it inhibits ACTH, paradoxially, in Cushing's disease, which suggests a potential therapeutic role for the use of long-acting opiate antagonists in this condition.

However, naloxone has no effect on GH levels in acromegalics or on PRL in patients with hypersecreting PRL adenomas. Thus, it appears that endogenous opiates play an important role in the regulation of ACTH secretion and a minor role in the regulation of GH and PRL.

The effects of opioids on ACTH in rats are believed to be exerted at the hypothalamic level because they can be reproduced by intrahypothalamic injections of opioids or blocked by focal lesions. In addition, the stimulatory effects of opioids on GH and PRL in rats can be blocked by interruption of nonadrenergic or adrenergic and serotoninergic neurotransmission, respectively. Thus, the effects of opioids on pituitary hormone secretion may be mediated through monoaminoergic systems. However, the possibility of effects exerted directly at the pituitary gland is not entirely excluded. The physiologic significance of these findings is not clear.

## Epilogue

Recent discoveries in basic and clinical neuroendocrine research have provided insights into the pathophysiology of hypothalamic-pituitary disorders. This research has produced new pharmacologic agents for the diagnosis and treatment of neuroendocrine disorders, and promises more.

### REFERENCES
1. Moore R.Y., Bloom F.E.: Central catecholamine neuron systems: Anatomy and physiology of the dopamine systems. *Annu. Rev. Neurosci.* 1:129, 1978.
2. Moore R.Y., Bloom F.E.: Central catecholamine neuron systems: Anatomy and physiology of the norepinephrine and epinephrine systems. Annu. Rev. Neurosci. 2:113, 1979
3. Iversen L.I., Iversen S.D., Snyder S.H.: *Chemical Pathways in the Brain: Handbook of Psychopharmacology.* New York: Plenum Press, 1978, vol. 9.
4. Hökfelt T., et al.: Aminergic and peptidergic pathways in the nervous

system with special reference to the hypothalamus, in Reichlin S., et al. (eds): *The Hypothalamus.* New York: Raven Press, 1978, vol. 56.

5. Muller E., Nistico G., Scapagnini U.: *Neurotransmitters and Anterior Pituitary Function,* ed 1. New York: Academic Press, 1977.
6. Martin J.B., Reichlin S., Brown G.M.: *Clinical Neuroendocrinology.* Philadelphia: F.A. Davis, Co., 1977, Contemporary Neurology Series, vol. 14.
7. Tolis G., Labrie F., Martin J.B., et al.: *Clinical Neuroendocrinology: A Pathophysiological Approach,* ed 1. New York: Raven Press, 1979.
8. Martini L., Besser G.M.: *Clinical Neuroendocrinology,* ed 1. New York: Academic Press, 1977.
9. Frohman L.A.: Neurotransmitters as regulators of endocrine function, in Krieger D.T., et al. (eds): *Neuroendocrinology.* Sunderland, Mass.: Sinauer Associates, 1980.
10. Frohman L.A.: Neuroendocrine pharmacology, in DeGroot L., et al.(eds): *Endocrinology.* New York: Grune & Stratton, 1979, vol 1.
11. Reichlin S.: Anatomical and physiological basis of hypothalamic-pituitary regulation, in Post K.D., et al. (eds): *The Pituitary Adenoma.* New York: Plenum Press, 1980.
12. del Pozo E., Lancranjan I.: Clinical use of drugs modifying the release of anterior pituitary hormones, in Ganong W.F., et al. (eds): *Frontiers in Neuroendocrinology.* New York: Raven Press, 1978, vol 5.
13. Cooper J.R., Bloom F.E., Roth R.H.: *The Biochemical Basis of Neuropharmacology,* ed 3. New York: Oxford University Press, 1978.
14. Tolliver J.M., Taylor R.L., Burt D.R.: Muscarinic receptors in the posterior pituitary gland. *Neuroendocrinology* 32:33, 1981.
15. Burt D.R., Taylor R.L.: Muscarinic receptor binding in sheep anterior pituitary. *Neuroendocrinology* 30:344, 1980.
16. Taylor R.L., Burt D.R.: Is acetylcholine a releasing hormone? Evidence for muscarinic receptors in anterior pituitary. *Soc. Neurosci. Abstr.* 5:460, 1979.
17. Schaeffer J.M., Hsueh A.J.W.: Acetylcholine receptors in the rat anterior pituitary gland. *Endocrinology* 106: 1377, 1980.
18. Beaulac-Baillargeon L., et al.: α-Adrenergic binding sites in bovine anterior pituitary gland and control of ACTH secretion in rat anterior pituitary cells in culture. *Soc. Neurosci Abstr.* 6:29, 1980.
19. Schally A.V., et al.: Isolation of γ-amino butyric acid from pig hypothalami and demonstration of its prolactin release-inhibiting (PIF) activity in vivo and in vitro. *Endocrinology* 100:681, 1977.
20. Grandison L., Guidotti A.: γ-Aminobutyric acid receptor function in rat anterior pituitary: Evidence for control of prolactin release. *Endocrinology* 105:754, 1979.
21. Enjalbert A., et al.: Independent inhibition of prolactin secretion by dopamine and γ-aminobutyric acid in vitro. *Endocrinology* 105:823, 1979.
22. Martin J.B., et al.: Neuroendocrine organization of growth hormone regulation, in Reichlin S., et al. (eds): *The Hypothalamus.* New York: Raven Press, 1978, vol 56.
23. Boyar R.M.: Sleep-related endocrine rhythms, in Reichlin S., et al. (eds): *The Hypothalamus.* New York, Raven Press, 1978, vol 56.
24. Krulich L.: Central neurotransmitters and the secretion of prolactin GH, LH, and TSH. *Annu. Rev. Physiol.* 41:603, 1979.

25. Martin J.B.: Functions of central nervous system neurotransmitters in regulation of growth hormone secretion. *Fed. Proc.* 39:2902, 1980.
26. Falkner B., et al.: Growth hormone release in hypertensive adolescents treated with clonidine. *J. Clin. Pharmacol.* 21:31, 1981.
27. Mendelson W.B., et al.: Methscopolamine inhibition of sleep-related growth hormone secretion. *J. Clin. Invest.* 61:1683, 1978.
28. Mendelson W.B., et al.: Piperidine enhances sleep-related and insulin-induced growth hormone secretion: Further evidence for a cholinergic secretory mechanism. *J. Clin. Endocrinol. Metab.* 52:409, 1981.
29. Terry L.C., et al.: Regulation of episodic growth hormone secretion by the central epinephrine system: studies in the chronically cannulated rat. *J. Clin. Invest.* 69:104, 1982.
30. McCann S.: Control of anterior pituitary hormone release by brain peptides. *Neuroendocrinology* 31:355, 1980.
31. Molitch M.: Medical therapy of pituitary tumors, in Post K.D., et al. (eds): *The Pituitary Adenoma.* New York: Plenum Press, 1980.
32. Clemens J.A., Shaar C.J., Smalstig E.B.: Dopamine, PIF, and other regulators of prolactin secretion. *Fed. Proc.* 39:2907, 1980.
33. Gonzalez-Villapando C., Szabo M., Frohman L.A.: Central nervous system-mediated stimulation of prolactin secretion by cimetidine, a histamine $H_2$-receptor antagonist: Impaired responsiveness in patients with prolactin-secreting tumors and idiopathic hyperprolactinemia. *J. Clin. Endocrinol. Metab.* 51:1417, 1980.
34. Thorner M.D., et al.: A broad spectrum of prolactin suppression by bromocriptine in hyperprolactinemic women: A study of serum prolactin and bromocriptine levels after acute and chronic administration of bromocriptine. *J. Clin. Endocrinol. Metab.* 50:1026, 1980.
35. Thorner M., et al.: Rapid regression of pituitary prolactinomas during bromocriptine treatment. *J. Clin. Endocrinol. Metab.* 51:438, 1980.
36. Vale W. et al.: Characterization of a 41-residue ovine hypothalamic peptide that stimulates secretion of corticotropin and β-endorphin. *Science* 214:1394, 1981.
37. Ganong W.F.: Neurotransmitters and pituitary function: Regulation of ACTH secretion. *Fed. Proc.* 39:2923, 1980.
38. Lanberts S.W.J., et al.: The mechanism of the suppressive action of bromocriptine on adrencorticotropin secretion in patients with Cushing's disease and Nelson's syndrome. *J. Clin. Endocrinol. Metab.* 51:307, 1980.
39. Morley J.E.: The endocrinology of the opiates and opioid peptides. *Metabolism* 30:195, 1981.
40. Meites J.: Relation of endogenous opioid peptides to secretion of hormones. *Fed. Proc.* 39:2531, 1980.
41. Demura R., et al.: Plasma pituitary hormone responses to the synthetic enkephalin analogue (FK 33–824) in normal subjects and patients with pituitary disease. *J. Clin. Endocrinol. Metab.* 52:263, 1981.

# Metabolic Effects of Neuropeptides

## ABBAS E. KITABCHI, Ph.D., M.D.

*Professor of Medicine and Biochemistry Director, Division of Endocrinology and Metabolism Program Director, Clinical Research Center The University of Tennessee Center for the Health Sciences Memphis, Tennessee*

THE DISCIPLINE OF NEUROBIOLOGY has made great strides since 1935, when Dale first advanced the concept of one neuron-one neurotransmitter.[1] It is now well established, however, that neurotransmitter and neuropeptide may reside in the same neuron. The list of these neuropeptides according to the latest account amounts to about 30 as enumerated by Cooper and Martin[2] and shown in Table 1.

Research in the area of neurobiology is characterized by an inter-disciplinary cooperation and pooling of the talents of biologists, chemists, physicists and clinicians. This has brought to fruition the most dramatic advances in the area of neuroendocrinology. Probably among the most prominent and exciting advances are the following: (1) the concept of precursor molecule in peptide biosynthesis; (2) behavior-modifying effects of neuropeptides; and (3) pluripotential effect of neuropeptides at the peripheral tissue.

For the purpose of this discussion, I will not delve into the fascinating area of peptide biosynthesis in detail; suffice it to say that the brilliant work of Donald Steiner in insulin biosynthesis in 1967 (for review see refs. 3–5) set the pace for all subsequent studies regarding synthesis of polypeptide hormones in general. The obvious implication that these precursor molecules may have in certain geneti-

---

NOTE: This work was supported in part by USPHS grants AM07088 and RR00211.

45

0-8151-3530-0/82/006-45-62-$03.75

TABLE 1.—Peptides Found in the Central Nervous System*

Hypophysiotropic hormones
1. Thyrotropin-releasing hormone (TRH)
2. Luteinizing hormone/follicle-stimulating hormone releasing hormone, or gonadotropin releasing hormone (GnRH)
3. Growth hormone release-inhibiting hormone (somatostatin)
Adenohypophysial hormones (including opiocortins)
1. Growth hormone
2. Prolactin
3. Thyroid stimulating hormone (TSH)
4. Luteinizing hormone
5. Follicle-stimulating hormone
6. Opiocortins
   a. Adrenocorticotropic hormone (ACTH)
   b. β-Lipotropic hormone (β-LPH)
   c. Endorphins
   d. Enkephalins
   e. α-Melanocyte stimulating hormone (α-MSH)
   f. β-Melanocyte stimulating hormone (β-MSH)
Neurohypophysial hormones
1. Vasopressin or antidiuretic hormone (ADH)
2. Oxytocin
3. Neurophysins
Brain-gut hormones
1. Cholecystokinin (CCK)
2. Gastrin
3. Insulin
4. Vasoactive intestinal polypeptide (VIP)
5. Motilin
6. Bombesin
7. Substance P (SP)
8. Neurotensin
9. Glucagon
Others
1. Bradykinin
2. Isorenin-angiotensin
3. Sleep peptide
4. Carnosine
5. Calcitonin

*Reproduced from Cooper and Martin.[2] Used by permission.

cally directed diseased states is fascinating and presents challenging topics of research. For an updated review of neuropeptide synthesis in the brain, particularly in reference to the opiocortin, see Krieger's recent review on the subject.[6] A graphic demonstration of these processes is presented in Figure 1, which is reconstructed mainly from the studies of bovine intermediate lobe and mouse pituitary tissue.[7]

I will briefly review the metabolism of various nutrients in the fed and fasted states as this topic becomes the central theme in the discussion on the role of neuropeptides in metabolism.

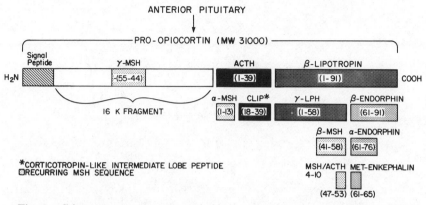

Fig 1.—Schematic representation of the bovine precursor molecule for ACTH, MSH, lipotropins and endorphins. (Adapted from Krieger et al.[6])

Figure 2 depicts the sources and metabolism of glucose.[8] Glucose production is enhanced by ingestion of glucose, glycogenolysis, and gluconeogenesis. Three major ways to dispose of glucose are through glycogen production, Kreb's cycle oxidation, or fat deposition. Obviously, any acceleration of synthetic pathway or decrease in rate of disposition brings about hyperglycemia, whereas opposite processes produce hypoglycemia.

Figure 3 depicts multiple factors that bring about euglycemic state when a meal is taken. Interaction of carbohydrate, protein and fat with intestinal mucosa leads to production of glucose, amino acids

**Fig 2.**—Sources and fate of glucose.

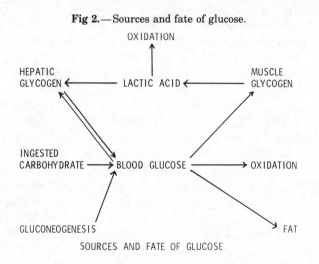

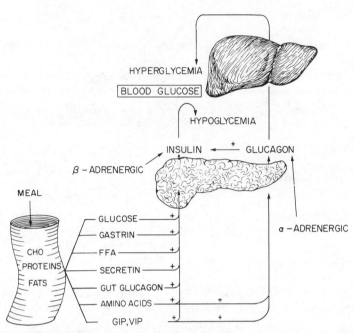

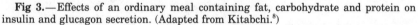

**Fig 3.**—Effects of an ordinary meal containing fat, carbohydrate and protein on insulin and glucagon secretion. (Adapted from Kitabchi.[8])

and free fatty acids, respectively, as well as certain GI hormones (gastrin, gut glucagon, GIP and VIP), which in turn facilitate insulin secretion. During this period, insulin is secreted and glucose is taken up by the insulin-sensitive cells for energy production. However, some of these hormones (GIP + VIP) as well as amino acids also stimulate glucagon secretion. Glucagon's effect mediated through the liver phosphorylase stimulates glycogenolysis, leading to increased glucose production and thus combatting the potential hypoglycemic effect of insulin.

During the postprandial state certain metabolic alterations occur in certain organs. Figure 4 depicts representative organs, with the major role played by the pancreas and liver. As can be seen from this figure, the metabolic changes during the fed state are insulin-induced. Insulin is the major anabolic hormone in the body assimilating glucose in the liver to glycogen, FFA in the fat tissue to triglyceride and amino acids in the muscle to protein. Glucagon plays a minor role in the fed state, and its level is quite low. In this period, an adequate amount of glucose is available to the brain, the organ that depends exclusively on glucose for its metabolism.

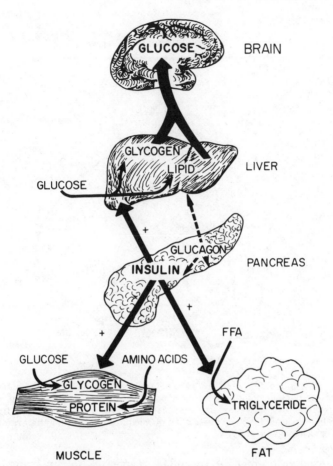

**Fig 4.**—The role of insulin in the utilization of substrates in the fed state. An adequate amount of insulin ensures assimilation of glucose to lipid and glycogen in the liver, amino acid to protein in muscle and free fatty acid (FFA) into triglyceride in fat tissue. (Reproduced from Kitabchi.[8])

On the other hand, the fasted state (Fig 5) is characterized by hyperglucagonemia (albeit transient) as insulin level is decreased with a longer period of fast. Unlike insulin, which is anabolic, glucagon is catabolic. The fasting state might be compared to an alarmed state such as stress, severe infection, surgery or diabetic ketoacidosis (DKA), all of which are accompanied by increase in counter-regulatory hormones, such as catecholamines, glucagon and glucocorticoids. In the absence of the opposing effect of insulin, the influence of catabolic hormones predominates. Thus catecholamines stimulate lipoly-

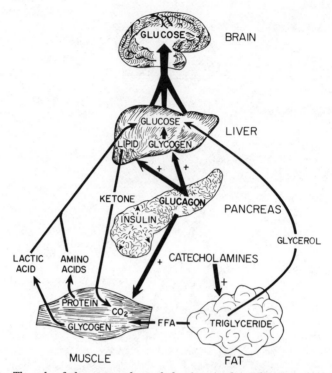

**Fig 5.**—The role of glucagon and catecholamines in the utilization of substrates in the fasted state. Catecholamines bring about glycogenolysis with ensuing hyperglycemia as well as increased free fatty acids as a result of increased lipolysis from depot fat. Glucagon ensures further availability of adequate glucose for the brain through increased gluconeogenic activity.

sis and production of FFA from TG. Hypercortisolism leads to catabolic states including proteolysis, and hyperglucagonemia leads to ketogenesis and further gluconeogenesis (excessive FFA production is used as fuel for energy in muscle as well as a source of ketogenic substrate whereas alanine serves as a substrate for stimulated gluconeogenesis in the liver). The brain, however, continues to use glucose exclusively up to 3–4 weeks of starvation. In general, gluconeogenesis thus ensures adequate supply of glucose to the brain.

Returning now to the neuroanatomy of the pancreas, it is important to note that islets of Langerhans are richly supplied by both fibers from vagi and sympathetic fibers, and individual axons enter the islet along with blood vessels to innervate many secretory cells (for review see ref. 9). There are also many afferent fibers within the islets. Four major cells and their products have been identified in the islet of Langerhans: α-cells with glucagon as their major secretion; β-cells, responsible for synthesis and release of insulin; D-cell, which produces somatostatin; and F-cells, producing pancreatic polypeptide. Cell-to-cell messages and modulations are apparently ensured by the presence of gap junction.

Tables 2 and 3 summarize many factors that stimulate or inhibit pancreatic insulin and glucagon secretion.

TABLE 2.—STIMULATORS AND INHIBITORS
OF INSULIN RELEASE*

| STIMULATORS | INHIBITORS |
|---|---|
| Carbohydrates | Carbohydrates |
| Glucose | 2-Deoxyglucose |
| Fructose | D-Mannoheptulose |
| Mannose | Hormones |
| Polypeptide hormones | Epinephrine |
| Glucagon | Norepinephrine |
| ACTH (not in man) | Somatostatin |
| Growth hormone | Miscellaneous |
| Amino acids | Starvation |
| Fatty acids | Diazoxide |
| Enteric hormones | Hypoxia |
| Secretin | Hypothermia |
| Pancreozymin | Vagotomy |
| Gastrin | |
| Gut glucagon | |
| Miscellaneous | |
| Cyclic 3′,5′-AMP | |
| Glucocorticoids | |
| Ketones | |
| Potassium | |
| Calcium | |
| Sulfonylurea | |
| Vagal stimulation | |
| Methyl xanthines | |

*Reproduced from Kitabchi.[8]

TABLE 3.—STIMULATORS AND INHIBITORS OF
GLUCAGON RELEASE*

| STIMULATORS | INHIBITORS |
|---|---|
| Pancreozymin | Glucose |
| Amino acids | Glucagon |
| Starvation | Secretin |
| Hypoglycemia | Somatostatin |
| Exercise | |
| D-Mannoheptulose | |

*Reproduced from Kitabchi.[8]

As to the role of neuropeptides in carbohydrate metabolism, suffice it to say that the role of the central nervous system (CNS) in control of glucose metabolism was first described about 130 years ago by Claude Bernard,[10] who demonstrated development of transient hyperglycemia and glycosuria in rabbits when he punctured the floor of the fourth ventricle in these animals ("piqure diabetes"). The effect was not countered by vagotomy but was prevented by spinal cord section or cutting the splanchnic nerves.[11] Cannon, about 50 years later, advanced the concept of hyperglycemia of stress as an adrenal-mediated phenomenon.[12] Gellhorn and co-workers[13] and Feldman and colleagues[14] in the 1940s developed the concept of sympathoadrenal axis and vagoinsulin axis.

In modern times the neural regulation of glucose metabolism was pioneered by Porte's demonstration of the inhibitory effect of epinephrine on insulin secretion[15] and subsequent demonstration by Frohman[16] and Kaneto[17] that insulin and glucagon secretions are changed following hypothalamic stimulation. Thus, stimulation of the ventrolateral hypothalamus (VLH) stimulates insulin secretion and lowers blood glucose and stimulation of the ventromedial hypothalamus (VMH) inhibits insulin secretion and elevates plasma level of glucagon and glucose.

Additional evidence for support of the role of CNS in glucose homeostasis is the observation that 2-deoxyglucose, a nonmetabolizable sugar, produces hyperglycemia when placed in the brain,[18] and demonstration of insulin receptors in the brain[19-20] and its sensitivity to insulin.[21]

The major GI neuropeptides and their action on the endocrine pancreas merit a brief discussion.

*Vasoactive inhibitory peptide (VIP)* is a 28-amino acid that was originally extracted from hog intestine and has properties of peripheral vasodilation.[22] Besides its location in the GI tract, it is also found in the cerebral cortex, hypothalamus (median eminence), amygdaloid nucleus, corpus striatum, peripheral nervous system, placenta, adrenal glands and nerves in the female and male genital organs. The H cells that produce VIP are in GI mucosa and the autonomic nervous system with identical structure. VIP stimulates insulin and glucagon release as well as several pituitary hormones, including prolactin and growth hormone.

*Gastric inhibitory peptide (GIP)* is a 43-amino acid residue that was extracted from duodenal mucosa.[23] It is produced by the K-cells, with highest concentration in the jejunum followed by the ileum and duodenum. K-cells are more numerous in patients with low gastric acidity and are more difficult to find in patients with duodenal ulcer disease. GIP inhibits secretion of pepsin, gastrin and GI motility. It stimulates intestinal secretion, insulin and glucagon. GIP, therefore, has an enterogastrone effect (inhibition of gastric acid secretion and motility), an incretin effect (insulin release) and an enterocrinin effect (stimulation of insulin secretion). It has been suggested that the enhancement of insulin secretion when glucose is taken orally as compared to the lesser secretion induced by intravenous administration is the result of the production of GIP in the gut with oral glucose.

*Pancreatic polypeptide (PP)* is a 36-amino acid (Mwt. 4,200) peptide originally isolated from chicken pancreatic extract.[24] It is produced by $D_2$ cells of pancreas, the fundus of stomach and the upper small intestine. This material increases after meals, opposes CCK effect, and is elevated in diabetic patients.[25]

*Bombesin* is a tetradecapeptide first isolated from amphibian skin. Bombesin-producing cells have been localized in the GI tract, lung and brain of man.[26] In large doses, it stimulates the smooth muscle of the intestine, urinary tract, uterus and afferent arterioles, the last effect resulting in angiotensin activation, hypertension and antidiuresis. In smaller doses, it elevates gastric and pancreatic secretions. Bombesin also increases glucagon secretion in man, which will be discussed in detail later.

*Substance P* was originally found in extracts of equine brain, intestine, and also in the spinal cord.[27] It is an unidecapeptide that stimulates salivary secretion and inhibits insulin secretion from the pancreas.[27, 28] Systemic vasodilation and contraction of nonvascular smooth muscle are among its other actions.

*Neurotensin* is a tridecapeptide isolated from the hypothalamic region.[29] It produces gut contraction, hyperglycemia and also stimulates glucagon following systemic injection.[30] It is also found in mammalian ileum and its level is said to be increased in patients with dumping syndrome in the postprandial state. Neurotensin stimulates glucagon and glucose and the effect is blocked by $H_1$ receptor.[31]

*Cholecystokinin (CCK)* is a 33-amino acid peptide first isolated from GI tract.[32] At least three forms of CCK and a large precursor molecule of 15,000 daltons have been found in the brain. Recent studies in which a reduced amount of CCK has been found in the brain of obese hyperphagic mice[32] as well as its inhibitory effect on feeding when given into the lateral ventricle of sheep[33] suggest that CCK may play a role in the "set point" of appetite through the CNS.

*Somatostatin (SRIF)* was first isolated from the hypothalamus by

Guillemin and co-workers at the Salk Institute in 1973. It was found to be a growth hormone (somatotropin) releasing inhibitor polypeptide[34] (SRIF). It is also found in the GI tract and in the D-cells of the pancreas. This is a 14-amino acid compound with cystine bridge. Somatostatin is not only a potent inhibitor of gastrin release in both the fasting and the meal-stimulated state but is also an inhibitor of gastric motility and secretion, of gallbladder contraction and of pancreatic secretion.[35] SRIF inhibits GH release,[34] lowers ACTH in Nelson's syndrome,[36] and inhibits furosemide-induced renin,[37] prolactin,[38] TRH-induced TSH release[39] as well as insulin and glucagon.[40-42] It is sometimes called an "All American" blocker! Although its relationship to diabetes has not been established, it is possible that excess SRIF in the pancreas may be responsible for some cases of diabetes mellitus and that lack of it may cause excessive HCl production and duodenal ulcer. Somatostatin and some of its analogs have been shown to act on the CNS to modulate glucoregulation.[43]

Table 4 summarizes the effect of neuropeptides on insulin and glucagon secretion based on present evidence in both human and animal studies.

One of the most interesting and significant advances in the understanding of neuropeptide activity and glucoregulation has been in the area of hypothalamic-mediated hyperglycemia. Although neurotensin and β-endorphin produce CNS-dependent hyperglycemia in rats, bombesin exemplifies the type of influence these neuropeptides may have in overall hypothalamic-directed glucoregulation and will be discussed in more detail. As discussed before, bombesin was originally isolated from frog skin but a mammalian bombesin, gastrin-releasing peptide, has also been isolated and characterized.[44] Bombesin-like peptide[45, 46] and receptors[47] have been demonstrated in the hypothalamus and brain stem nuclei.

When injected intracisternally (IC) or intracerebroventricularly (ICV), bombesin causes sustained increase in plasma glucose without a change in peripheral glucose turnover. This hyperglycemia is not prevented by hypophysectomy but is by adrenalectomy, and it is associated with a concomitant elevation of plasma epinephrine and glucagon and a reduction of plasma insulin[48] and body temperature.[49] It thus appears that bombesin-induced hyperglycemia is the result of catecholamine-induced changes in pancreatic insulin and glucagon secretion.

Studies by Brown and co-workers have shown that bombesin's inhibition of insulin secretion and stimulation of glucagon and glucose levels are time-dependent phenomena.[50] Carbachal, a cholinester,

TABLE 4.—NEUROPEPTIDE EFFECT ON PANCREATIC
HORMONES

| HORMONE | INSULIN | GLUCAGON |
|---|---|---|
| Vasoactive intestinal polypeptide (VIP) | + | + |
| Gastric inhibitory polypeptide (GIP) | + | + |
| Pancreatic polypeptide (PP) | 0 | + ? |
| Bombesin | − | + |
| Substance P | − | + |
| Neurotensin | 0 | + |
| Somatostatin (SRIF) | − | − |
| β-Endorphin | + | ? |

+ = stimulation; − = inhibition; 0 = no effect.

also induces hyperglycemia and hyperglucagonemia but, unlike bombesin, its effect is blocked by atropine.[51]

Thyrotropin-releasing factor (TRF) also produces hyperglycemia and hypercatecholaminemia but, unlike bombesin, raises body temperature.[52] TRF's effect is independent of the pituitary-thyroid axis but is CNS-mediated. Therefore, it is evident that while both bombesin and TRF produce elevation of adrenomedullary epinephrine secretion, they have different general patterns of influence on the autonomic nervous system.

To further determine whether these effects are mediated through plasma glucagon and insulin, nerve-mediated glucogenic signals to the liver, or epinephrine, Brown and associates administered somatostatin analog (ODT8-SS) systemically or centrally to animals receiving bombesin intracisternally. ODT8-SS, which is 10-fold more potent than SRIF, does not cross into the systemic circulation when injected IC. ODT8-SS reduced hyperglycemia and hyperglucagonemia after IC bombesin administration,[51] suggesting that bombesin acted on hormonal pathways in the CNS rather than peripherally. It also elevated body temperature and counteracted the adrenomedullary activity induced by bombesin, carbachal, β-endorphin and 2-deoxyglucose.[43]

These effects reported by Brown and co-workers[43] are graphically demonstrated in Figure 6. Based on these and other findings, Brown formulated a hypothesis (Fig 7) proposing that a parallel response to activation of nutrient-mobilizing components of the sympathetic nervous system is activation of adaptive hypothermia. By activating the adrenomedullary component of the sympathetic nervous system (AMSNS), hepatic glucose production is increased with concomitant lowering of body temperature, which may lead to reduction of sub-

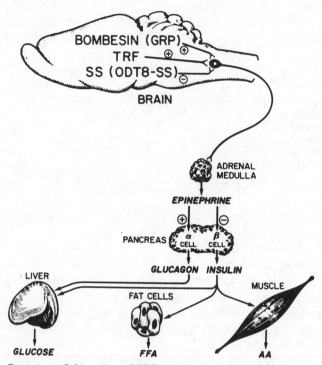

**Fig 6.**—Summary of the action of TRF, bombesin and somatostatin (somatostatin analogues) to act within the CNS to influence peripheral nutrient metabolism. (Reproduced from Brown.[52])

strate utilization by the cell. Such a neural pathway activation would ensure adequate entry of substrate to the brain. A similar phenomenon may also be operating in another form of nutrient deprivation, such as insulin deficiency of diabetic ketoacidosis.[53, 54]

In this regard it is interesting to note that bombesin given to rats, IC or ICV, reversibly lowers body temperature and activates AMSNS. To determine whether the decrease in body temperature following the above treatments is due to irreversible inhibition of thermoregulation, Brown and associates assessed the ability of animals made hypothermic with bombesin, 2-deoxyglucose, insulin and fasting to respond to a neurochemical stimulus that increases body temperature, SRIF or ODT8-SS. ODT8-SS acutely reversed the hypothermia and increased AMSNS activity induced by bombesin, 2-deoxyglucose, insulin-induced hypoglycemia and fasting. The animals receiving these treatments exhibited no impairment of their

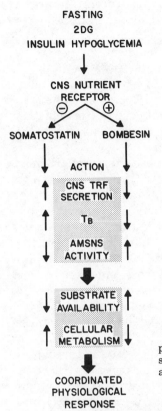

FASTING
2DG
INSULIN HYPOGLYCEMIA

CNS NUTRIENT
RECEPTOR
⊖   ⊕

SOMATOSTATIN   BOMBESIN

ACTION

CNS TRF
SECRETION

T$_B$

AMSNS
ACTIVITY

SUBSTRATE
AVAILABILITY

CELLULAR
METABOLISM

COORDINATED
PHYSIOLOGICAL
RESPONSE

Fig 7.—Suggested model for coordination of physiologic responses to nutrient deprivation by somatostatin and bombesin. (Reproduced from Brown and Fisher.[43])

thermoregulatory response to the hyperthermia-producing stimulus of this somatostatin analog. These results show that several neural stimuli reversibly activate the AMSNS and lower body temperature as an adaptive mechanism to conserve energy and ensure adequate substrate for CNS function. Furthermore, somatostatin and bombesin exert acutely opposing CNS actions on the thyrotropin-releasing factor (TRF) control. These effects complement the potential actions of SRIF and bombesin on temperature regulation and nutrient metabolism.[55]

These data, according to Brown and associates,[43] support the hypothesis that changes in body temperature may potentially subserve neurally induced mechanisms to reduce nutrient utilization in states that may pharmacologically or physiologically mimic nutrient deprivation. Furthermore, the neuropeptides bombesin and SRIF are capable of inducing changes in the adrenomedullary component of the sympathetic nervous system (AMSNS) and body temperature in qualitatively opposite fashions and may constitute coordinated physiologic responses, as shown in Figure 7. It thus appears that hypothalamic secretions affect the control of metabolism (for review see ref. 56).

It is interesting that many states of nutrient deprivation, including DKA, are associated with hypothermia and hypercatecholinemia;[57] thus, changes in body temperature and AMSNS activity may play an important role in conservation of energy and maintenance of CNS cellular functions in nutrient-deprived states.

The role of hormones and obesity has been the subject of extensive investigation and review in recent literature.[58] Unfortunately, most of the work in this area is either in experimental animals, or the evidence of a hormonal role in obesity in humans has been indirect or inferential. There is experimental evidence from animal studies that the opioid peptides may participate in the nutritional economy of the body by regulating appetite and/or satiety. For example, pituitary β-endorphin is elevated in genetically obese mice (ob/ob) and rats (fa/fa), and naloxone administration decreases the amount of food eaten, and hypothalamic injections of β-endorphin induce overeating in the nonobese rats.[59,60] These data have led to the hypothesis that there is abnormal opioid metabolism in the ob/ob mice and that β-endorphin is involved in the regulation of food intake through interactions of peripheral as well as central opiate receptors. However, a careful evaluation of the time-course relationship between weight gain and β-endorphin increase in the pituitary of the ob/ob mouse reveals that an excessive increase in weight occurs prior to the increase in β-endorphin levels, suggesting that the β-endorphin and ACTH increases in the pituitary gland of ob/ob mice are a secondary phenomenon.[61] In support of this is the finding that fasting decreases the level of pituitary ACTH in obese animals.[62]

Increased pituitary-adrenal activity is present in at least some obese humans, and weight reduction reduces the activity, which suggests that it is a secondary phenomenon. Givens et al.[63] in our laboratory have demonstrated increased β-endorphin and LPH plasma levels in obese, hirsute females, proportionate to their body weight. These findings may simply reflect the increased pituitary-adrenal activity in obesity as a secondary phenomenon. However, CNS opiate activity may be involved in the overeating. Further studies are needed to define the relationship between opiate activity and appetite or satiety in obesity.

## REFERENCES

1. Dale H.H.: Reizuberragung durch chemische Mittel im peripheren Nervensystem. Sammlung der von der Nothnagel—Stiftung veranstalteten Vortrage 4, in *Adventures in Physiology: A Selection of Scientific Papers* (London: Pergamon, 1953).
2. Cooper P.E., Martin J.B.: Neuroendocrinology and brain peptides. *Ann. Neurol.* 8:551, 1980.
3. Steiner D.F., Clark J.L., Nolan C., Rubenstein A.H., Margo-Liash E., Oyer P.E.: Proinsulin and the biosynthesis of insulin. *Recent Prog. Horm. Res.* 25:207, 1969.
4. Kitabchi A.E.: Proinsulin and C-peptide: a review. *Metabolism* 26:547, 1977.
5. Chan S.J., Kwok C.M., Steiner D.F.: The biosynthesis of insulin: some genetic and evolutionary aspects. *Diabetes Care* 4:4, 1981.
6. Krieger D.T., Liotta A.S., Brownstein M.J., Zimmerman E.A.: ACTH β-lipotropin and related peptides in brain, pituitary, and blood. *Recent Prog. Horm. Res.* 36:277, 1980.
7. Mains R.E., Eipper B.A.: β-Endorphin and Related Peptides, in Martin R.E., Reichlin S., Bick K. (eds): *Neurosecretion and Brain Peptides: Implications for Brain Function and Neurological Disease* (New York: Raven Press, 1980).
8. Kitabchi A.E.: Hormonal control of glucose metabolism. *Otolaryngol. Clin. North Am.* 8:335, 1975.
9. Woods S.C., Smith P.H., Porte D.: The Role of the Nervous System in Metabolic Regulation and Its Effects on Diabetes and Obesity, in Brownlee M. (ed.): *Handbook of Diabetes Mellitus* (New York: Garland STPM Press, 1981), vol. 5.
10. Bernard C.: Chiens rendus diabetiques. *C. R. Soc. Biol.* 1:60, 1849.
11. Bernard C.: *Leçons sur la Physiologie et al Pathologie du Système Nerveus* (Paris: Bailliere, 1858), vol. 1.
12. Cannon W.B., McIver M.A., Bliss S.W.: Studies on the conditions of activity in endocrine glands. *Am. J. Physiol.* 69:46, 1924.
13. Gellhorn E., Cortell R., Feldman J.: The effect of emotion, shame, rage and hypothalamic stimulation on the vagoinsulin system. *Am. J. Physiol.* 133:532, 1941.
14. Feldman J., Cortell R., Gellhorn E.: On the vagoinsulin and sympathetic-adrenal system and their mutual relationship under conditions of central excitation induced by anoxia and convulsant drugs. *Am. J. Physiol.* 131:281, 1940.
15. Porte D.: A receptor mechanism for the inhibition of insulin release by epinephrine in man. *J. Clin. Invest.* 46:86, 1967.
16. Frohman L., Muller E.E., Cocchi D.: Central nervous system mediated inhibition of insulin secretion due to 2-deoxyglucose. *Horm. Metab. Res.* 5:21, 1972.
17. Kaneto A.: The Role of the Autonomic Nervous System in Glucagon Secretion, in Foa P.O., Bajaj J.S., Foa N.L. (eds.): *Glucagon: Its Role in Physiology and Clinical Medicine* (New York: Springer-Verlag, 1977).
18. Himsworth R.L.: Compensatory reaction to a lack of metabolizable glucose. *J. Physiol. (Lond.)* 198:451, 1968.

19. Havrankova J., Roth J., Brownstein M.: Insulin receptors are widely distributed in the central nervous system of the rat. *Nature* 272:827, 1978.
20. Storlien L.H., Bellingham W.P., Martin G.P.: Localization of CNS glucoregulatory insulin receptors within the ventromedial hypothalamus. *Brain Res.* 06:156, 1975.
21. Szabo O., and Szabo A.J.: Neuropharmacological characterization of insulin-sensitive CNS glucoregulator. *Am. J. Physiol.* 229:663, 1975.
22. Said S.I., Mutt V.: Polypeptide with broad biological activity: isolation from small intestine. *Science* 169:1217, 1970.
23. Brown J.C., Pederson R.A., Jorpes E., Mutt V.: Preparation of a highly active enterogastrone. *Can. J. Physiol. Pharmacol.* 47:113, 1969.
24. Kimmel J.R., Pollok H.G., Hazelwood R.C.: Isolation and characterization of chicken insulin. *Endocrinology* 83:1323, 1968.
25. Floyd J.D., Jr., Fajans S.S.: A newly recognized human pancreatic islet polypeptide: concentration in healthy subjects and in patients with diabetes mellitus. *Diabetes 25,* Suppl. 1:330, 1976.
26. Brown M., Vale W.: Bombesin: putative mammalian neurogastrointestinal peptides. *Trends in Neuroscience* 2:95, 1979.
27. Euler V.S., Von Gaddem J.H.: An unidentified depressor substance in certain tissue extracts. *J. Physiol. (Lond.)* 72:74, 1931.
28. Efendic S., Lutt R., Pernour B.: Effect of substance P on arginine induced insulin and glucagon release from isolated perfused rat pancreas. *Nobel Symposium Abstract,* Jan. 14–16, 1976, p. 37.
29. Carraway R., Leeman S.E.: The isolation of a new hypotensive peptide, neurotensin, from bovine hypothalami. *J. Biol. Chem.* 248:6854, 1973.
30. Nagai K., Frohman L.A.: Hyperglycemia and hyperglucagonemia following neurotensin administration. *Life Sci.* 19:273, 1976.
31. Nagai K., Frohman L.A.: Neurotensin hyperglycemia: evidence for histamine mediation and the assessment of a possible physiologic role. *Diabetes* 27:577, 1978.
32. Mutt V., Jorpes J.E.: Isolation of aspartyl-phenylalanine amide from cholecystokinin-pancreosymin. *Biochem. Biophys. Res. Commun.* 26:393, 1967.
33. Della-Fera M.A., Baile C.A.: Cholecystokinin octapeptide: continuous picomole injections into the cerebral ventricles of sheep suppress feeding. *Science* 206:471, 1979.
34. Brazeau P., Vale W., Burgus R., Ling N., Butcher M., Rivier J., Guillemin R.: Hypothalamic polypeptide that inhibits the secretion of immunoreactive pituitary growth hormone. *Science* 179:77, 1973.
35. Le Roith D., Vinik A.I., Epstein S., et al.: Somatostatin and serum gastrin in normal subjects and in patients with pernicious anemia, chronic liver and renal disease. *South Afr. J. Med. Sci.* 49:1601, 1975.
36. Tyrrell J.B., Orenzi M., Gerich J.E., et al.: Inhibition by somatostatin of ACTH secretion in Nelson's syndrome. *J. Clin. Endocrinol. Metab.* 40:1125, 1975.
37. Rosenthal J., Raptis S., Escobar F.: Inhibition of furosemide-induced hyperreninemia by growth hormone releasing inhibitory hormone in man. *Lancet* 1:772, 1976.
38. Yen S.C., Siler J.M., DeVane G.W.: Effect of somatostatin in patients

with acromegaly: suppression of growth hormone, prolactin, insulin and glucose level. *N. Engl. J. Med.* 290:935, 1974.

39. Luche G., Hoffken B., Von Zen Muhlen X.: The effect of somatostatin in TSH levels in patients with primary hypothyroidism. *J. Clin. Endocrinol. Metab.* 41:1082, 1975.

40. Alberti K.G.M.M., Christensen S.E., Iversen J., et al.: Inhibition of insulin secretion by somatostatin. *Lancet* 2:1299, 1974.

41. Koerker D., Rich, W., Chideckel E., et al.: Somatostatin: hypothalamic inhibitor of the endocrine pancreas. *Science* 184:482, 1974.

42. Gerich J.E., Lorenzi M., Schneider V., et al.: Effects of somatostatin on plasma glucose, and glucagon levels in human diabetes mellitus. *N. Engl. J. Med.* 291:544, 1974.

43. Brown M.R., Fisher D.A.: Glucoregulation and Sympathetic Nervous System: CNS Control by Brain Peptides, in Bloom F.E. (ed): *Peptides: Integrators of Cells and Tissue Function* (New York: Raven, 1980).

44. McDonald T.J., Jornvall H., Nilsson G., Vagne M., Ghatei M., Bloom S.R., Mutt V.: Characterization of a gastrin releasing peptide from porcine non-antral gastric tissue. *Biochem. Biophys. Res. Commun.* 90:227, 1979.

45. Brown M.R., Allen R., Villarreal J., Rivier J., Vale W.: Bombesin-like activity: radioimmunologic assessment in biological tissues. *Life Sci.* 23:2721, 1978.

46. Moody T.W., Pert C.B.: Bombesin-like peptides in rat brain: quantitation and biochemical characterization. *Biochem. Biophys. Res. Commun.* 90:7, 1979.

47. Moody T.W., Pert C.B., Rivier J.E., Brown M.R.: Bombesin: specific binding to rat brain membranes. *Proc. Natl. Acad. Sci. USA* 75:5372, 1978.

48. Brown M., Tache Y., Fisher D.: Central nervous system action of bombesin: mechanism to induce hyperglycemia. *Endocrinology* 105:660, 1979.

49. Pittman Q.J., Tache Y., Brown M.: Bombesin acts in preoptic area to produce hypothermia in rats. *Life Sci.* 26:725, 1980.

50. Brown M., Rivier J., Vale W.: Bombesin affects the CNS to produce hyperglycemia in rats. *Life Sci.* 22:1729, 1977.

51. Fisher D.A., Brown M.R.: Somatostatin analog: plasma catecholamine suppression mediated by the central nervous system. *Endocrinology* 107:714, 1980.

52. Brown M.: Neuropeptides: CNS effects on nutrient metabolism. *Diabetologia* 20:1, 1981.

53. Kitabchi A.E.: The Definition and Current Concepts of the Pathogenesis of Diabetes Mellitus, in Givens J.R. (ed); *Gynecological Endocrinology* (Chicago: Year Book Medical Publishers, 1977), vol. 1.

54. Kitabchi A.E., Fisher J.N.: Insulin Therapy of Diabetic Ketoacidosis: Physiologic vs. Pharmacologic Doses of Insulin and Their Routes of Administration, in Brownlee M. (ed): *Handbook of Diabetes Mellitus* (New York: Garland STPM Press, 1981), vol. 5.

55. Brown M., Rivier J., Vale W.: Somatostatin: central nervous system actions on glucoregulation. *Endocrinology* 104:1709, 1979.

56. Frohman L.A.: Hypothalamic Control of Metabolism, in Morgane P.J.,

Panksepp J. (eds): *Handbook of the Hypothalamus* (New York: Marcel Dekker, 1980), vol. 2.
57. Kitabchi A.E.: Hypercatecholinemia and hypothermia in diabetic ketoacidosis. In preparation.
58. Salans L.B., Cushman S.W.: Relationship of Adiposity and Diet to the Abnormalities of Carbohydrate Metabolism in Obesity, in Katzen H.M., Mahler R.J. (eds): *Diabetes, Obesity, and Vascular Disease* (Washington: Hemisphere Publishing Corporation, 1978).
59. Margules D.L., Moisset B., Lewis M.J., Shibuya H., Pert C.B.: β-Endorphin is associated with overeating in genetically obese mice (ob/ob) and rats (fa/fa). *Science* 202:988, 1978.
60. Grandison L., Guidotti A.: Stimulation of food intake by muscimol and β-endorphin. *Neuropharmacology* 16:533, 1977.
61. Rossier J., Rogers J., Shibasaki T., Guillemin R., Bloom F.E.: Opioid peptides and alpha-melanocyte-stimulating hormone in genetically obese (ob/ob) mice during development. *Proc. Natl. Acad. Sci. USA* 76(4):2077, 1979.
62. Chowers I., Einat R., Feldman S.: Effects of starvation on levels of corticotrophin releasing factor, corticotrophin and plasma corticosterone in rats. *Acta Endocrinol.* 61:687, 1969.
63. Givens J.R., Wiedemann E., Andersen R.N., Kitabchi A.E.: β-Endorphin and β-lipotropin plasma levels in hirsute women: correlation with body weight. *J. Clin. Endocrinol. Metab.* 50(5):975, 1980.

# Panel I: Basic Physiology of Pituitary Function

*Moderator:* RICHARD M. BERGLAND, M.D.
*Panelists:* C. SEYMOUR REICHLIN, M.D., PH.D., L. CASS TERRY, M.D., PH.D., ABBAS E. KITABCHI, PHD., M.D.

BERGLAND: *Dr. Reichlin, would you comment on what we just heard?*

REICHLIN: I told Dr. Kitabchi that he needs another hour to explain what he said in the first hour, and that if I talk I will need another hour to explain what I said. But anyway, I can't comment on the whole talk because he covered an awful lot of stuff—the biosynthesis of all peptides, the integrated metabolic control of glucose metabolism by the pancreas, and finally the role of the brain in glucose homeostasis. I think that is what you were talking about. Let me talk about the role of the brain in glucose homeostasis because that is the most novel and exciting recent material. It also fits in quite a bit with what I was talking about. It looks as though there are integrated systems that regulate major homeostatic functions, the guts of surviving—food intake, water intake, sex drive, sleep, body temperature, glucose homeostasis. There are integrated systems that maintain all of that, and the important new information that Dr. Kitabchi discussed is about the way certain brain systems are organized to fit into that network. The ones that strike me as being extremely interesting, and for which there is a lot of work, are integrated systems for regulation of appetite. In these types of control systems food drive is a behavioral response and feeding into that are substrates. There are signals coming from the gut, such as cholecystokinin, and signals coming from the periphery, such as insulin or insulin modulation, or hormonal modulation by fat depots, and that is all integrated in the brain by neuronal networks that have specific peptide markers. As I

0-8151-3530-0/82/006-63-72-$03.75

interpret Marvin Brown's work, there are bombesin or bombesinergic pathways (to be really precise) that are involved in glucose homeostasis. So that a lot of these signals that impinge on the brain impinge on neurons that are either bombesinergic or intimately related with them. I put that together in a big network. But then that is part of a much bigger picture that includes the angiotensinergic system, which regulates water intake, and maybe the LH-RH system, which regulates the pituitary glands and the sex drive. Obviously, the details are not in yet, but people are putting together these vast multiple phenomena and trying to simplify them into certain circuits of which the brain is one part.

BERGLAND: *Earlier today you showed us somatostatin neurons that were very close to the ventricle. Interpret that for me in light of what I just heard—that this is the "all-American" blocker.*

REICHLIN: Well, you know somatostatin is diffused into the spinal fluid. The dye is very remarkably constant, though Martin's group has recently found that it fluctuates with the diurnal rhythm in monkeys. It is less important that these neurons put somatostatin into the ventricle than that they are so close to the ventricle they are reading what is going on inside the spinal fluid. If you put a small molecule of a chemical into the third ventricle, it goes right to those somatostatin neurons, so that that system and all periventricular systems are being informed, they are getting information constantly by the spinal fluid. Whatever is in the spinal fluid is going to impinge on those neurons.

KITABCHI: *Is there a somatostatin receptor in the brain?*

REICHLIN: I am glad that you bring this up. There is another point I want to make. Cass showed some very classic ideas about somatostatin or biogenetic amine fibers ending on another fiber to form what is called an axoaxonic synapse, so that would be an organized synapse. But I think that one of the things in neurobiology that is becoming more evident is that nerve cells have receptors in two ways: one on organized synapses, which are very restricted, and receptors everywhere, perhaps not condensed into a synapse but on their dendrites, their bodies, and their axons. And the whole state of function of the neuron can be modified by the milieu in which it is bathed. So that the norepinephrine-secreting cell can leak out both at the nerve endings and along the sides, and at the same time it can get information from receptors that are stuck all along the neuron from top to the bottom. In the median eminence, which is really what Cass was showing, electronmicroscopy suggests that there are no organized synapses, that most of the interactions are naked neurons coming into contact with other neurons in a bath of biogenetic amines and other bioactive compounds, and that the action is through receptors on these cells, which are not organized into synapses. These ideas are changing a lot. It is different from two years ago.

BERGLAND: *Are the receptors on the neuronal surface or on the nucleus of the neuron?*

REICHLIN: There are classical nuclear receptors, such as estrogens, progesterone, testosterone, and thyroxin. What holds true for the liver holds true for the brain. You have cellular receptors, I mean you have membrane receptors for peptides and biogenetic amines and nuclear receptors for estrogen and thyroxin. Every neuron does not have or do everything, but there are enough neurons that have specialized functions.

BERGLAND: *Everyone this morning has commented about the prohormone that has traveled under the name of 31K. Is that still a good enough name for this?*

REICHLIN: The β-lipotropin precursor molecule is found in many places. It is found in the anterior pituitary in those species that have intermediate lobes, it is found in the intermediate lobe. Although man has a rudimentary intermediate lobe, it is diffusely scattered through the neurohypophysis. There is a selected population of nerve cells that has a beta-lipotropin. It may actually exist in the adrenal medulla and is also found in the lung. A member of the staff at this school mentioned to me that there are cells in the lung which, when they become neoplastic, form oat cell tumors, and become ectopic ACTH producers. Now in all of these places you have the gene for 31K, and in some cells, the gene is turned on and in other cells it is not. Or the gene can be turned on in the lung to produce ACTH. Now how these cells differ is, first, that the processing is very different. In some cells the only secretion it gets out is ACTH; in others, a piece of ACTH, in others β-lipotropin β-endorphin, and ACTH. So that the cells differ in their machinery for processing and also in how much they store as compared with how much they secrete. And those regional differences, I presume, are related to their functions in different places.

KITABCHI: About six or eight months ago some fascinating studies were published in *Lancet*. When they took apudoma and various materials, they took the messenger RNA and injected it into the frog egg because they cannot convert any further. What they found was

65K and then in some of the tumor tissue, the tumor tissue could not convert, their microsome could not convert to what we know as calcitonin ACTH, while normal tissue could convert as if the last message were somehow missing in this tumor tissue and everybody made 65K. It looks as though that is the way apudoma is.

REICHLIN: The gene for the sequences is there in any cell that makes these peptides, but the processing and packaging and control of secretion is very, very different. We know for a fact that the machinery for making ACTH is turned off by cortisone as part of the feedback loop. That is not true for tumors that make ACTH, like the bronchogenic carcinoma or the oat cell carcinoma. The ACTH secretion by those cells is autonomous. Furthermore, there is a predominance of large ACTH, which is precursor ACTH in tumors of the lung, as compared with pituitary ACTH production. So the processing is a very crucial difference in tissues.

BESSER: We have to be very careful about assuming that what happens in rats happens in the human being. I have been trying to stop myself from talking about it. The evidence in the human being is now very good that the ACTH-related peptides are made on the pro-opiocortone precursor that has been isolated in rats and mice, and it is important to understand the discrepancy in the human being from what we were shown, which really applied mostly to rodents. It would appear that the pro-opiocortone—we just take the corticotropin first, the anterior pituitary cell. You can take human anterior pituitary ACTH-secreting cells in isolation and you can demonstrate in vitro by a perifusion system. That molecule never comes out and it is never found in the blood of the human being, only do you get the fragments and the fragments consist of what we call pro-γ-MSH, which is the front end (for which we have an assay), ACTH (for which we have several assays of different parts of the molecule), and β-lipotropin. Now that is also made in the intermediate lobe in those species where there is an intermediate lobe. Now, Dr. Reichlin and I disagree slightly about the presence of the intermediate lobe in the human adult. It is certainly there in the fetus. You certainly can find a few residual cells in the human adult, but the secretory products identified as being those of the intermediate lobe are never found in the adult human, except, perhaps, in pregnancy. I am not talking about ectopic production by tumors because they can act catalystically, as it were. We can forget those for the moment. No one has ever convincingly shown the intermediate lobe products to occur in the adult human, because the intermediate lobe products consist of what we were shown, which is a breakdown of ACTH into α-MSH and corticotropin-like intermediate lobe peptide (CLIP) that was found and described in our laboratory. Now CLIP is certainly insulinotropic in the obese mouse, but it would be quite wrong to suggest that it is an insulinotropic factor in the human being, because it does not exist in man. Because the cells that can package this part of the molecule do not exist in sufficient quantity anywhere to produce CLIP or α-MSH. So that generation only occurs in subhuman species or as an artifact in the peptide chemist's laboratory. So you get out of the anterior pituitary those three fragments plus a degradation of β-lipotropin into γ-lipotropin and β-endorphin. Now those are the fractions that you find in blood in the human being, going up and down with ACTH; if you have specific assays for all of these, as we do, you can find the dispersed anterior pituitary cells of man coming out of the effluent. β-Endorphin is not and never is converted subsequently into met-enkephalin. Although it contains a sequence of met-enkephalin, there are no data now to support that concept. You do not find met-enkephalin coming from the pituitary. In the human being, met-enkephalin comes from the adrenal medulla from its own precursor, which has nothing to do with this molecule. We have isolated the mean assay constituent of the precursor of met-enkephalin; we have identified met-enkephalin from the adrenal gland of human beings. It also comes from the autonomic ganglion, so it is an antinergic peptide that comes from the autonomic ganglion and not from pro-opiocortone. So that does not occur. Nor do you get MSH, which does not occur in humans except in the ectopic syndromes. Beta-2MSH (β2MSH) is an artifact of a breakdown of the lipotropin molecule because the first people who worked on it boiled the human pituitary in weak acid for 16 hours. So that conversion does not occur in an artifact. Now the brain seems to make pro-opiocortone and to secrete it into the cerebrospinal fluid (CSF), because we have never failed to find the intact molecule in human CSF. It reacts with large 21K fragment, it reacts with pro-γ MSH antiserum, all the MSH antiserums, and all the lipotropin antiserums. So that thing is thrown out in a big parcel. You also find the fragments but that does not happen in blood, another illustration of the difference. Presumably this big parcel is divided up into little bits according to the different parts of the neuraxis that the precursor gets to. Again, met-enkephalin, which does come from the brain, does not come from this precursor. So I think of met-enkephalin as separate. That has lots of interesting effects, for example, on met-enkephalin, in terms of mediating acupuncture relief of the heroin withdrawal syndrome. Acupuncture seems to pinpoint the β-endorphin. Met-enkephalin modulates much of the anterior pituitary hormone secretion. You saw the results; there are a lot more. But this seems to be the cascade in the human being and it does not involve CLIP, which is not insulinotropic in the human being. It does not involve α-MSH that leaks corisportin. β2MSH does not exist. Met-enkephalin does, but it comes from a different source.

BERGLAND: *You're measuring the behaviorally important hormone in the wrong place. Maybe you can never measure it in the right place, because if it is behaviorally important it is probably within the neuron someplace. Given the fact that this is a very long peptide and given my understanding of a neuron, this stuff has got to be made in the reticular substance—endoplasmic reticulum—within the neuron. This cell has a thousand tails. This peptide is going down to many different places in that cell. And do we know anything about whether it is CLIP or not within the neuron, and can we ever know that?*

BESSER: All we can do is extract human brain and spinal cord tissue, which we are doing. The evidence to date suggests that precisely that process goes on and that there are relatively different concentrations in different parts of the brain. You can find the whole molecule and you can find bits of it, and you can find the relative portions of bits of that molecule. In other words, you can find the little parcels made up from the big package in different proportions in different parts of the brain.

BERGLAND: So within the brain it might be important for insulin.

KITABCHI: These points must be made regarding prohormones: (1), just because they are not found in the peripheral circulation does not mean they do not exist. A classic example is the study of preproinsulin and insulin: the former has such a fast turnover rate that it goes undetected in normal human blood. (2), studies on perfused organ or organ extraction of the hormone must be done to establish the tissue's ability to synthesize a hormone or its precursor. Cleavage of precursor to an active hormone may occur at a different subcellular site than that of synthesis. (3), most normal pathways in prohormone synthesis have been studied in abnormal tissue. Again, I refer you to the classic work of Steiner (1969) on proinsulin synthesis first noted in an islet cell adenoma. In similar studies by Oki A.L. (*J. Clin. Endometab.* 52:32, 1981), dispersed pituitary cells from tissues with Cushing's disease were found to secrete ACTH, in β-endorphin, β-lipotropin and α-MSH. Addition of lysovasopressin or TRH and LRH elicited release of these peptides in one case. Thus, we must elucidate the normal biochemical pathways for hormone synthesis in an exaggerated state, e.g., a diseased tissue, rather than in circulation.

BESSER: The point that I am trying to make is that there is a difference between the brain and the extraneural tissues. The precursor hormone is present in CSF. That must have significance. We have never failed to find it. Whereas it is not present in blood. I agree with you that tumors sometimes practice things differently, but unless we understand the normal, we can't interpret the abnormal, we can't use it for clinical purposes.

BERGLAND: Let me put this anecdote before the panel and before everybody. Imagine that a student gets thirsty (there is a new class of hormones that we want to correlate with thirst); he stops studying, goes to a local bar, meets his girlfriend, and suddenly gets hungry. (Now there is a new kind of hormone involved with hunger.) They have a nice meal and suddenly they are filled. (Now we have hormones concerned with satiety.) They return to a room and are lovers. (Now, at the height of this excitement, a new kind of hormone comes to the fore.) She announces that this is the last time and he is filled with rage. (Another class of hormones is involved in his behavioral pattern.) He goes to the top of a tall building, jumps from a window and, as he looks at the sidewalk coming up, he is suddenly filled with fear. (A new class of hormones is involved.) As he passes the tenth floor he recites the 23rd Psalm and it is all joy and peace. (Another kind of hormone is involved.) When he hits the sidewalk there is incredible pain. (Still another kind of hormone!)

The point of my story is, if we were to look at his brain at that time, we would not be able to make any correlations with any of these kinds of hormones. My guess is that most of the time when endocrinologists are looking at an animal's brain, the animal has just had his head in the guillotine for the first time, I really wonder what it means. And yet, if you were to go back and try to make a correlation between any of these hormones and any of these behavioral things that we wish to study, I am not sure where you can sample from to make these kinds of correlations. I don't think you can sample from blood, given the fact that many of these important hormones do not cross the blood-brain barrier and are going to be trapped in brain, and I'm not sure that you can sample from the ventricle, either. It might be that we are never going to be able to make these kinds of correlations that I would like to make.

REICHLIN: I would like to make two comments. You did not ask me but I am going to make them. One is that you are trying to impose a Galen-like simplicity on brain function, which I know you are just doing to make a point, so I will pass over it. The other point I would make is that, when he smashes into the ground, the student is not going to feel anything. There has been a quite fascinating correspondence in the *Lancet* over the last few years about what people feel like when they are about to die. There is a famous quotation by Stanley, the British explorer, who described having been attacked by a lion in Africa. Having his head in the lion's mouth, he felt that he was about to have his head crunched. He felt extreme peace, tranquility, and euphoria. The gist of that correspondence has been that, under such circumstances, the endorphin effect is so profound that you really get a morphine-like high. So I would say that if this fellow did really have a moment before his brains were scattered on the sidewalk, he would be feeling euphoric as he went down.

BERGLAND: *Are there other questions?*

BESSER: There is another thing in *Lancet* that says that one thing that is certain about β-endorphin is that it induces euphoria, both in the recipient and in the research workers.

QUESTION FROM THE AUDIENCE: *Dr. Besser, did the microadenomas of the pituitary have the same breakdown products?*

BESSER: You mean the tumors associated with Cushing's disease, right? We haven't studied very many, but we have not found either the met-enkephalin or MSH or CLIP coming out of those tumors that we have studied.

QUESTION FROM THE AUDIENCE: *Dr. Reichlin, how many prohormones are there going to be found in the brain a century from now? Are there thousands, are there ten, how many are there?*

REICHLIN: Right now, everybody has been bandying around the word, so they numb your mind, but there are hundreds that are recognized and there must be many, many other brain compounds that regulate function that no one has looked for because no one knows how to measure them. A good example is diazepam, that is Valium. Valium receptors have now been identified in the brain. There must be an endogenous Valium like an endogenous endorphin and people have been looking for it.

QUESTION FROM THE AUDIENCE: *Does there have to be a receptor for every hormone for it to be effective?*

REICHLIN: I think that is pretty doctrinal now. If you find an effect, there is a receptor. No there are some other issues, like there are some things like alcohol which don't have receptors, but if you find a receptor, it is most likely there because there is an endogenous compound. If there is an endogenous compound, then it has a precursor. Could someone comment further on somatotropin, that is somatostatin and TRH? Why does it stimulate TRH?

BESSER: Somatostatin is not, by the way, the All-American inhibitor. I think that is quite the wrong impression to allow people to go away with. Somatostatin has a very specific inhibitory profile. It does not inhibit everything. It only inhibits two out of all the anterior pituitary hormones, for example, TSH and gross hormone. It is not in the normal pituitary and it does not do prolactin gonadotropins, either. It has a specific profile although it is fairly broad. I do not think we know what somatostatin does to TRH itself.

REICHLIN: Charlie Hollander reported in one confirmation that somatostatin turns off TRH secretion and there are a couple of reports that somatostatin turns off somatostatin secretion. I like those, those are particularly nice. You know, whose script is responsible for that, makes a very nice statement that somatostatin is ubiquitous but not promiscuous.

BESSER: Somatostatin in human beings certainly can turn off somatostatin. We had a patient who had ectopic production of somatostatin from a carcinoid tumor of the mediastinum, and postoperatively and also preoperatively, the patient had a suppressed GH level. Postoperatively the GH levels were in the acromegalic range and went up paradoxically with glucose and took some 8 to 10 weeks to come down to normal. We have to presume that the somatostatin produced ectopically from a carcinoid tumor of the thymus suppressed the hypothalamic somatostatin, given the paradoxical GH responses of an acromegalic pituitary.

BERGLAND: *We have one minute left. Mike, I would like to put this question to you. So much of the pituitary and our understanding of the pituitary hinges on our ability to measure reliably hormone levels, usually in blood. Would you comment on how well it is done or how poorly it is done?*

BESSER: It is particularly relevant in the ACTH-related peptides. There are common sequences, which we must call beta-MSH, gamma- and beta-lipotropin, met-enkephalin, and beta-endorphin. Anybody who claims to be measuring one in the presence of the other has a very hard job to prove that he can. There are innumerable papers in literature claiming to have specifically measured beta-endorphin, for example. It is theoretically just possible but practically impossible to get a specific beta-endorphin assay that will not also measure beta-lipotropin. There is one described from Sam Yen, who has published several papers on it. He now says that it shows total modal cross reactivity. We checked it in our laboratory and Dorothy Krieger checked it in hers. His specific Y10 antiserum shows 100% cross reactivity with beta-lipotropin. There is no assay that will specifically detect beta-endorphin in the presence of lipotropin. You have to take extraordinary precautions in the collection of the sample to prevent breakdown of that molecule. We collect all our blood samples and cold syringes, immediately cold spin, add the plasma to glycinate cells, and set the pH to 1.5 to stop proteolysis. Everything is chromatographed in formic acid to prevent aggregation of the molecules. We do all the assays using two antisera, one to the N terminal end of the lipotropin and one to the C terminal end of the lipotropin, because one will measure endorphin plus lipotropin and the other only measures gamma- and beta-lipotropin. It is very complicated. It is equally complicated to measure met-enkephalin. You have to do a high-pressure liquid chromatography extraction and convert it all to met-enkephalin sulfoxide, then use an antiserum to the sulfoxide. It sounds complicated because it is.

# Pretreatment Endocrine Evaluation of Patients With Functional Pituitary Tumors

PETER O. KOHLER, M.D.
RICHARD JORDAN, M.D.

*Department of Medicine, University of Arkansas for Medical Sciences, Little Rock, Arkansas*

## Introduction

THE ABILITY OF THE CLINICIAN to assess pituitary function has improved dramatically over the past 15 years. New and constantly improving assays for peripheral blood levels of hormones have been developed and great advances have been made in understanding the hypothalamic control of pituitary function. The isolation and synthesis of several of the hypothalamic hypophysiotropic hormones have provided additional tools for clinical testing. Each newly identified releasing or inhibiting factor or analogue developed provides a potential technique for testing pituitary function.

Endocrine testing used to evaluate pituitary function includes direct assay of pituitary or target hormone levels in the blood and on occasion assay of urine for these hormones or their metabolites. Measurement of basal blood hormone concentration is of somewhat limited usefulness because of the wide fluctuation in such levels. For this reason a variety of tests have been designed to either stimulate or suppress secretion of the trophic hormones.

Types of stimulation tests for pituitary function are shown schematically in Figures 1 and 2. Direct stimulation tests (see Fig 1) may be nonspecific, such as hypoglycemia, which causes release of ACTH, GH, and prolactin. Stimulation tests may be directed to specific hor-

73

0-8151-3530-0/82/006-73-95-$03.75

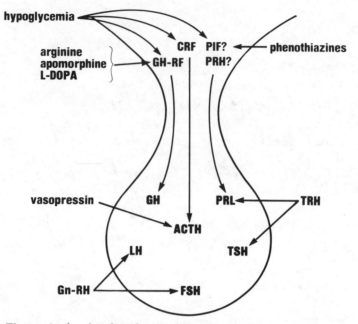

**Fig 1.**—Agents that directly stimulate release of pituitary hormones.

mones by the use of physiologic releasing hormones such as thyrotropin-releasing hormone (TRH) which also releases prolactin, or gonadotropin-releasing hormone (GnRH). At one time it had been hoped that the releasing hormones could accurately differentiate between the secondary pituitary hormone deficiencies caused by pituitary disease and deficits caused by hypothalamic disorders, which are termed "tertiary" hormone deficiencies. Unfortunately, the types of response in the secondary pituitary hormone deficiency and the tertiary or hypothalamic type are not specific enough to clearly distinguish between these forms of hormone deficiency.[1]

In addition to using direct tests for stimulating pituitary hormone release, the normal feedback regulation can be altered (see Fig 2). This can be used not only to attempt to suppress excess secretion, but also to block feedback regulation by a target organ such as the adrenal gland so that greater amounts of the trophic hormone are secreted. In addition to blocking the normal target gland hormone synthesis (as with metyrapone, to block cortisol synthesis and stimulate ACTH release), a competitive analogue can be used to block the feedback at the hypothalamic or pituitary level (see Fig 2). An example

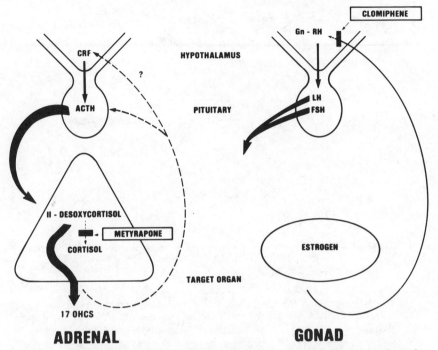

**Fig 2.**—Two methods are illustrated for stimulating pituitary hormone release by interfering with target organ feedback. Metyrapone decreases cortisol synthesis by blocking 11-β-hydroxylase. As a result, ACTH secretion is increased. Compound S (11-desoxycortisol) levels are increased in blood, and urinary 17OHCS levels which include metabolites of Compound S, are increased. In contrast, clomiphene citrate blocks the feedback of sex steroids at the hypothalamic level and results in increased gonadotropin secretion. (Figs 1–3 after Jordan & Kohler: *approach to laboratory diagnosis in internal medicine.* Stein J., ed, Little, Brown and Co, 1982.)

of this is clomiphene citrate, an estrogen analogue that increases gonadotropin release.

Suppression tests (Fig 3) are most commonly used to evaluate disease resulting from pituitary hormone hypersecretion, such as acromegaly and pituitary dependent Cushing's disease. In these disorders hormone overproduction results from autonomous secretion by a tumor or from a state of altered feedback regulation of the hypothalamic-pituitary axis. The hypersecreted hormone does not respond quantitatively or qualitatively to physiologic stimuli that normally suppress hormone secretion. Thus, failure of appropriate suppression during testing procedures that normally inhibit pituitary hormone secretion strongly suggests a disorder of pituitary hormone overproduction. Table 1 lists the endocrine tests used for this evaluation.

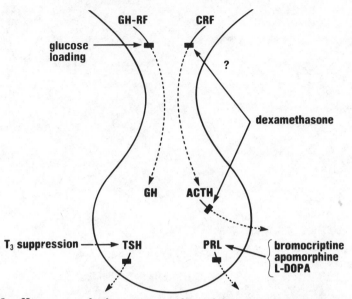

**Fig 3.**—Hormones and other agents used to inhibit pituitary hormone secretion. These agents will normally suppress the hormone indicated. In pituitary hypersecretory states such as acromegaly or Cushing's disease, suppression to appropriate agent may be absent, incomplete, or occur at a higher dose than normal. Prolactinomas, however, generally respond to agents that suppress prolactin secretion in a manner similar to other hyperprolactinemic states.

The endocrine evaluation of patients with pituitary disease should depend on the particular goal in the individual patients. Pituitary tumors usually produce morbidity by a combination of hormone hypersecretion and/or local mass effects of the expanding adenoma. Therefore, the problems of hypersecretion of one hormone may be combined with deficiencies of other "innocent bystander" hormones from destruction of normal pituitary tissue. This combination is obviously more likely to occur in patients with large tumors. These patients with hormone deficiencies are also more likely to have an enlarged sella and possible visual field defects. However, even in a patient with an obvious hypersecretory syndrome such as prolactinoma, acromegaly, or Cushing's disease, the endocrine status should be evaluated prior to treatment. The reasons for this evaluation include confirmation of the diagnosis to establish the extent of pretreatment hormone excess, determination of the degree of pretreatment pituitary hormone deficiencies so that they can be managed before and during definitive therapy, and gathering of baseline data with which to judge the effect of treatment or to document subsequent tumor progression.

The extent of the endocrine evaluation in patients with functioning pituitary tumors varies considerably with the type and size of the tumor. A reasonable evaluation does not require an excessive amount of hospital time. Certain historical data, such as the presence of cyclic menses or a normal semen analysis, are a better indication of normal gonadotropin function than the usual laboratory tests. Therefore, the endocrine evaluation should be composed of a judicious selection of available tests for the hypersecreted hormone, in the case of a functional tumor, as well as for the adequacy of the other pituitary hormones. The following discussion will first consider specific tests for each hormone and then potential tests for patients with specific diseases.

## Endocrine Evaluation of Pituitary Function

The evaluation of pituitary function will be divided into two major sections. The first will deal with tests for hormone excess associated with specific disorders such as prolactinoma, acromegaly, and Cushing's disease. Tests to establish these diagnoses will be discussed (Table 1). The second section will deal with testing for endocrine deficiencies. These can occur as the result of a nonfunctioning pituitary tumor or other mass lesions. However, deficiencies of one or more anterior pituitary hormones can also occur as a result of a hormone-secreting pituitary adenoma. Therefore, evaluation in a patient with

TABLE 1.—TYPES OF ENDOCRINE TESTS USED IN EVALUATION OF
PITUITARY FUNCTION

| TYPES | COMMENT |
|---|---|
| Basal blood levels | Frequent temporal variation |
| Urinary excretion of hormone or metabolites | Integrates 24-hour period, but may be difficult to collect accurately on general hospital unit |
| Stimulation tests | Usually used to determine if secretion is adequate, as in hypopituitarism, but may be useful in some hypersecreting adenomas such as prolactinomas |
| Direct | Examples: TRH, GnRh |
| Indirect | Utilize block of feedback inhibition |
| Suppression tests | Usually used to determine if excessive secretion is normally or appropriately suppressed |
| Other | Imaging techniques such as CT scanning and adrenal radionuclide scanning are sometimes valuable in pituitary disorders |

a disease such as acromegaly should also include an assessment of the "innocent bystander" pituitary hormones, which may be deficient as a result of compression of the normal pituitary tissue by an expanding adenoma.

## TESTS FOR HORMONE EXCESS

These will be considered according to the suggested clinical condition.

### *Prolactinoma*

The evaluation of a patient with a suspected prolactinoma is usually designed to differentiate the patient with a true prolactinoma from patients with the multiple other causes of hyperprolactinemia listed in Table 2. The diagnosis of a prolactinoma is often suspected in the young woman with galactorrhea and/or amenorrhea, the young man with decreased libido or impotence, or in a patient of either sex with a large pituitary tumor.[3] The following tests are useful.

BASAL BLOOD LEVELS.—Prolactin blood levels by radioimmunoassay are a reasonably reliable method of determining prolactin excess.[2] Levels above 20 μg/ml in man and 25 μg/ml in women are

TABLE 2.—CAUSES OF
HYPERPROLACTINEMIA*

Physiologic
  Newborn
  Pregnancy
  Nursing mothers
  Stress
  Sleep
  Drugs (estrogens, TRH,
      dopamine antagonists such as
      phenothiazines,
      metoclopramide, reserpine,
      methyldopa)
Pathologic
  Prolactinoma
  Hypothalamic disorders
  Pituitary stalk damage or lesion
  Primary hypothyroidism
  Renal disease
  Idiopathic

*Adapted from Cowden: *Ann. Clin. Biochem.*
16:113, 1979.

generally believed to be abnormal. However, stress, many drugs and other factors will also elevate prolactin levels. Table 2 lists various known causes of prolactin elevations. To avoid possible problems related to stress, several authorities recommend three fasting basal samples drawn at least 20 minutes apart or on separate days. Since there is some diurnal prolactin variation,[2, 3] the levels should probably be drawn at a constant time or between 9:00 A.M. and noon, when levels are lowest. Once complicating factors such as stress or drugs have been excluded by history and appropriate evaluation, there remains the clinical problem of identifying patients with pituitary adenomas and separating them from patients with idiopathic galactorrhea. The latter condition in some instances is related to the presence of a microadenoma too small to be identified by current radiographic techniques, including the very important computerized tomography (CT), with or without enhancement techniques.

SUPPRESSION TESTS FOR PROLACTINOMA.—Although dopaminergic agonists suppress prolactin levels,[4] these tests, including L-dopa and bromocriptine, usually suppress elevated prolactin levels regardless of etiology. Therefore, these agents generally have not been useful in differentiating patients with adenoma from those with hyperprolactinemia from other causes. Water loading has been reported to suppress prolactin levels[5] but confirmation has been difficult and the test has not been found to be clinically useful.[6]

STIMULATION TESTS FOR PROLACTIN.—Since prolactin suppression tests are nonspecific at present, stimulation tests have been used in an effort to differentiate adenomas from nontumorous causes of hyperprolactinemia.[7–10] These tests represent an exception to the more common use of stimulation tests to document adequate hormone levels. Although prolactin levels have been increased during the insulin tolerance test, the major forms of prolactin stimulation have been TRH, which acts directly on prolactin-secreting cells to stimulate prolactin release, and the antidopaminergic drugs metoclopramide and chlorpromazine (CPZ), which presumably block the dopaminergic suppression of prolactin release. Although normal people usually show at least a doubling of basal prolactin values, patients with prolactinomas generally have a blunted response with less than a 50% increase in prolactin levels after the stimulatory tests.

CPZ increases prolactin levels in normal people. The mechanism appears to consist of an alteration of the normal hypothalamic suppression of prolactin secretion through a presumptive decrease in the prolactin inhibiting factor (PIF). The test is performed by giving

25 mg of CPZ intramuscularly and obtaining blood specimens immediately and one, two, and three hours afterward. The CPZ test has some risks[11] and does not allow clear differentiation between prolactinoma and patients with idiopathic galactorrhea-amenorrhea.[8, 9]

METOCLOPRAMIDE TEST.—Metoclopramide is perhaps the most potent stimulator of prolactin secretion in normal adults. A dose of 10 mg given intravenously produces at least a doubling of prolactin levels in normal men and women. Blood samples for prolactin should be drawn at 0, 15, 60, and 120 minutes.[10] Patients with prolactinomas usually show a considerably blunted response with less than a 50% increase in prolactin levels. This test has been used in conjunction with the TRH test by some authorities to diagnose small prolactinomas in patients with a normal sella turcica.[10]

TRH TEST.—This test is performed by giving 400 μg of TRH intravenously and obtaining blood at 0, 15, 30, 60, and 90 minutes. The two most important samples—those taken at once and 30 minutes later—are usually adequate for prolactin. A normal response is at least a doubling of prolactin values in women and an increase greater than 50% of basal levels in men. The side effects include occasional increases or decreases in blood pressure, urinary urgency, sweating, and palpitations. These are fairly frequent (they appear in 50% of patients) but usually mild and transient. The response in tumor patients appears to be blunted[8-10] but this type of response may also be seen in idiopathic galactorrhea-amenorrhea.

## Conclusions

Although there is some disagreement regarding the role of dynamic tests, basal prolactin levels over 100 ng/ml frequently, and over 300 ng/ml usually, indicate a pituitary adenoma. Prolactin levels of less than 100 ng/ml also are commonly associated with prolactinomas. However, the absolute level is not diagnostic, since in this range there is considerable overlap with other hyperprolactinemic disorders. This information should be used in conjunction with radiographic information, including the improved CT scans or tomography to identify patients with adenomas or hypothalamic lesions. In difficult patients with modest prolactin elevations, the blunted prolactin response to TRH and metoclopramide have been used to identify patients with small adenomas in radiographically normal sella.[10] The assessment of patients with prolactinomas for deficiencies of other pituitary hormones is discussed below.

## Acromegaly and Gigantism

The diagnosis of acromegaly can usually be made by using the combination of characteristic signs and symptoms. The major laboratory finding in acromegaly has been the documentation of inappropriately elevated GH levels. Since GH may be elevated as a result of stress, the failure to suppress normally after a glucose load has provided a more reliable laboratory test in most series. Normal people suppress GH levels to essentially unmeasurable levels by 30 to 90 minutes after an oral glucose load.

SUPPRESSION TESTS.—Glucose suppression of GH is performed in the same manner as a standard glucose tolerance test. Fifty to 100 gm of glucose is given by mouth in the fasting state. Blood for glucose and GH is drawn at 0, 30, 60, 90, and 120 minutes. At some point between 30 to 90 minutes the GH levels should be less than 2 to 3 ng/ml. Failure to suppress below this level is an abnormality found in acromegaly. Patients with acromegaly or gigantism may show a partial suppression, no change, or a paradoxical rise in GH levels.[12] Patients with a few other conditions such as acute intermittent porphyria, anorexia, starvation, cirrhosis, or renal failure may also show a failure to suppress GH levels.[13] However, the clinical differentiation of these conditions from acromegaly does not usually present any problem.

### STIMULATORY TESTS

*TRH tests.*—Patients with acromegaly show a variety of abnormal responses to normal releasing factors. TRH does not provoke a GH release in normal people, but will release GH in approximately 80% to 90% of acromegalic patients. This may be used as a diagnostic test with TRH injected as described above and GH levels measured.[14, 15] However, this test also has some false positive responses in nonacromegalic patients with psychiatric disorder or diabetes mellitus.[16] GnRH also may release GH abnormally in acromegalic patients and may be used as an ancillary diagnostic maneuver.[15] Dopaminergic agents such as L-dopa and bromocriptine depress GH levels in acromegalic patients.[17] Bromocriptine has had more therapeutic than diagnostic usefulness, and in most medical centers these tests are rarely used for diagnostic purposes.

*Somatomedin assay.*—Since GH acts at least in part through the stimulation of somatomedins by the liver, the new radioreceptor and radioimmunoassays for the somatomedins have been proposed as a less labile means of measuring GH excess. This has theoretical potential and the measurment of somatomedin-C has had promising results in some series.[18] However, in our own experience the currently available commercial assay for somatomedin-C has not been of value in determining the postoperative GH activity in acromegalic patients.[19] Newer assays for the somatomedins may be of greater value.

The visual field measurement and CT scanning or tomography of the sella turcica are also important in the preoperative evaluation of the acromegalic patient.

## Conclusions

The diagnosis of acromegaly rests on the clinical features and the measurement of elevated GH levels that fail to suppress after a glucose load. Other endocrine tests, such as the TRH stimulation of GH release, may provide diagnostic or confirmatory information. The mass effects of the pituitary adenoma should be evaluated by CT scanning. In some instances tomography may be useful. Ophthalmologic evaluation should be performed in most patients prior to surgery or irradiation.

## Cushing's Disease

The patient with findings suggestive of Cushing's syndrome must have the existence of hypercortisolism established by biochemical means. The screening tests most commonly used are the overnight dexamethasone suppression test, urine free cortisol measurement, and the determination of the diurnal variation of cortisol (assuming the P.M. value is obtained in the late evening). If one or more of these screening tests indicate that Cushing's syndrome is present, the source of the hypercortisolism must be found. The major considerations are pituitary-dependent Cushing's disease (Cushing's disease usually secondary to an ACTH-secreting pituitary tumor), an adrenal adenoma, an adrenal carcinoma, or ectopic ACTH secretion.

A useful diagnostic protocol is that of measuring baseline urine 17-hydroxycorticosteroids (17OHCS), plasma cortisol, and the plasma ACTH concentration, and then determining the patient's response of the urine 17OHCS to metyrapone, 2 mg of dexamethasone, and 8 mg of dexamethasone.[20] The plasma cortisol response to dexamethasone should also be measured. The protocol is performed as follows: Basal urines are collected on days one and two. On day 3, the patient is given metyrapone, 750 mg orally, every 4 hours for 6 doses. Since the increase of urinary 17OHCS in response to metyrapone can occur on the day of or the day following administration of this agent, urine is collected on day 4 without any manipulations being performed. On days 5 and 6, the patient receives 0.5 mg of dexamethasone every 6 hours (2 mg dexamethasone test) and on days 7 and 8 the patient is given 2 mg of dexamethasone every 6 hours (8 mg dexamethasone test). Although some physicians are now advocating an abbreviated workup for Cushing's syndrome, relying heavily upon the plasma ACTH value,[21] we believe that until such an approach is fully validated the standard workup probably should be routinely used.

The response of the various types of Cushing's syndrome to these manipulations and the expected basal plasma ACTH concentration in each entity is shown in Table 3. Thus, the 2-mg dexamethasone test is used to confirm Cushing's syndrome because normals will suppress with this dose whereas patients with Cushing's syndrome will not. The 8-mg dexamethasone test is used to separate pituitary-dependent Cushing's disease from the other varieties of Cushing's syndrome because only patients with the pituitary-dependent form will show suppression. It should be noted, however, that some patients with pituitary-dependent Cushing's disease have only mild or equivocal suppression with 8 mg of dexamethasone, but usually such patients will suppress when given 32 mg of dexamethasone.[20] Metyrapone is useful since only patients with pituitary-dependent Cushing's disease will respond with an increase of the urinary 17OHCS. Although many experienced endocrinologists do not use metyrapone in the workup of Cushing's syndrome, we have found it very helpful in diagnosis, especially in patients with equivocal suppression with dexamethasone. During sequential urine collections it is prudent to save an aliquot from each 24-hour collection to allow retesting of specimens lost or mishandled by the laboratory. The plasma cortisol will not increase with metyrapone, which inhibits the conversion of 11 desoxycortisol to cortisol.

Plasma ACTH determinations are used to distinguish adrenal tumors from the ectopic ACTH syndrome. Patients with pituitary-dependent Cushing's disease have ACTH levels with normal to slightly elevated ranges. With an adrenal tumor the ACTH concentration should be undetectable, whereas patients with the ectopic ACTH syndrome generally have a very high plasma ACTH level. Adrenal tumors can be further delineated with CT scanning, adrenal venography, or adrenal arteriography. Adrenal scanning with iodocho-

TABLE 3.—RESPONSE TO TESTING PROCEDURE*

| VARIETY OF CUSHING'S SYNDROME | PLASMA ACTH | METYRAPONE (URINARY 17-OHCS) | DEXAMETHASONE 2 MG (URINE 17-OHCS) | DEXAMETHASONE 8 MG (URINE 17-OHCS) |
|---|---|---|---|---|
| Pituitary-dependent Cushing's disease | Normal or mildly elevated | Increase to as much as 2–3 times over baseline | No change or minimal suppressing from baseline | Definite† suppression |
| Adrenal neoplasm (Adenoma or carcinoma) | Undetectable | No change or fall | No change | No change |
| Ectopic ACTH | Usually very elevated | No change | No change | No change |

*Characteristic basal plasma ACTH concentration and the expected response of the urinary 17OHCS to dynamic testing with metyrapone and dexamethasone in patients with Cushing's syndrome of various etiologies.

†Some patients with ACTH-secreting pituitary tumors will not suppress with 8 mg of dexamethasone but will suppress with 32 mg of dexamethasone.

Paradoxical response to dexamethasone or metyrapone suggests the presence of cyclic Cushing's syndrome.

lesterol will also visualize benign tumors; however, carcinomas usually will not concentrate sufficient radiolabeled cholesterol to be detected.[22]

A caveat in the diagnostic workup of Cushing's syndrome is the increasingly recognized entity of cyclic Cushing's syndrome.[23] Such patients demonstrate rhythmic fluctuations of adrenal cortisol production, which is largely independent of the diagnostic manipulation being performed. Cycles have varied from 4.5 to 86 days. Thus, one may obtain very confusing test results with totally unexpected results, such as a paradoxical increase with dexamethasone administration. Patients described with periodic Cushing's syndrome usually have had ACTH-secreting pituitary tumors, but bronchial carcinoids causing this syndrome have also been described. Another potentially confusing situation is the development of a "pseudo"-Cushing's syndrome in which some alcoholic patients have physical findings and biochemical evidence of hypercortisolism.[24] Discontinuing alcohol results in resolution of the disorder. Drugs can also affect test results for Cushing's syndrome. Diphenylhydantoin accelerates the metabolism of both metyrapone and dexamethasone, which can alter testing results.[25, 26] Details of the endocrine testing procedures for Cushing's syndrome are discussed below.

TESTS FOR ACTH SECRETION

*The hypothalamic-pituitary-adrenal axis in the basal state.*—Detecting perturbations of ACTH secretion in the basal state includes blood determinations of ACTH, cortisol, and excretion of cortisol and its metabolites in urine. This type of measurement is most helpful in states of ACTH excess, although very low blood levels of cortisol in the morning (8:00 A.M.) are very suggestive of hypocortisolism.

*Diurnal variation of cortisol.*—The 8:00 A.M. cortisol varies between 8 and 22 µg/dl and the 10:30 P.M. cortisol should be less than 10 µg/dl. Loss of this diurnal rhythm is a strong indication of hypercortisolism.[27] A common error is to obtain the evening specimen too early, which can lead to an incorrect diagnosis of Cushing's syndrome. Loss of this variation is also seen in depression and in patients with liver disease. Presumably the abnormality in liver disease occurs because of a reduced rate of cortisol removal from plasma.

*Plasma ACTH.*—Plasma ACTH measurement has only recently become available to the clinician. Unfortunately, many commercial assays are of questionable reliability in regard to reproducibility of results. In addition, ACTH secretion is quite pulsatile, and like the gonadotropins it requires at least three specimens obtained several minutes apart in order to be confident that the level obtained is truly a representative value.[20] The conditions for collection of ACTH are extremely important. The specimen needs to be immediately placed in an ice bath and maintained in chilled state until the plasma is separated and frozen. Deviation from this procedure will result in destruction of the ACTH molecule and artificial lowering of the ACTH level. Basal plasma ACTH levels are most useful in the diagnostic workup of Cushing's syndrome in the instances in which very high concentrations are seen in the ectopic ACTH syndrome and uniformly suppressed levels are present in patients with an adrenal tumor (Fig 4). Patients with pituitary-dependent Cushing's syndrome have ACTH values that hover at or just above the upper limit of normal.[20] The normal 8:00 A.M. value ranges from 20 to 110 pg/ml. In patients with Nelson's syndrome ACTH levels may become extraordinarily elevated; values as high as 100,000 pg/ml are sometimes seen.

*Urine-free cortisol.*—The urine-free cortisol is a measurement of the cortisol secreted in urine that is neither metabolized nor conjugated. It represents approximately 0.2% of the cortisol secreted by the adrenal glands. In normal people the total free cortisol in urine is virtually always less than 100 μg per 24 hours. In a well-validated assay, this type of measurement is an especially good means to document hypercortisolism.[27] Elevated values do, however, occur in uncomplicated pregnancy.[28]

*Urinary 17-hydroxycorticosteroids (17OHCS).*—The urinary 17OHCS measures the conjugated steroids that have a 17-21-dihydroxy-20-ketone structure. Approximately 25% to 30% of the total cortisol is metabolized in this fashion. Many drugs can lead to interference with urinary 17OHCS determinations, and large urine volumes can cause difficulty in extraction. The normal range is from 3 to 10 mg per 24 hours or per gm creatinine. However, results may differ somewhat from laboratory to laboratory.

*Stimulatory testing.*—Metyrapone is a useful test in the evaluation of Cushing's syndrome because only patients with an intact hypothalamic-pituitary-adrenal axis show a brisk increase of the urinary 17OHCS in response to this drug. Patients with a cortisol-secreting adrenal tumor (adenoma or carcinoma) or ectopic ACTH secretion do not respond to metyrapone because high levels of circulating cortisol have suppressed the hypothalamic-pituitary axis in regard to ACTH secretion. Details of the mechanism of action by which metyrapone works are discussed later in the chapter. To perform the test 750 mg of metyrapone is given at four-hour intervals over 24 hours. Urine is

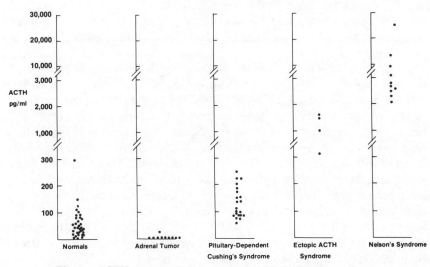

**Fig 4.**—ACTH concentration in patients with Cushing's syndrome.

collected the day of and the day after administration of metyrapone, since the maximum increase of urinary 17OHCS can occur on either day.

*Suppression tests.*—Dexamethasone, a potent synthetic glucocorticoid, will readily suppress ACTH secretion in normal individuals. This testing is used to document the presence of Cushing's syndrome and, by administering graded increases of dexamethasone, hypercortisolism resulting from pituitary-dependent Cushing's disease can be separated from other varieties of Cushing's syndrome.

*Overnight dexamethasone suppression.*—The overnight dexamethasone suppression test is a screening procedure used to diagnose hypercortisolism.[27] The dosage used is small, such that almost all normal individuals show suppression of plasma cortisol, whereas the plasma cortisol level in those patients with hypercortisolism, regardless of the etiology, is not suppressed. To perform the test, 1 mg of dexamethasone is given at 11:00 P.M. and the plasma cortisol is measured at 8:00 A.M. It should be suppressed to less than 5 µg/dl. Occasionally there are false positive results with low-dose dexamethasone. This is most commonly seen in depression, chronically ill patients, and obesity.[27] Thus, the diagnosis of Cushing's syndrome should be confirmed with standard dexamethasone testing, as discussed below.

*Dexamethasone 2 mg and 8 mg suppression.*—To assess the patient's response to dexamethasone, urinary 17-hydroxycorticosteroids

(17OHCS) are collected during the period of administration. With 2 mg of dexamethasone per day the urinary 17OHCS of normal adults will suppress to less than 3 mg per 24 hours. Patients with Cushing's syndrome of any variety will not demonstrate normal suppression, thus separating normals from patients with Cushing's syndrome. Given 8 mg of dexamethasone the great majority of patients with pituitary-dependent Cushing's disease will show significant suppression of the urinary 17OHCS but not necessarily to less than 3 mg for 24 hours. Occasionally a patient with pituitary-dependent Cushing's disease will not show any suppression with 8 mg of dexamethasone but usually will suppress when given 32 mg of dexamethasone. This suggests that there may be a spectrum of gradations in disordered cortisol feedback in pituitary-dependent Cushing's disease. Dexamethasone suppression is usually accomplished by giving 0.5 mg every six hours for two days (2 mg test), which is followed by giving 2 mg every six hours for two days (8 mg test).[29] This testing sequence is often combined with metyrapone, as discussed above.

## Conclusions

The presence of Cushing's syndrome is usually suggested by characteristic physical findings, some of which are central obesity, hirsutism, hypertension, and glucose intolerance. To confirm the suspicion of Cushing's syndrome, screening tests using either an overnight dexamethasone test or determinations of the diurnal variation of cortisol should be performed. If the screening tests are indicative of hypercortisolism, the patient needs to be hospitalized for a standard workup, including baseline measurements for urinary 17OHCS and plasma cortisol levels, followed by dynamic studies employing metyrapone and the 2-mg and 8-mg dexamethasone suppression tests. Greatly abbreviated versions of the Cushing's syndrome workup probably should not be routinely performed until they have been validated as superior to the standard testing protocol.

## TSH-, LH-, or FSH-Secreting Tumors

Although hypersecreting adenomas producing the glycoprotein hormones (TSH, LH, and FSH) have been described, they are extremely uncommon. Frequently, gonadotropin or TSH hypersecretion occurs as the result of primary gonadal or thyroid deficiency, respectively. In these instances the feedback of target organ hormones is reduced and subsequent increased secretion of the appropriate trophic hormone occurs. This may progress to actual pituitary and sella enlargement. The enlarged sella of primary hypothyroidism has been recognized in children and adults.[30] Similarly, gonadal insufficiency such as occurs in Turner's or Klinefelter's syndrome may lead to increased gonadotropins and sella enlargement.[31] The important clinical aspect is to recognize that the sella enlargement is the result of a response to the target organ failure. This is one reason for measuring the glycoprotein hormones in patients with an enlarged sella. At times, this "secondary" hypertrophy or hyperplasia of the pituitary may become autonomous and fail to suppress after administration of the appropriate target hormone. Rarely, hypersecretory tumors producing glycoprotein hormones appear to arise in the absence of target organ failure. These will be found during the screening tests for hormone deficiency suggested below.

## Tests for Hormone Deficiencies in Patients with Pituitary Tumors

PROLACTIN.—Since prolactin deficiency causes no clinically recognizable syndrome except failure to lactacte in the postpartum woman, prolactin stimulatory tests such as the TRH test or metoclopramide test described above are not usually necessary in patients with pituitary lesions. However, basal prolactin levels should always be measured in patients with suspected nonsecreting pituitary tumors because of the relatively high incidence of prolactin secretion in "functionless" pituitary adenomas.[32]

### Tests of GH Secretion

*Stimulation tests.*—GH levels may be valuable in the assessment of pituitary function. GH deficiency is a "silent" lesion in adults. To adequately evaluate GH reserve, GH provocative tests must be performed. There are multiple possible GH stimulation tests.[33] Some of the more commonly used are listed below.

*Insulin-induced hypoglycemia.*—Hypoglycemic stress activates hypothalamic pathways that presumably cause a stimulation of GH-releasing factor that then acts on the pituitary to cause GH release. Insulin at 0.1–0.2 μ/kg of body weight is injected intravenously and blood is drawn for GH (and cortisol) at 0, 30, 60, and 120 minutes. The blood sugar must decrease to below 45 mg/dl for an adequate test. In normal individuals the GH will exceed at least 7 ng/ml during the test. The presence of either hypothyroidism or hypogonadism may cause a subnormal GH increase that reverts to normal once the deficiencies are corrected. Obesity will also blunt the GH response. The test is usually safe but should be performed with utmost caution or avoided in patients over 65 years of age and patients with cardiac or cerebrovascular disease.[34]

*L-dopa.*—L-dopa, a precursor of both dopamine and norepinephrine, is a stimulatory agent for GH secretion.[35] It is presumed that α-stimulation within the hypothalamus mediates the formation and/or release of GH-releasing factor, which then causes GH secretion. A normal response is a GH value of 7 ng/ml or greater. The test is performed by oral administration of 500 mg of L-dopa and collecting blood at 0, 30, 60, 90, and 120 minutes.

*Apomorphine.*—Apomorphine, a dopamine agonist, stimulates GH release through α-stimulation via apparent hypothalamic activation of GH-releasing factor.[36] A subemetic dose of 750 μg is administered subcutaneously. Although a value of 7 ng/ml is considered a normal response, most normal people increase their growth concentration to considerably higher levels.

*Arginine.*—Arginine stimulates GH secretion presumably through the hypothalamus.[37] A solution of 30 gm of arginine in 100 ml of sterile water is given over 30 minutes and the blood is sampled at 0, 30, 60, 90 and 120 minutes. In children, the dose is 0.5 μg/kg of body weight. A normal response is an increase of GH to greater than 7 ng/ml.

TESTS FOR GONADOTROPIN SECRETION.—The possibility of hypogonadotropic hypogonadism is one reason for evaluation of the hypothalamic-pituitary-gonadal axis in patients with pituitary disease. Although many women come to the physician with the complaint of amenorrhea, men seem less likely to volunteer problems in the area of decreased libido and impotence. Laboratory assessment of gonadotropin function is less important in the women with normal cyclic menses (once it is certain she is not taking oral contraceptives) or in the man with a normal sperm count. The latter is infrequently used, but is a cost-effective method for screening men for hypogonadism.

Basal levels of FSH and LH measured in the blood can provide important information in both men and women. These should be measured on three occasions at least 10–20 minutes apart to avoid the problem of fluctuating blood levels.[38] Unfortunately, there is still a problem in distinguishing low from normal blood levels of the gonadotropins. The serum testosterone value is very helpful in the male to exclude hypogonadotropic hypogonadism. Testosterone is low in hypogonadotropic states in men. Plasma estradiol levels are less useful in women because of the greater fluctuations. Vaginal smears for estrogen activity and cervical mucus patterns can provide some information of biologic effect of estrogen. Twenty-four hour urine values for gonadotropin by radioimmunoassay or bioassay are still useful in certain situations. However, normal people can have low values by either measurement, so that distinguishing low and normal values may be difficult.[39]

GONADOTROPIN STIMULATION TESTS.—GnRH is a stimulatory agent for both LH and FSH.[40] To perform the test 100 to 150 μg of GnRH is injected intravenously or subcutaneously and blood samples are drawn at 0, 30, 45, 60, and 90 minutes. LH levels usually increase by at least 10 mIU/ml over baseline values in normal people. The FSH response is considerably less. The test does not reliably separate hypothalamic from pituitary disease since both hypopituitarism and diseases in which there is a GnRH deficiency, such as Kallmann's syndrome or a craniopharyngioma, may have a blunted response to GnRH. Therefore, this test is not presently a positive one for gonadotropin evaluation. GnRH has not as yet been released by the FDA for commercial use.

Another approach to evaluation of gonadotropin function is the Clomid or clomiphene citrate test. Clomiphene is widely used as a fertility drug and the clinical test works on the same principle of feedback inhibition of sex steroids on the hypothalamic-pituitary unit. Clomiphene is an estrogen antagonist, but works on both males and females.[41] The test can be performed on an outpatient basis with 50 to 100 mg a day for seven days. A normal response is a doubling of LH values. In women, a menstrual period may also be used as an indication of a normal pituitary response.

### TESTS FOR TSH SECRETION

*Basal thyroxine (T₄) and TSH.*—In any patient with a pituitary mass lesion it is important to measure the levels of thyroid hormone in blood. This is most easily performed by determining the blood levels of the $T_4$, the $T_3$ resin uptake, and the TSH. The $T_3$ resin uptake is helpful because it can be used to adjust the $T_4$ level for abnormalities of thyroid-binding proteins in blood. Measurement of the TSH will allow the physician to distinguish between primary (dysfunction of the thyroid) and secondary (dysfunction of the hypothalamic-pituitary unit) forms of hypothyroidism. In primary hypothyroidism the TSH levels are greatly elevated with a low $T_4$, whereas in secondary hypothyroidism TSH levels are low or normal in the face of a low $T_4$.

Although mildly hypothyroid patients may tolerate anesthesia and surgery well, it is important to identify severely hypothyroid patients prior to operation so that such deficits can be replaced before surgery. Patients with moderate to severe hypothyroidism tend to develop respiratory difficulties postoperatively and generally have less tolerance for stress. In addition, primary hypothyroidism in some instances can mimic a pituitary neoplasm.[42] This occurs because hypothyroidism results in hypertrophy and hyperplasia of thyrotropic cells in the pituitary. This can occur to such an extent there is enlargement of the sella turcica with extension of the mass into the basilar cisterns. Since hyperprolactinemia and galactorrhea can also occur as a result of hypothyroidism, the clinical picture may closely resemble a pituitary tumor. Such patients must be recognized because thyroid hormone replacement results in virtual total involution of the hyperplastic cells even when there is considerable suprasellar extension, thus making a surgical procedure unnecessary.[42]

TESTS FOR ADEQUACY OF ACTH SECRETION.—Basal levels of plasma cortisol drawn at 7:00 A.M. to 8:00 A.M. are useful in screening for ACTH deficiency. Morning blood levels are preferable to evening levels when testing for adequate function. Urinary 17OHCS steroids are also valuable as a screening test. Where there is a question of inadequate function, ACTH stimulation may be necessary.

## ACTH STIMULATION TESTS

*Insulin-induced hypoglycemia.*—Insulin-induced hypoglycemia causes hypothalamic activation with subsequent pituitary secretion of ACTH.[34] It is usually cortisol that is measured rather than ACTH, since cortisol is more readily available and more reliable than current commercial ACTH assays. With a fall of glucose to below 40 to 45 mg/dl, the plasma cortisol value should normally increase to an absolute value of 20 μg/dl or greater. In some instances the anticipated stress of venipuncture will result in basal testing values of 20 μg/dl higher with little further increase of the plasma cortisol at subsequent times. This type of response is not indicative of hypocortisolism. Hypoglycemic stress should not be performed in patients with ischemic heart or cerebrovascular disease or those with a seizure disorder. The test is performed as described in the section on GH stimulation.

*Vasopressin.*—Lysine vasopressin acts directly on the pituitary to cause release of ACTH.[43] Although this test is less well standardized than other tests of adrenal function, a patient who has a subnormal rise of plasma cortisol levels to insulin-induced hypoglycemic stress and a normal response to vasopressin can be presumed to have a hypothalamic deficit. The plasma cortisol levels in normals should increase to 20 μg/dl or greater. The test can be accomplished by either giving 10 units of vasopressin intramuscularly and measuring blood for cortisol at 0, 30, 60, 90, and 120 minutes, or by infusing vasopressin at two units per hour over two hours and collecting blood at the same time intervals as listed above. The intravenous route is preferable, since the infusion can be quickly stopped if the patient becomes overly symptomatic. Like the insulin tolerance test, this study should not be done in patients with ischemic heart disease. It is also contraindicated in patients with moderate or severe hypertension.

*ACTH stimulation.*—Use of the ACTH stimulation in patients with suspected hypothalamic-pituitary disease is based on the assumption that loss of ACTH reserve will result in a blunted cortisol response to ACTH. The majority of published data supports this notion.[44] In patients with significant hypothalamic-pituitary dysfunction the cortisol level will rarely increase to greater than 12 μg/dl. The test is performed by giving 0.25 mg of synthetic ACTH (Cortosyn) and measuring blood for cortisol at 0, 30, 60, and 90 minutes.

*Metyrapone stimulation (evaluation of feedback regulation).*—Metyrapone inhibits the adrenal enzyme 11-β-hydroxylase, thereby blocking the conversion of 11-deoxycortisol (Compound S) to cortisol.[45] The concentration of Compound S increases as the blood cortisol levels fall. Because the cortisol levels fall and because Compound S is not an effective inhibitor of ACTH secretion, ACTH levels in the blood increase, causing a further increase in Compound S. Compound S can be measured directly in blood or as a urine 17OHCS, since it is converted to this metabolite. Only the patients with an intact hypothalamic-pituitary-adrenal axis respond with increased blood levels of Compound S or an increase of the urinary 17OHCS after metyrapone administration. A subnormal response indicates that there is defect in cortisol secretion but does not localize the level of the defect. Because the long test, as described in the workup for Cushing's syndrome, can cause a precipitous fall of blood cortisol level, patients with decreased adrenal reserve may be tipped into an adrenal crisis. Therefore, if the clinician strongly suspects adrenal insufficiency the long test should not be used and an ACTH test can be performed. A shorter variation of the metyrapone test, however, can be used.[46] It is performed by administering a single dose of metyrapone (30 mg/kg of body weight) at midnight and measuring the 8:00 A.M. blood Compound S level. In normals the level should exceed 10 μg/dl. To assure that the block in conversion of Compound S to cortisol is complete, the blood cortisol level should be concurrently measured. An adequate block is present if the cortisol level is below 5 μg/100 ml. No conclusion can be made concerning a subnormal rise in the blood Compound S concentration if the cortisol level is above 5 μg/dl. Even though the risk of this test is much less than the long test, patients should be under close observation during the procedure.

*Antidiuretic hormone (ADH, vasopressin).*—Hormone-secreting tumors of the adenohypophysis rarely enlarge to the degree that ADH deficiency and diabetes insipidus are produced. However, craniopharyngiomas and other suprasellar lesions may produce diabetes insipidus, and extensive surgical procedures, such as transfrontal craniotomy for resection of very large pituitary tumors, not uncommonly result in diabetes insipidus.

In the preoperative patient with a small pituitary tumor, the diagnosis of diabetes insipidus can usually be excluded on the basis of the patient's medical history and measurement of an overnight urine specific gravity level or osmolality that indicates an ability to concentrate urine. If the patient has a history of polyuria and polydypsia, a dilute urine, and/or a high serum sodium level or osmolality, a water deprivation test can be performed after the method of Miller and Moses.[47]

## Summary

The extent of the pretreatment endocrine evaluation in patients with functioning pituitary tumors varies considerably with the type

TABLE 4.—Tests for Hormone Excess (Depending on Hypersecreted Hormone)

| DISEASE | PRIMARY TESTS | OPTIONAL TESTS |
|---------|---------------|----------------|
| Prolactinoma | Basal prolactin levels<br>Radiographic studies<br>CT scan | TRH test<br>Metoclopramide test |
| Acromegaly (gigantism) | Basal and glucose<br>Suppressed GH<br>Appropriate x-ray studies | Somatomedin C<br>TRH test |
| Pituitary Cushing's syndrome | Basal cortisol and dexamethasone suppression test (P.M. cortisol or diurnal variation, or urine-free cortisol) | ACTH levels<br>Metyrapone test |

TSH, LH-FSH, or ADH-secreting tumors are rare, but these hormones should be measured as part of the routine evaluation of an enlarged sella.

TABLE. 5.—TESTS FOR HORMONE DEFICIENCIES IN PATIENTS
WITH FUNCTIONING TUMOR

| HORMONE | MINIMAL EVALUATION | COMMENT |
|---|---|---|
| GH | (ITT)<br>(L-Dopa)<br>(Arginine) | GH testing is not always necessary but may be a clinically "silent" lesion in adults |
| Prolactin | Basal levels | Always measure because many "nonfunctioning" tumors secrete prolactin |
| LH-FSH | (Basal levels)<br>(Testosterone in men)<br>(LRH test) | A history of normal menses in women or a normal ejaculate in men is excellent biologic evidence of adequate function |
| TSH | T4<br>$RT_3U$<br>(TSH)<br>(TRH test) | Severe hypothyroidism should be corrected before surgery |
| ACTH | A.M. Cortisol<br>(ITT)<br>(Metyrapone) | The A.M. cortisol test is better than the P.M. test in determining if ACTH function is adequate |
| ADH | Urine sp. gr.<br>(Urine osmolality)<br>(Dehydration test) | ADH assays are not generally available |

and size of tumor and the specific goals of therapy. However, prior to either surgery or irradiation, an endocrine evaluation should be performed. The reasons for the hormone evaluation include: (1) to confirm the diagnosis and need for therapy, and (2) to provide baseline information about the other pituitary hormones that might be compromised by progression of the tumor or by treatment. Judicious selection of appropriate tests from the multitude of available possibilities should be the goal of the pretreatment assessment. Evaluation should include appropriate testing of the hypersecreted hormone as well as an evaluation of the adequacy of the other pituitary hormones. Depending on the specific disease process (i.e., prolactinoma, acromegaly, etc.), a minimal appropriate endocrine evaluation can be performed with the tests listed in Tables 4 and 5.

If a provocative test such as the insulin tolerance test is done, releasing factors such as TRH and GnRH can be combined into a single infusion. Without extensive provocative tests, the pretreatment pituitary function can be evaluated adequately.

References available upon request from the author.

# Pathology of Pituitary Adenomas

KALMAN KOVACS, M.D., PH.D., F.R.C.P.(C) AND
EVA HORVATH, PH.D.

*Department of Pathology, St. Michael's Hospital,
University of Toronto, Toronto, Canada*

PITUITARY ADENOMAS are usually benign, slowly growing, common epithelial neoplasms deriving from and consisting of adenohypophysial cells.[1, 2] Previous attempts to correlate their morphologic features with endocrine activity provided ambiguous results, primarily because reliable methods had not yet been developed to determine hormone concentrations in blood and tissue. Histologic techniques were also inadequate; they failed to reveal the composition and derivation of tumors. The use of radioimmunoassay, electron microscopy, and immunocytology brought about substantial progress and opened new avenues in the investigation of endocrine organs, including the pituitary gland. Radioimmunoassay permitted the measuring of minute quantities of hormones in blood and tissue. Electron microscopy disclosed the subcellular features of nontumorous and adenomatous adenohypophysial cells, shed light on various steps of the secretory process, and helped to elucidate the morphogenesis of adenomas. Immunocytology made it possible to localize specifically various hormones stored in the cell cytoplasm. The usefulness of the immunoperoxidase technique in both academic and diagnostic pathology cannot be overemphasized. This procedure can reveal the presence of immunoreactive hormones in formalin-fixed and paraffin-embedded material; even autopsy tissue kept in paraffin for many years is suitable for study.[3-5] It can also be applied at the electron microscopic level[6, 7]; i.e., it can unveil the subcellular sites where hormones are localized.

Previous hypophysial tumor classifications hinged on the staining affinity of the cell cytoplasm and distinguished three adenoma types: chromophobic (Figs 1 and 2), acidophilic, and basophilic (Fig 3) ad-

0-8151-3530-0/82/006-97-119-$03.75

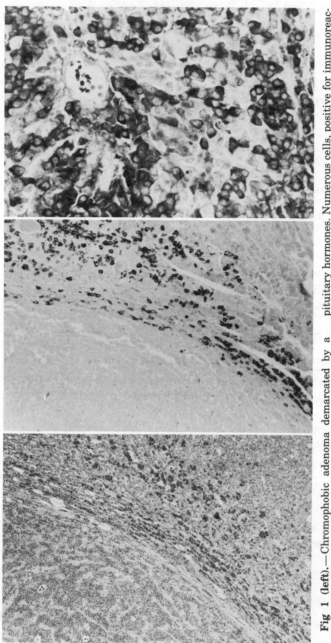

Fig 1 (left).—Chromophobic adenoma demarcated by a "pseudocapsule" consisting of compressed nontumorous adenohypophysial cells. The nontumorous gland (right) contains numerous basophilic cells. Periodic acid-Schiff-hematoxylin stain; original magnification × 40.

Fig 2 (center).—Chromophobic adenoma, unassociated with endocrine symptoms and containing no immunoreactive pituitary hormones. Numerous cells, positive for immunoreactive GH, are present in adjacent nontumorous gland (right). Immunoperoxidase technique for GH; original magnification × 100.

Fig 3 (right).—Basophilic adenoma associated with Cushing's disease. Lead hematoxylin stain; original magnification × 250.

enomas. Acidophilic adenomas, frequently associated with acromegaly or gigantism, were assumed to secrete GH. Basophilic adenomas, implicated in the genesis of Cushing's disease, were believed to produce ACTH. Chromophobic adenomas were interpreted as tumors unaccompanied by hypersecretion of any hormones.

Recent studies[1, 2, 8–11] provided strong evidence that pituitary adenoma classifications, depending on the tinctorial properties of the cell cytoplasm, have only limited usefulness; they cannot distinguish clearly various cell types, provide no information on the cytogenesis or biologic behavior of the tumors, and fail to take into account structure-function relationships. It became increasingly obvious that acidophilic adenomas did not always produce GH; some of these tumors synthesized prolactin or exhibited no endocrine activity. Basophilic adenomas were either associated with increased ACTH release resulting in the development of Cushing's disease or Nelson's syndrome, or were silent, unaccompanied by hormone discharge. Chromophobic adenomas were found to produce various hormones such as GH, prolactin, ACTH, FSH, LH, and TSH.

With the extensive use of immunocytology and electron microscopy, a new pituitary tumor classification has been introduced that divides hypophysial adenomas into well-defined entities.[1, 2, 10, 11] It is based on the immunocytologic findings, i.e., the presence of immunoreactive hormones stored in the cell cytoplasm. It relies mainly on the ultrastructural features of the adenoma cells and attempts to identify the cell type from which the tumor derives. It aims to correlate the morphologic findings with clinical history, biochemical results, biologic behavior, and endocrine activity.

Table 1 shows the pituitary adenoma classification used at St. Michael's Hospital, a major teaching hospital of the University of Toronto. The incidence of various adenoma types is also included. The results are based on the histologic, immunocytologic, and electron microscopic study of 480 surgically removed pituitary adenomas.

It can be seen from Table 1 that sparsely granulated prolactin cell adenomas represent, in our material, the most frequently occurring type of adenoma. This is a remarkable finding, since this type of tumor could not have been diagnosed by morphologic techniques two decades ago and was only recognized recently. If mixed GH cell-prolactin cell adenomas, acidophil stem cell adenomas, and mammosomatotroph cell adenomas are included, it becomes obvious that almost every other pituitary adenoma consists of, or at least contains, prolactin-producing cells. These results underline the significance of prolactin cell adenoma in endocrine pathology.

TABLE 1.—CLASSIFICATION AND INCIDENCE OF
PITUITARY ADENOMAS

| TYPE | INCIDENCE (%) |
| --- | --- |
| Densely granulated GH cell adenoma | 8 |
| Sparsely granulated GH cell adenoma | 10 |
| Densely granulated prolactin cell adenoma | <1 |
| Sparsely granulated prolactin cell adenoma | 31 |
| Mixed GH cell-prolactin cell adenoma | 6 |
| Acidophil stem cell adenoma | 4 |
| Mammosomatotroph cell adenoma | 1 |
| Corticotroph cell adenoma associated with Cushing's disease | 4 |
| Corticotroph cell adenoma associated with Nelson's syndrome | 4 |
| Silent corticotroph cell adenoma | 7 |
| Gonadotroph cell adenoma | 2 |
| Thyrotroph cell adenoma | <1 |
| Null cell adenoma | 15 |
| Oncocytoma | 6 |
| Unclassified | 2 |

It can also be concluded from Table 1 that sparsely granulated GH cell adenomas are somewhat more common than densely granulated GH cell adenomas; the difference between these two types is insignificant. However, there is a striking preponderance of sparsely granulated adenomas among tumors containing prolactin-producing cells. In our material, only one tumor consists solely of densely granulated prolactin cells. Unlike prolactin cell adenomas, the majority of hormonally active corticotroph cell adenomas are classified as densely granulated tumors. Silent corticotroph cell adenomas are not infrequently-occurring tumors. Although their structural features are insufficiently investigated, they should be separated from corticotroph cell adenomas that secrete ACTH in excessive amounts and that are accompanied by Cushing's disease or Nelson's syndrome. Gonadotroph cell adenomas, as well as thyrotroph cell adenomas, are tumors occasionally diagnosed clinically, biochemically, or by morphologic techniques. Tumors with increased production of FSH, LH, or TSH can only be detected rarely even if many patients are examined by several sophisticated methods. Null cell adenomas constitute a commonly found type of tumor. Pituitary oncocytomas are not infrequent tumors and must be considered in the differential diagnosis, especially in cases unaccompanied by increased secretion of any of the known adenohypophysial hormones.

It is also evident that adenomas originating in the acidophilic cell line, i.e., in GH cells and prolactin cells, are diagnosed more commonly than those arising in basophilic cells, i.e., in corticotrophs, gonadotrophs, and thyrotrophs. These findings indicate that acidophilic cells are more prone to undergo neoplastic transformation than other cell types. Null cell adenomas and oncocytomas lack immunologic markers and their cellular derivation remains to be established. These tumors are unassociated with increased hormone secretion and contain no adenohypophysial hormones on immunocytology, although several membrane-bound secretory granules can be detected in the cytoplasm of every adenoma cell. They may originate in immature precursor cells or resting cells, whose structural features are not sufficiently distinctive to permit their identification by electron microscopy.

## Morphologic Features of Various Pituitary Adenoma Types

### GROWTH HORMONE CELL ADENOMAS

GH cell adenomas[1, 12–16] are accompanied by acromegaly or gigantism. Two morphologically distinct subtypes, densely and sparsely granulated adenomas, can be distinguished.

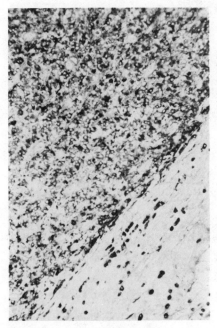

**Fig 4.**—GH cell adenoma exhibiting strong positivity for immunoreactive GH. The nontumorous GH cells *(right bottom corner)* show normal staining pattern and morphology. Immunoperoxidase technique for GH; original magnification × 100.

Densely granulated GH cell adenomas are diagnosed as acidophilic adenomas by light microscopy. The cytoplasm of adenoma cells exhibits a positive staining with various acidic dyes and shows a diffuse positivity for GH by the immunoperoxidase technique (Figs 4 and 5). By electron microscopy (Fig 6), densely granulated adenomatous GH

**Fig 5 (top).**—Immune precipitate, indicating presence of GH, is exclusively located over secretory granules in this densely granulated GH cell adenoma. Immunoelectron microscopy for GH; × 8,300.

**Fig 6 (bottom).**—Fine structure of a densely granulated GH cell adenoma. × 5,800.

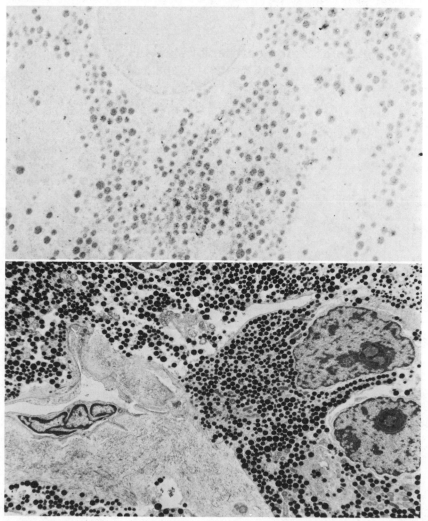

cells are similar to GH cells of the nontumorous adenohypophysis; they are characterized by well-developed, rough-surfaced endoplasmic reticulum membranes and Golgi complexes as well as numerous spherical, evenly electron-dense secretory granules, and measure 300 to 600 nm.

Sparsely granulated GH cell adenomas are identified as chromophobic adenomas by light microscopy. The immunoperoxidase method reveals the presence of GH in the cytoplasm of adenoma cells. The fine structural features of sparsely granulated adenomatous GH cells differ from those of nontumorous GH cells (Fig 7). They possess irregular nuclei, rough-surfaced endoplasmic reticulum profiles, aggregates of smooth-surfaced endoplasmic reticulum membranes, conspicuous Golgi complexes, several centrioles and cilia, as well as fibrous bodies composed of type II microfilaments and smooth-walled tubules. The secretory granules are sparse, spherical, evenly electron-dense, and usually measure not more than 100 to 300 nm.

## PROLACTIN CELL ADENOMAS

Prolactin cell adenomas[1, 4, 17-20] coexist with amenorrhea, infertility, and in many patients with galactorrhea, loss of libido and impotence. In some patients, however, mainly in men, the endocrine manifestations are not apparent and only elevated blood prolactin

**Fig 7.**—Ultrastructural features of a sparsely granulated GH cell adenoma with fibrous bodies *(FB).* × 10,300.

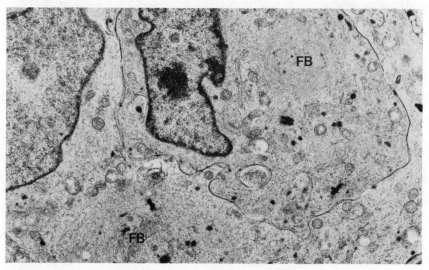

concentrations may pinpoint prolactin secretion by the adenoma cells. It should be understood, however, that hyperprolactinemia itself yields no direct proof that prolactin is produced by the adenoma cells, since injury of certain hypothalamic structures or the hypophysial stalk may interfere with the synthesis or discharge of hypothalamic prolactin-inhibiting factors or their transport to the adenohypophysis via the portal vessels, and can result in hyperprolactinemia. A careful morphologic study can provide strong evidence as to whether prolactin is released from the adenoma cells or from the nontumorous portion of the anterior lobe. The usefulness of the immunoperoxidase technique and electron microscopy, in these conditions, underlines the importance of morphologic investigation in the differential diagnosis of pituitary adenomas.

Prolactin cell tumors can be separated into densely and sparsely granulated adenomas.

Densely granulated prolactin cell tumors are uncommon; there is only one adenoma in our material that consists solely of densely granulated prolactin cells. Light microscopy shows this tumor to be an acidophilic adenoma indistinguishable from those of densely granulated GH cell adenomas. The adenoma cells contain many cytoplasmic secretory granules that show positive staining with Herlant's erythrosin and Brookes' carmoisin techniques. The immunoperoxidase technique demonstrates the presence of prolactin in the cytoplasm of adenoma cells. The fine structural features of densely granulated adenomatous prolactin cells resemble those of resting prolactin cells seen in the nontumorous adenohypophysis: they possess well-developed rough-surfaced endoplasmic reticulum membranes and conspicuous Golgi complexes, as well as numerous, spherical, oval, or irregular, evenly electron dense secretory granules measuring 400 to 1,200 nm.

Sparsely granulated prolactin cell adenomas are identified as chromophobic adenomas by light microscopy. Herlant's erythrosin and Brookes' carmoisin methods usually reveal a few small secretory granules in the cytoplasm of adenoma cells. The immunoperoxidase technique is of foremost importance in the diagnosis of this type of tumor, since it invariably reveals the presence of prolactin in the cytoplasm of adenoma cells (Fig 8). Sparsely granulated prolactin cell adenomas show characteristic features and can be recognized without any difficulty on electron microscopy (Figs 9 and 10). The adenoma cells contain prominent rough-surfaced endoplasmic reticulum membranes and conspicuous Golgi complexes. Nebenkern formations, i.e., concentric whorls of endoplasmic reticulum membranes, and mis-

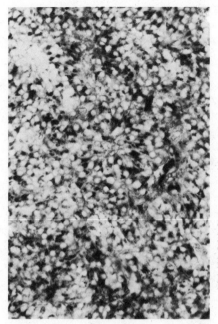

**Fig 8.**—Prolactin cell adenoma containing immunoreactive prolactin. The positivity is present mainly in a circumscribed juxtanuclear area representing the Golgi apparatus. Immunoperoxidase technique for prolactin. × 250.

placed exocytoses are evident. The secretory granules are sparse, spherical, oval, or irregular, evenly electron-dense, and measure 150 to 350 nm.

## MIXED GH CELL-PROLACTIN CELL ADENOMAS

Mixed GH cell-prolactin cell adenomas[1, 14, 16, 21-23] are accompanied by acromegaly. In some patients, amenorrhea and galactorrhea are also apparent. Blood GH and prolactin concentrations are elevated. Morphologic study reveals that mixed GH cell-prolactin cell adenomas consist of two different cell types: GH cells and prolactin cells. On light microscopy these tumors represent acidophilic-chromophobic adenomas, and the immunoperoxidase technique demonstrates the presence of GH in the cytoplasm of some adenoma cells, whereas prolactin is detected in the cytoplasm of some other adenoma cells. Electron microscopy has a substantial role in the diagnosis of mixed GH cell-prolactin cell adenomas. The fine structural features of the tumor cells are identical to those of GH cells or prolactin cells seen in adenomas producing only GH or prolactin. Every combination may occur; densely or sparsely granulated GH cells can be interspersed

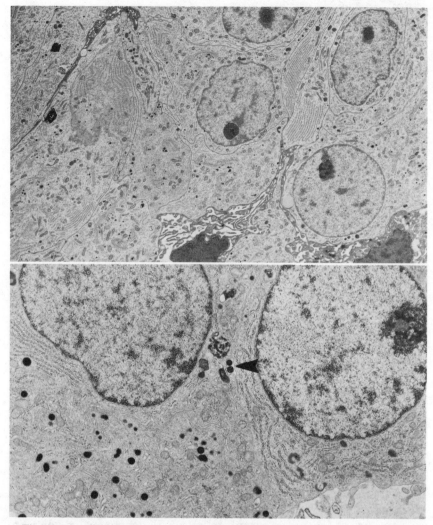

**Fig 9 (top).**—Fine structure of a sparsely granulated prolactin cell adenoma. Note the large nuclei with conspicuous nucleoli and the prominence of rough-surfaced endoplasmic reticulum (RER) and Golgi apparatus. × 4,400.

**Fig 10 (bottom).**—Sparsely granulated prolactin cell adenoma. Note extrusion of secretory granules into intercellular space ("misplaced exocytosis," *arrowhead*). × 10,900.

with densely or sparsely granulated prolactin cells. Cells of the same type frequently form smaller or larger nests. In some areas, however, single cells of different origin are intermingled.

## ACIDOPHIL STEM CELL ADENOMAS

Acidophil stem cell adenomas[2, 24, 25] are usually unaccompanied by acromegalic features and often appear as nonfunctioning tumors. Blood GH levels are within the normal range; hyperprolactinemia, however, is evident in the majority of patients. Morphologically, acidophil stem cell adenomas are composed of immature cells and exhibit features reminiscent of sparsely granulated adenomatous GH cells and prolactin cells. The histologic and fine structural characteristics of the tumor cells are consistent with the assumption that they originate in a common precursor of the two types of acidophil cell. On light microscopy, they represent chromophobic adenomas, although in some cases, the Brookes' carmoisin method demonstrates positively staining granules in the cytoplasm of adenoma cells. The immunoperoxidase technique shows the presence of prolactin in the cytoplasm of many adenoma cells. In some cases, GH and prolactin can be demonstrated in the cytoplasm of the same adenoma cell. On electron microscopy, the adenoma cells are closely apposed, elongated, attenuated, and possess irregular nuclei. The rough-surfaced endoplasmic reticulum consist of dispersed short profiles and may be abundant in some cells. The Golgi complexes are, in general, inconspicuous. In many cases, the volume density of mitochondria is increased, indicating oncocytic transformation. Giant mitochondria may also be formed. The secretory granules are sparse, spherical, oval, or irregular, evenly electron-dense, and measure 150 to 300 nm. Fibrous bodies, misplaced exocytosis, and multiple centrioles may be noted in the cytoplasm of the same cells.

## MAMMOSOMATOTROPH CELL ADENOMAS

Mammosomatotroph cell adenomas[26, 27] are accompanied by acromegaly. Blood GH concentrations are increased and, in some patients, hyperprolactinemia is also present. Morphologically, these tumors are acidophilic or partly acidophilic, partly chromophobic adenomas and are composed of one cell type, the mammosomatotroph cell. The immunoperoxidase technique demonstrates GH and some prolactin in the cytoplasm of adenoma cells. Electron microscopy shows well differentiated adenoma cells that exhibit ultrastructural features similar to those of densely granulated GH cells and possess prominent rough-surfaced endoplasmic reticulum membranes and Golgi apparatuses. The secretory granules are spherical, oval, or irregular, evenly electron-dense, vary in size and number, and measure 200 to 1,000 nm. Exocytoses are apparent. Large extracellular deposits of secretory material is a distinct subcellular finding in this adenoma type. Mammosomatotroph cell adenomas have a slow growth rate as well as benign biologic behavior and appear to represent the well-differentiated variant of acidophil stem cell adenoma.

## CORTICOTROPH CELL ADENOMAS

Corticotroph cell adenomas[1, 28-31] are endocrinologically active or silent tumors. The latter type is unassociated with clinical and biochemical evidence of increased hormone secretion.

Hormonally functioning corticotroph cell adenomas produce ACTH, β-LPH, and endorphins and are accompanied by Cushing's disease or Nelson's syndrome. On light microscopy, the majority of corticotroph cell adenomas represent basophilic adenomas and possess cytoplasmic secretory granules that stain positively with basic dyes, the periodic acid, Schiff (PAS) technique, and lead hematoxylin (see Fig 3). A few corticotroph cell adenomas are chromophobic and show little or no PAS or lead hematoxylin positivity. The immunoperoxidase technique reveals the presence of ACTH, β-LPH, and endorphins (Fig 11) in the cytoplasm of adenoma cells. The biologic and clinical significance of the presence of various ACTH related peptides in corticotroph cell adenomas has yet to be elucidated. On electron microscopy (Fig 12), in the adenomas, corticotroph cells are similar to those of the nontumorous adenohypophysis, possessing well-developed rough-surfaced endoplasmic reticulum stacks and prominent Golgi apparatuses. The secretory granules are spherical or slightly irregular, vary in electron density, frequently line up along the cell membranes, and measure 250 to 700 nm. In corticotroph cell adenomas removed from patients with Cushing's disease, bundles of type I microfilaments are frequently noted. They represent the fine structural manifestations of Crooke's hyaline material, revealed in nontumorous corticotroph cells of patients treated with pharmocologic doses of cortisol or its derivatives, and of those with cortisol-producing adrenocortical tumors or with the ectopic ACTH syndrome. Type I microfilaments are inconspicuous or absent in adenomatous corticotroph cells of patients with Nelson's syndrome. These patients had undergone bilateral adrena-

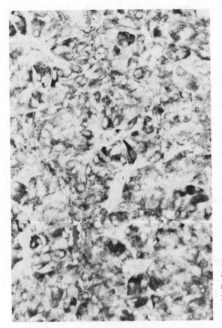

**Fig 11.**—Immunoreactive α-endorphin is shown in cells of a corticotroph cell adenoma associated with Nelson's syndrome. Immunoperoxidase technique for α-endorphin. × 250.

**Fig 12.**—Ultrastructure of a typical corticotroph cell adenoma associated with Cushing's disease. Note bundles of type I microfilaments *(arrowheads).* × 10,300.

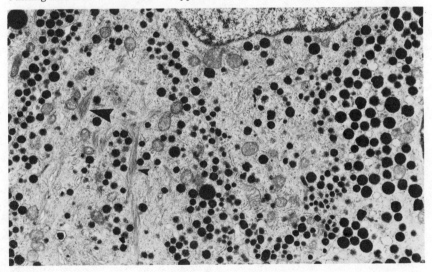

lectomy because of preexisting hypercorticism; their ACTH-producing pituitary neoplasm was diagnosed only after the removal of the adrenal glands.

## SILENT "CORTICOTROPH" CELL ADENOMAS

Silent "corticotroph" cell adenomas[11, 32–35] are clinically unassociated with increased ACTH production. On light microscopy, they represent basophilic or chromophobic adenomas and the immunoperoxidase technique reveals the presence of ACTH and related peptides in the cytoplasm of adenoma cells. In some cases, the subcellular features are indistinguishable from those of ACTH-secreting neoplasms. In other cases, however, ultrastructural investigation reveals substantial differences between silent and endocrinologically functioning tumors (Fig 13), indicating morphologic heterogeneity of silent corticotroph cell adenomas. The mechanisms implicated in the causation of hormonal inactivity are unknown. The study of more cases and the introduction of new techniques may result in further subdivisions of this adenoma type. The relationship between hormonally inactive and endocrinologically active corticotroph cell adenomas remains also to be clarified.

## GONADOTROPH CELL ADENOMAS

Gonadotroph cell adenomas[11, 36–40] usually produce FSH and LH. The discharge of these two gonadotroph hormones is not always comparable and, in some patients secretion of FSH prevails. Adenomas arising from gonadotroph cells are rare. They differ markedly in their differentiation and may develop in patients with long-standing primary hypogonadism. The question whether protracted reduction of gonadal function plays a role in the genesis of these tumors is obscure. In some cases, the adenoma cells are so immature that their origin cannot be clarified, not even by detailed electron microscopic study. On light microscopy, gonadotroph cell adenomas represent chromophobic tumors. The PAS method, in general, reveals a few positive granules and the immunoperoxidase technique demonstrates FSH and/or LH in the cytoplasm of several adenoma cells. Immunocytologic procedures are valuable in the differential diagnosis, since the subcellular features of the adenomas are, in some cases, not sufficiently distinctive to disclose their cellular derivation. It must be emphasized that for the immunocytologic diagnosis, anti β-FSH and anti β-LH must be applied. The α-subunits of FSH, LH, and TSH are

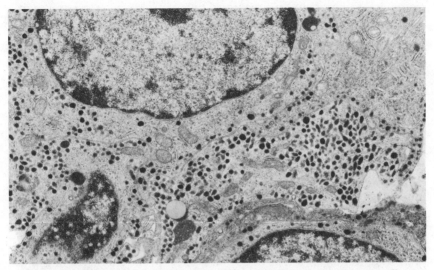

**Fig 13.**—Silent "corticotroph" adenoma. The well-differentiated adenoma cells contain numerous spherical and teardrop-shaped secretory granules. × 12,800.

immunologically very similar, and antibodies raised against the entire FSH or LH molecule cross-react with TSH produced by thyrotroph cells. Thus, the use of antisera generated against α-subunits or the whole FSH or LH molecule may lead to erroneous results. In some cases, the fine structural features of adenomatous gonadotroph cells resemble those of nontumorous gonadotroph cells. In others, adenomatous gonadotroph cells appear to be undifferentiated and differ markedly from those found in the nonadenomatous anterior lobe. In the cytoplasm of adenomatous gonadotroph cells, moderately developed rough-surfaced endoplasmic reticulum, conspicuous Golgi apparatus, and many microtubules are observed. The secretory granules are spherical, evenly electron-dense, often line up along the cell membranes, and measure 100 to 250 nm. So far only a few cases of gonadotroph cell adenomas have been described. Hence, more cases have to be investigated to assess the real incidence of this newly recognized type of adenoma and to correlate the morphologic features of the tumor cells with secretory activity.

## THYROTROPH CELL ADENOMAS

Thyrotroph cell adenomas[11, 41–45] are uncommon tumors. So far, only a few cases have been reported that have been investigated by sophisticated morphologic techniques. They are found mainly in patients with long-standing primary hypothyroidism, consistent with the assumption that deficiency of thyroid hormones stimulates thyrotroph cells, leading to thyrotroph cell hyperplasia and, subsequently, to the formation of thyrotroph cell adenoma. Occasionally, thyrotroph cell adenomas are accompanied by hyperthyroidism. In these patients, hyperthyroidism is attributed to excessive TSH secretion by adenoma cells. On light microscopy, thyrotroph cell adenomas are diagnosed as chromophobic tumors. They possess a few small PAS-positive, aldehyde fuchsin-positive and aldehyde thionin-positive cytoplasmic secretory granules that may exhibit positivity for β-TSH by the immunoperoxidase technique. Some tumors, however, cannot be immunostained. The causes accounting for the absence of TSH immunoreactivity are obscure. Further work is required to assess the value of immunocytologic procedures in the differential diagnosis of thyrotroph cell adenoma. On electron microscopy, thyrotroph cell adenomas consist of elongated or angular cells with long cytoplasmic processes, scanty rough-surfaced endoplasmic reticulum membranes, and moderately developed Golgi apparatus. Secretory granules are sparse, spherical, often line up along the cell membrane, and measure 100 to 200 nm. The limiting membranes of the secretory granules are frequently separated from the electron dense core by a wide, prominent electron-lucent halo. Microtubules are abundant in many adenoma cells.

## Null Cell Adenomas

Null cell adenomas[8, 11, 46-48] are unassociated with clinical or biochemical evidence of increased hormone secretion. In our material, they are not found in patients under 30 years of age and are diagnosed more frequently in older people. Large tumors may press the nontumorous portion of the pituitary, and by obstructing the portal vessels may block adenohypophysial blood flow. Injury of adenohypophysial tissue can cause various degrees of hypopituitarism. Null cell adenomas are occasionally accompanied by the elevated blood prolactin levels. Interference by the growing tumor with the production, release, or transport of hypothalamic prolactin-inhibiting factors may provide an explanation for the hyperprolactinemia. On light microscopy, null cell adenomas represent chromophobic tumors. In some adenoma cells, the cytoplasm exhibits a granular acidophilic appearance. The acidophilia is due to the affinity of mitochondria for acidic dyes. Since mitochondria markedly increase in number in some cells, acidophilic staining of the cytoplasm may become conspicuous. Most null cell adenomas do not store biologically active hormones, and exhibit negative staining for GH, prolactin, ACTH, FSH, LH, and TSH with the immunoperoxidase technique. A few tumors, however, may contain scattered cells showing positive immunostaining for one or more pituitary hormones, most commonly for α-subunit. By electron microscopy, null cell adenomas consist of closely apposed, polyhedral or irregular cells with pleomorphic and frequently indented nuclei and poorly developed scanty cytoplasm (Fig 14). The rough-surfaced endoplasmic reticulum membranes are composed of randomly scattered short stacks and are, in general, inconspicuous. The Golgi complexes may be prominent and the microtubules are abundant in the cytoplasm of many adenoma cells. The secretory granules are spherical and measure 100 to 250 nm. They are detected in every adenoma cell, often line up along the cell membrane, and have an electron-dense core, separated from the limiting membrane by a prominent electron lucent halo. No exocytoses are noted. Oncocytic transformation, i.e., increase in the volume density of mitochondria, is evident in some cells, and it may be so extensive that almost the entire cytoplasm is occupied by mitochondria and the other cytoplasmic organelles are obscured. Tumors composed of cells with marked mitochondrial abundance are termed "oncocytomas." They may originate in the pituitary, and in other organs as well, such as thyroid, parathyroid, salivary glands, kidney, etc.

## ONCOCYTOMAS

Oncocytomas[11, 49-53] are variants of null cell adenomas and are unassociated with increased secretion of any known pituitary hormone. They are most likely to occur in elderly patients. By the immunoperoxidase technique, no hormone storage can be demonstrated in the adenoma cells. In a few oncocytomas, however, the presence of α-subunit or other adenohypophysial hormones is detectable in the cytoplasm of some adenoma cells, a fact that suggests that these tumors may originate in various hormone-producing cells of the adenohypophysis that gradually transform to oncocytes and lose their endocrine potential. Electron microscopy is indispensable for the diagnosis of this tumor type. The identifying fine structural feature of oncocytoma is the abundance of mitochondria (Fig 15). The underlying mechanisms accounting for the accumulation of mitochondria are unknown.

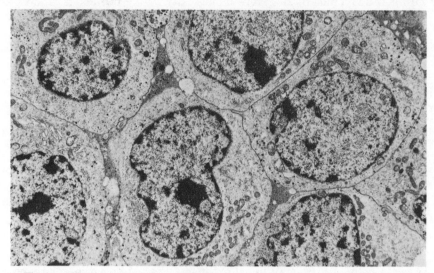

**Fig 14.**—Fine structure of a null cell adenoma consisting of small, incompletely differentiated cells. Note paucity of cytoplasmic organelles and secretory granules. × 6,800.

**Fig 15.**—Pituitary oncocytoma. The cells contain a large number of slender *("dark")* or swollen and partially cavitated *("light")* mitochondria. × 6,800.

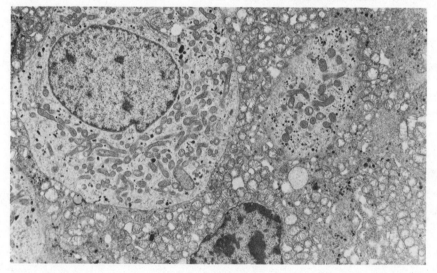

## UNCLASSIFIED PITUITARY ADENOMAS

Unclassified pituitary adenomas[1, 54] are uncommon tumors, representing approximately 2% of hypophysial adenomas in our material. They consist of cells that cannot be classified even by ultrastructural investigation. In general, the adenoma cells seem to be well differentiated, but their structural features are different from any known adenohypophysial cell type. The endocrine activities of these unclassified adenomas may be atypical. Some tumors may produce two or more hormones markedly different in chemical structure, immunoreactivity, and biologic action. Adenomas that produce GH and TSH; or GH, prolactin, and TSH; or GH, prolactin and ACTH; or prolactin and FSH; or prolactin and TSH; or prolactin, endorphin, and α-subunit may rarely be recognized. According to the single cell-single hormone theory, adenohypophysial cells secrete one hormone only, with the exception of gonadotroph cells, which produce the two gonadotroph hormones FSH and LH. The existence of multiple hormone-producing adenomas provides strong evidence that the single cell-single hormone theory is oversimplified, and that our present theories on the cytogenesis of pituitary adenomas have to be reconsidered. These tumors are unusual and further work is required to understand their endocrine function, cellular derivation and pathogenesis.

In the substantial majority of patients, pituitary adenomas are histologically and biologically benign tumors with a slow growth rate, no invasion of neighboring tissue, and absence of distant metastases. Some pituitary adenomas, however, are pleomorphic, contain numerous mitotic figures, and their invasion of surrounding structures is evident. These invasive adenomas[1,11] show a more rapid rate of growth than benign adenomas. They may produce GH, prolactin, or ACTH, or they may possess no endocrine activity.

## PRIMARY PITUITARY CARCINOMAS

Primary pituitary carcinomas[55-60] are very uncommon tumors and represent the malignant variants of adenomas. They derive from adenohypophysial cells and may produce GH, prolactin, or ACTH, or they may be silent, i.e., unaccompanied by secretion of any known hypophysial hormones. The diagnosis of pituitary carcinoma may be very difficult and is justified only when distant metastases can be found. Histologic examination may fail, in some cases, to verify the biologic behavior of the tumor.

## Summary

This chapter deals with the morphologic features of pituitary adenomas. Sophisticated methods, primarily the immunoperoxidase technique and electron microscopy, made possible the introduction of a new morphologic classification that separates adenohypophysial tumors into well-defined entities based on hormone storage, fine structural appearance, and cytogenesis. The histologic study combined with the immunoperoxidase technique and the fine structural analysis are valuable procedures in the differential diagnosis of pituitary adenomas and yield meaningful information to the clinical endocrinologist and neurosurgeon. Although a deeper insight has been obtained into the pathology of pituitary adenomas during the last decade, several aspects are still inadequately explored. Further investigations may result in a better understanding of the morphologic features, endocrine activity, and biologic behavior of these fascinating neoplasms.

## Acknowledgment

This work was supported in part by Grant MA-6349 of the Medical Research Council of Canada and Grant 1 RO1 CA 21905–01, awarded by the National Cancer Institute, Department of Health, Education and Welfare. The authors wish to thank Gezina Ilse, Donna McComb, Gerhard Penz, and Nancy Ryan for their excellent contribution to the morphologic studies, and Wanda Wlodarski for her invaluable secretarial work.

REFERENCES

1. Kovacs K., Horvath E., Ezrin C.: Pituitary adenomas. *Pathol. Annu.* 12 (part 2):341, 1977.
2. Kovacs K., Horvath E.: Pituitary adenomas: Pathologic aspects, in Tolis G., et al. (eds): *Clinical Neuroendocrinology: A Pathophysiological Approach.* New York, Raven Press, 1979, p 367.
3. Nieuwenhuyzen-Kruseman A.C., Bots G.T.A.M., Lindeman E.: The immunohistochemical identification of hormone-producing cells in formalin-fixed, paraffin-embedded human pituitary tissue. *J. Pathol.* 117:163, 1975.
4. Kovacs K., Corenblum B., Sirek A.M.T., et al.: Localization of prolactin in chromophobe pituitary adenomas: Study of human necropsy material by immunoperoxidase technique. *J. Clin. Pathol.* 29:250, 1976.
5. Halmi N.S.: Immunostaining of growth hormone and prolactin in paraffin embedded and stored or previously stained material. *J. Histochem. Cytochem.* 26:486, 1978.

6. Moriarty G.C.: Adenohypophysis: Ultrastructual cytochemistry. A review. *J. Histochem. Cytochem.* 21:855, 1973
7. Pelletier G., Robert F., Hardy J.: Identification of human anterior pituitary cells by immunoelectron microscopy. *J. Clin. Endocrinol. Metab.* 46:534, 1978.
8. Landolt A.M.: Ultrastructure of human sella tumors: Correlations of clinical findings and morphology. *Acta Neurochir.* (suppl)22:1, 1975.
9. Saeger W.: Licht- und elektronenmikroskopische Untersuchungen zur Klassifikation von Hypophysenadenomen. *Z. Krebsforsch.* 84:105, 1975.
10. Horvath E., Kovacs K.: Ultrastructural classification of pituitary adenomas. *Can. J. Neurol. Sci.* 3:9, 1976.
11. Horvath E., Kovacs K.: Pathology of the pituitary gland, in Ezrin C., et al. (eds): *Pituitary Diseases*. Boca Raton: CRC Press, 1980, p 1.
12. Kinnman J.: *Acromegaly: An Ultrastructural Analysis of 51 Adenomas and a Clinical Study of 80 Patients Treated by Transanthrosphenoidal Operation*. Stockholm: Norstädt and Söner, 1973, p 1.
13. Robert F.: L'adénome hypophysaire dans l'acromégalie-gigantisme:Étude macroscopique, histologique et ultrastructurale. *Neurochirurgie* 19 (suppl 2):117, 1973.
14. Halmi N.S., Duello T.: "Acidophilic" pituitary tumors: A reappraisal with differential staining and immunocytochemical techniques. *Arch. Pathol. Lab. Med.* 100:346, 1976.
15. Horvath E., Kovacs K.: Morphogenesis and significance of fibrous bodies in human pituitary adenomas. *Virchows Arch.* [*Cell Pathol.*] 27:69, 1978.
16. Trouillas J., Girod C., Lhéritier, M., et al.: Morphological and biochemical relationships in 31 human pituitary adenomas with acromegaly. *Virchows Arch.* [*Pathol. Anat.*] 389:127, 1980.
17. Horvath E., Kovacs K.: Misplaced exocytosis: Distinct ultrastructural feature in some pituitary adenomas. *Arch. Pathol.* 97:221, 1974.
18. Kovacs K., Horvath E., Corenblum B., et al.: Pituitary chromophobe adenomas consisting of prolactin cells : A histologic, immunocytological and electron microscopic study. *Virchows Arch.* [*Pathol. Anat.*] 366:113, 1975.
19. Robert F., Hardy J.: Prolactin secreting adenomas: A light and electron microscopical study. *Arch. Pathol.* 99:625, 1975.
20. Kovacs K.: Morphology of prolactin-producing adenomas. *Clin. Endocrinol.* 6 (suppl.):71s, 1977.
21. Guyda H., Robert F., Colle E., et al.: Histologic, ultrastructural, and hormonal characterization of a pituitary tumor secreting both hGH and prolactin. *J. Clin. Endocrinol. Metab.* 36:531, 1973.
22. Corenblum B., Sirek A.M.T., Horvath E., et al.: Human mixed somatotrophic and lactotrophic pituitary adenomas. *J. Clin. Endocrinol. Metab.* 42:857, 1976.
23. Kameya T., Tsumuraya M., Adachi I., et al.: Ultrastructure, immunohistochemistry and hormone release of pituitary adenomas in relation to prolactin production. *Virchows Arch.* [*Pathol. Anat.*] 387:31, 1980.
24. Horvath E., Kovacs K., Singer W., et al.: Acidophil stem cell adenoma of the human pituitary. *Arch. Pathol. Lab. Med.* 101:594, 1977.
25. Horvath E., Kovacs K., Singer W., et al.: Acidophil stem cell adenoma of the human pituitary: Clinico-pathological analysis of 15 cases. *Cancer* 47:761, 1981.

26. Landolt A.M., Rothenbuhler V.: Extracellular growth hormone deposits in pituitary adenomas. *Virchows Arch.* [*Pathol Anat.*] 378:55, 1978.
27. Horvath E., Kovacs K., Killinger D.W., et al.: Mammosomatotroph cell adenoma of the human pituitary. *Proc. 38th Ann. Meet. Electr. Micr. Soc. Amer.* Baton Rouge: Claitor's Publ., 1980, p. 726.
28. Saeger W.: Zur Ultrastruktur der Hypophysenadenome beim Cushing-Syndrome nach Adrenalektomie. *Virchows Arch.* [*Pathol. Anat.*] 361:39, 1973.
29. Garcia J.H., Kalimo H., Givens J.R.: Human adenohypophysis in Nelson syndrome: Ultrastructural and clinical study. *Arch. Pathol. Lab. Med.* 100:253, 1976.
30. Kovacs K., Horvath E., Kerenyi N.A., et al.: Light and electron microscopic features of a pituitary adenoma in Nelson's syndrome. *Am. J. Clin. Pathol.* 65:337, 1976.
31. Robert F., Pelletier G., Hardy J.: Pituitary adenomas in Cushing's disease. *Arch. Pathol. Lab. Med.* 102:448, 1978.
32. Kovacs K., Horvath E., Bayley T.A., et al.: Silent corticotroph cell adenoma with lysosomal accumulation and crinophagy: A distinct clinicopathologic entity. *Am. J. Med.* 64:492, 1978.
33. Tramu G., Beauvillain J.C., Mazzuca M., et al.: Adénome hypophysaire à cellules à 17–39 ACTH et β-, MSH sans hypercorticisme. *Ann. Endocrinol. (Paris)* 39:51, 1978.
34. Hassoun J., Charpin C., Jaquet P., et al.: Analogies immunocytochimiques des adénomes hypophysaires de la maladie Cushing et des adénomes "non fonctionelles" (adénomes chromophobes) de l'hypophyse. *Ann. Endocrinol. (Paris)* 40:559, 1979.
35. Horvath E., Kovacs K., Killinger D.W., et al.: Silent corticotropic adenomas of the human pituitary gland : A histologic, immunocytologic and ultrastructural study. *Am. J. Pathol.* 98:617, 1980.
36. Woolf P.D., Schenk E.A.: An FSH-producing pituitary tumor in a patient with hypogonadism. *J. Clin. Endocrinol. Metab.* 38:561, 1974.
37. Friend J.N., Judge D.M., Sherman B.M., et al.: FSH-secreting pituitary adenomas: Stimulation and suppression studies in two patients. *J. Clin. Endocrinol. Metab.* 43:650, 1976.
38. Snyder P.J., Sterling F.H.: Hypersecretion of LH and FSH by a pituitary adenoma. *J. Clin. Endocrinol. Metab.* 42:544, 1976.
39. Kovacs K., Horvath E., Van Loon G.R., et al.: Pituitary adenomas associated with elevated blood follicle-stimulating hormone levels: A histologic, immunocytologic and electron microscopic study of two cases. *Fertil. Steril.* 29:622, 1978.
40. Kovacs K., Horvath E., Rewcastle N.B., et al.: Gonadotroph cell adenoma of the pituitary in a woman with long-standing hypogonadism. *Arch. Gynecol.* 229:57, 1980.
41. Leong A.S.Y., Chawla J.C., Teh E.C.: Pituitary thyrotropic tumour secondary to long-standing primary hypothyroidism. *Pathol. Eur.* 11:49, 1976.
42. Samaan N.A., Osborne B.M., Mackay B., et al.: Endocrine and morphologic studies of pituitary adenomas secondary to primary hypothyroidism. *J. Clin. Endocrinol. Metab.* 45:903, 1977.
43. Tolis G., Bird C., Bertrand G., et al.: Pituitary hyperthyroidism: Case report and review of the literature. *Am. J. Med.* 64:177, 1978.

44. Afrasiabi A., Valenta L., Gwinup G.: A TSH-secreting pituitary tumour causing hyperthyroidism: presentation of a case and review of the literature. *Acta Endocrinol. (Copenh.)* 92:448, 1979.
45. Katz M.S., Gregerman R.I., Horvath E., et al.: Thyrotroph cell adenoma of the human pituitary gland associated with primary hypothyroidism: Clinical and morphological features. *Acta Endocrinol. (Copenh.)* 95:41, 1980.
46. Schelin U.: Chromophobe and acidophil adenomas of the human pituitary gland: A light and electron microscopic study. *Acta Pathol. Microbiol. Scand.* (suppl) 158:1, 1962.
47. Schechter J.: Electron microscopic study of human pituitary tumors: I. Chromophobic adenomas. *Am. J. Anat.* 138:371, 1973.
48. Kovacs K., Horvath E., Ryan N., et al.: Null cell adenoma of the human pituitary. *Virchows Arch.* [*Pathol. Anat.*] 387:165, 1980.
49. Kovacs K., Horvath E., Pituitary "chromophobe" adenoma composed of oncocytes: A light and electron microscopic study. *Arch. Pathol.* 95:235, 1973.
50. Landolt A.M., Oswald U.W.: Histology and ultrastructure of an oncocytic adenoma of the human pituitary *Cancer* 31:1099, 1973.
51. Kovacs K., Horvath E., Bilbao J.M.: Oncocytes in the anterior lobe of the human pituitary gland: A light and electron microscopic study. *Acta Neuropathol. (Berl.)* 27:43, 1974.
52. Saeger W.: Vegleichende licht- und elektronenmikroskopische Untersuchungen an onkocytären Hypophysenadenomen. *Virchows Arch.* [*Pathol. Anat.*] 369:29, 1975.
53. Bauserman S.C., Hardman J.M., Schochet S.S. Jr., et al.: Pituitary oncocytoma: Indispensable role of electron microscopy in its identification. *Arch. Pathol. Lab. Med.* 102:456, 1978.
54. Heitz P.U.: Multihormonal pituitary adenomas. *Hormone Res.* 10:1, 1979.
55. Sheldon W.H., Golden A., Bondy P.K.: Cushing's syndrome produced by a pituitary basophil carcinoma with hepatic metastases. *Am. J. Med.* 17:134, 1954.
56. Salassa R.M., Kearns T.P., Kernohan J.W., et al.: Pituitary tumors in patients with Cushing's syndrome. *J. Clin. Endocrinol. Metab.* 19:1523, 1959.
57. Scholz D.A., Gastineau C.F., Harrison E.G.: Cushing's syndrome with malignant chromophobe tumor of the pituitary and extracranial metastases: Report of a case. *Proc. Staff Meet. Mayo Clin.* 37:31, 1962.
58. D'Abrera V.S.E., Burke W.J., Bleasel K.F., et al.: Carcinoma of the pituitary gland. *J. Pathol.* 109:335, 1973.
59. Queiroz L.S., Facure N.O., Facure J.J., et al.: Pituitary carcinoma with liver metastases and Cushing syndrome: Report of a case. *Arch. Pathol.* 99:32, 1975.
60. McCarty K.S. Jr., Bredesen D.E., Vogel F.S.: Neoplasms of the anterior pituitary. *Neurosurgery* 3:96, 1978.

# Radiation Therapy of Pituitary Tumors

GLENN E. SHELINE, Ph.D., M.D.

*Department of Radiation Oncology, University of California, San Francisco, Moffitt Hospital, San Francisco, California*

UNTIL THE MID 1960S, pituitary tumors generally were classified as eosinophilic, basophilic, chromophobic, or mixed adenomas. With improved diagnostic techniques, including multiple dyes, electron microscopy, immunohistologic staining techniques, and new serum hormone assays, it has been established that the various pituitary hormones are secreted by specific cell types.[1-6] An elevated serum hormone level of a pituitary hormone generally is associated with a pituitary adenoma composed of cells appropriate for that particular hormone. Hyperprolactinemia, of course, may result either from a prolactinoma or one of numerous other endogenous or exogenous causes. In addition to the functional adenomas, there are those for which no function is identifiable even with modern laboratory techniques. Anatomic extent together with functional status determine the clinical syndrome associated with a given tumor; both influence the choice of therapy. At present, there is no completely satisfactory system for categorizing anatomical extent. Hardy and Vezina[7] developed a one-to-four grading system based primarily on the extent of expansion or erosion of the sellar floor. Use of the term "Grade" is unfortunate in that it usually is applied to degree of malignancy, whereas "Stage" is used to designate anatomic extent. Hardy and Vezina adopted secondary designations, types A to D, to denote suprasellar or parasellar extension. Wilson[8] proposed a modification in which Grade 5 and categories O and E were added. Tumors that metastasized via cerebrospinal fluid or the bloodstream were Grade 5.

0-8151-3530-0/82/006-121-143-$03.75

Category (type) O indicated no extension above the diaphragma sellae, and category E, extension into or beneath the cavernous sinus. The present author proposed a modification attempting to incorporate the features of the Hardy-Vezina-Wilson approach and yet conform with the T, N, and M system widely used for classification of anatomical extent and spread.[9] Unfortunately, in most reported series, especially in the radiotherapy literature, pituitary tumors have not been classified according to anatomical extent and it is impossible to compare results of various types of therapy for anatomically similar adenomas.

The reported incidence of pituitary adenomas is as high as 22%,[10] but most are microscopic in size, nonsymptomatic and are found only at postmortem examination. They may be diagnosed premortem because of an incidental skull radiograph, excessive hormone secretion, and/or mass effects. Functional tumors may be small and without clinically significant mass effects, or relatively large. Probably due to earlier recognition, the incidence of large tumors associated with acromegaly appears to be decreasing in acromegalic patients seen in recent years. For example, at the University of California, San Francisco (UCSF), 44% of acromegalic patients seen prior to 1959 had visual field deficits[11]; but more recently only three of 43 had suprasellar extension sufficient to deform the third ventricle.[12] Landolt[4] reported visual symptoms in 11% of patients with acromegaly compared to 77% for those with endocrinologically inactive tumors. Hyperprolactinemia often is produced by a microadenoma but can be associated with a relatively large tumor with extension outside the sella and local mass effects. Since the mechanisms by which ionizing radiation effect secretion and cell replication may differ, there is no reason to expect irradiation to be equally effective in the control of excessive endocrine function and of mass effects. In fact, experience has shown that the effectiveness of conventional photon radiotherapy differs for control of tumor growth and for secretory suppression and that production of some hormones, either by normal or adenomatous pituitary glands, is more readily influenced than is that of other hormones.

## Acromegaly

Prior to the growth hormone (GH) assay, in the absence of a major visual deficit, conventional fractionated photon radiotherapy (CFPRT) was widely accepted as the treatment of choice for acromegaly. Sheline et al.[11] reported 37 patients treated at UCSF with evaluation based on skeletal changes, visceral hypertrophy, hypermetabolism, carbohydrate tolerance, serum phosphorus level, adrenal hyperactivity, visual fields, headaches, and roentgenograms of the sella turcica. The acromegaly was controlled in 78% of the 18 patients who received doses of 4,400 rad. With such doses, visual field deficits disappeared in six of the eight patients who had pretreatment deficits. Lower doses were less effective for control of acromegaly or visual field deficits. There was no major complication associated with a single course of radiation. Other authors have reported similar results. In 19 patients, Pistenma et al.[13] reported a 90% control rate with CFPRT. Six patients had pretreatment visual field deficits. The average dose to the pituitary was 5,800 rad fractionated over six weeks. Two patients required hypophysectomy for treatment failure and one developed hypothyroidism. Kramer[14] reported 29 patients given radiation dosages of approximately 4,500 rad in four and a half weeks. In 86% of the patients acromegaly was controlled, while four patients required hypophysectomy.

After the GH assay became available it was noted that GH levels were similar before and in the period shortly after irradiation.[15] However, if the interval was measured in many months or years, GH concentrations decreased. In 1972, 17 patients irradiated at UCSF prior to the GH assay were available for reevaluation.[16] This may not have been a representative group in that those with uncontrolled disease could have been disproportionately represented in patients who died in the intervening period of time. Of the 17, one patient, who refused further therapy, had clinically active acromegaly and a GH level of 200 ng/ml. Sixteen were clinically well and had fasting GH levels $\leq$ 7.5 ng/ml. Three of the 16 had postirradiation transsphenoidal cryohypophysectomy; however, in two of these, the surgical procedure was performed less than one year after irradiation, an interval now known to be too short for final evaluation of CFPRT. Excluding the two with early surgery, 13 of 15 (87%) were controlled by irradiation alone. Combining data for patients treated before the GH assay at UCSF, members of the Radiation Therapy Oncology Group (RTOG)[17] and Lawrence et al.[18] provided a pooled group of 53 patients. At the time of review, 44 (83%) had normal GH levels, two had been operated on within one year after irradiation and were not evaluable, and 7 had active acromegaly.

Lawrence et al.[18] reported on CFPRT of 12 acromegalic patients irradiated subsequent to the GH assay. The pretreatment GH levels ranged from 20 to 332 ng/ml. After irradiation, 9 (75%) had GH levels $\leq$ 10 ng/ml and 7 had levels $\leq$ 5 ng/ml. The two with concentrations between 5 and 10 ng/ml were evaluated only one year after treatment. Combining data from the RTOG survey,[17] Lawrence et al.[18] and Kramer[14] gave 40 patients treated with megavoltage conventional radiotherapy and who had both preirradiation and postirradiation fasting GH levels. After irradiation, fasting GH concentrations of ≤ 10 ng/ml were reached in 13 of 31 (42%) by one year and in 22 of 24 (92%) by three years. Although the numbers were small and the difference of questionable significance, the three-year control rate was 100% when the pretreatment GH was ≤ 45 ng/ml and 71% if it was ≤ 50 ng/ml.

Eastman et al.[19] reported 47 patients treated by megavoltage photon radiotherapy using dosages of 4,000 to 5,000 rad to the pituitary, usually given in doses of 200 rad per day (Table 1). Fasting GH levels decreased slowly over several years. By two, five, and ten years the GH concentrations were ≤ 10 ng/ml in 38%, 73%, and 81%, respectively. Concentrations ≤ 5 ng/ml were reached in 17%, 42%, and 69% at these time intervals. Other metabolic parameters showed a similar improvement with time. Serum phosphate, fasting plasma glucose, two-hour glucose levels (standard oral glucose test), maximum percent fall in glucose during insulin tolerance test, and subjective features such as acral and facial soft tissue changes reverted toward normal at a rate roughly parallel with the decrease in plasma GH. These authors found no correlation between pretreatment GH concentration and response to radiotherapy. Although 16 patients were followed at least ten years after irradiation, there was no recurrence of acromegaly nor increase in size of the adenoma. One patient who

TABLE 1.—ACROMEGALY: CONVENTIONAL RADIOTHERAPY*

| FINDING | BEFORE THERAPY | AFTER IRRADIATION | | |
|---|---|---|---|---|
| | | 2 YR. | 5 YR. | 10 YR. |
| Number of patients | 47 | 42 | 33 | 16 |
| Plasma GH: 10 ng/ml | 13% | 38% | 73% | 81% |
| Plasma GH: 5 ng/ml | 2% | 17% | 42% | 69% |
| Serum phosphate | 4.7±0.1 | 4.4±0.1 | 4.2±0.1 | 4.0±0.1 |
| Fasting plasma glucose | 118±6 | 107±6 | 100±5 | 92±3 |
| 2-hr. glucose† | 191±15 | 158±10 | 153±14 | 123±6 |
| Max.% fall glucose‡ | 39±2 | 44±2 | 57±4 | 53±4 |
| Hypothyroid | 9% | 14% | 12% | 19% |
| Hypoadrenal | 6% | 12% | 30% | 38% |
| Hypogonadal (M/F) | 13%/19% | 32%/29% | 41%/44% | 58%/50% |

*Adapted from Eastman R.C., et al.: J. Clin. Endocrinol. Metab. 48:931, 1979.
†100-gm oral glucose test.
‡After 0.1 unit/kg regular insulin given intravenously.

received an unusually high dosage, 5,600 rad in six weeks, developed bilateral optic atrophy; however, this patient also had severe progressive systemic sarcoidosis and the amblyopia was attributed to the sarcoidosis.

The chief complication of CFPRT for acromegaly is delayed hypopituitarism of varying degree. Goldfine and Lawrence[20] reported three patients in whom there was loss of trophic hormones following irradiation for acromegaly. Eastman et al.[19] found a progressive increase in hypothyroidism, hypoadrenalism, and hypogonadism (see Table 1). Hypothyroidism increased from 9% before therapy to 19% at ten years and hypoadrenalism from 6% to 38%. Since these authors attributed hypofunction to the postirradiation period whenever the date of onset was uncertain and interpreted equivocal laboratory tests as indicative of hypofunction, the incidence of clinically significant radiation induced hypofunction actually was less than these data suggest. For example, only four of the eight cases of hypoadrenalism attributed to irradiation were sufficiently severe enough to require corticosteroid replacement therapy.

CFPRT appears to be equally effective for treatment of acromegaly persisting or recurring after subtotal resection. Williams et al.[21] irradiated six patients after failure of transsphenoidal resection; GH levels returned to normal in four. Sheline[22] reported seven patients with GH levels of 17 to 48 ng/ml after cryohypophysectomy and four with posttransfrontal resection levels of 54 to 200 ng/ml. One year after irradiation, two patients had GH concentrations of less than 10 ng/ml. Two years postirradiation, GH levels had reached the normal range in seven of the 11 (64%) patients. Eastman et al.[19] irradiated five patients with GH concentrations of 12 to 70 ng/ml after transfrontal hypophysectomy. Levels of $\leq$ 10 ng/ml and $<$ 6 ng/ml were obtained in four patients by two and five years, respectively. Thus, 15 (68%) of the 22 patients in these three series were controlled by conventional radiotherapy. As with irradiation for previously untreated acromegaly, the control rate increases with time, at least up to five years.

High energy $\alpha$-particles (AP)[23] and proton (P)[24] beams have been used to irradiate pituitary tumors. These particle beams yield more sharply defined dose distributions than conventional photon beams, thus permitting higher doses to limited volumes. At the University of California in Berkeley (UCB), Linfoot[23] and co-workers employed an AP beam with a cross-section measured in millimeters. Treatment was delivered via a double pendulum motion. This technique produced a nonuniform dose distribution, maximized at the center of the sella but with lower doses toward the periphery and in adjacent extrasellar structures. The maximum total dosage at the center of the pituitary ranged from 5,000 to 15,000 rad. In the earlier UCB patients, the dose was delivered in three to six fractions; more recently, four fractions were given in four or five days. Because of the extremely large daily fractions and total doses, such AP irradiation must be limited to tumors contained within the sella or extending a very limited distance into the sphenoid. Therefore, the UCB group excluded patients with significant superior or lateral extension or with a pituitary diameter $\geq$ 2.5 mm. Linfoot reported results in terms of mean GH concentration for the entire group of patients rather than in terms of number of patients achieving a normal level. The mean preirradiation fasting plasma GH concentration was 37 ng/ml. This decreased to 12 ng/ml at one year, 9 ng/ml at two years, 8 ng/ml at three years, and 4 ng/ml five years postirradiation. In spite of the large radiation doses, response followed essentially the same time course as with conventional irradiation. Patients with tumors < 10 mm in maximal diameter responded more rapidly than did those with larger tumors; this may have been related to dose distribution rather than an inherent difference in radiosensitivity as a function of adenoma size. In the 233 patients treated by AP irradiation, irradiation induced hypofunction of a degree sufficient to require endocrine replacement was: hypoadrenalism, 34%; hypothyroidism, 33%; and hypogonadism, 25%. These rates for iatrogenic hypoadrenalism and hypothyroidism are higher than reported for conventional supervoltage irradiation.[19] The average time to beginning replacement therapy was approximately four years. Since Linfoot and co-workers adopted the biplanar, or double pendulum, rotation technique and utilized only the plateau portion of the depth dose curve, the incidence of central nervous system complications has been < 1%. Earlier patients treated with the Bragg peak portion of the curve, especially if previously exposed to photon irradiation, had an incidence of 13% to 43% injury to cranial nerves and/or temporal lobe. Although the data are reported in a different fashion and details of follow-up are uncertain, the results of Kjellberg and Kliman[24] using Bragg peak photon irradiation are similar to those of Linfoot with the AP plateau beam.

Thus, conventional photon radiotherapy and high dose α-particle or proton radiotherapy yield similar control rates and require about the same time to produce control. Time to control is measured in months or years rather than the minutes or hours associated with successful surgical intervention. Reported treatment-induced hypofunction is less with conventional therapy than with the particle beams, probably due to the lesser doses used for CFPRT. Conventional irradiation is applicable to all sizes of tumors, whereas the α-particle/proton irradiation is limited to tumors of relatively small volume. Radiotherapy is effective and is an appropriate method for treatment of acromegaly whenever rapid control is not essential, the patient is not a good candidate for the appropriate surgical procedure, or hyperfunction persists after subtotal resection.

## Cushing's Disease

Pituitary irradiation for Cushing's disease was described as early as 1932.[25] Subsequent reports of patients successfully treated with CFPRT have appeared periodically. At present, at least in North America, most patients with Cushing's disease are treated by transsphenoidal microdissection. A few patients, however, are inoperable and some fail to respond adequately to the surgical procedure. If radiotherapy is effective without an excessive complication rate, it is preferable to irradiate rather than perform total hypophysectomy or bilateral adrenalectomy for surgical failure.

Dohan et al.[26] reported 12 patients irradiated for Cushing's disease. Evaluation was based on disappearance of physical stigmata, improved glucose metabolism, lowered blood pressure, resumption of menses in females, and urinary excretion of 17-ketosteroid and corticoid. Little or no improvement occurred in six patients with dosages of 400 to 1,570 rad. With doses of 3,800 to 5,200 rad, five of the six had "excellent" responses. The one high-dose failure may have resulted from excessive protraction of the irradiation: the daily dose was only 54 rad and treatment was extended over a period of 85 days. For those who responded to irradiation, the average interval to improvement ranged from three to six months and no relapse occurred during the five and a half to seven years of follow-up.

Heuschele and Lampe[27] irradiated 16 patients with Cushing's disease. They gave a pituitary dose of 4,000 rad over four to four and a half weeks. Complete and permanent remission was achieved in ten (63%) patients. The average time to biochemical remission was five months, while for clinical remission it was seven and a half months. The mean age of patients with complete and permanent remission was 26 years, as compared with 45 years for those who either failed to respond or developed recurrences.

The most carefully studied and critically evaluated series of patients with Cushing's disease treated by CFPRT was reported by Orth and Liddle.[28] They irradiated 51 patients with total doses to the pituitary of 4,000 to 5,000 rad fractionated over about one month. Forty-four patients were observed for a mean of nine years posttherapy. Urinary 17-hydroxycorticosteroid excretion, mean plasma cortisol concentrations, and diurnal rhythm were used as criteria of control. "Cure" was defined as the achievement of a urinary 17-hydroxycorticosteroid excretion of < 7 mg/gm of creatinine and a mean plasma cortisol concentration < 13 μg/100 ml. If a normal diurnal rhythm was reestablished, the required low plasma cortisol value was < 7 μg/100 ml. For a patient to be classed as improved, the 17-hydroxycorticosteroid excretion had to be < 10 mg/gm creatinine and the mean plasma cortisol < 13 μg/100 ml. Using these criteria, ten of the 44 patients followed one to 14 years were cured and an additional 13 improved to the extent that further therapy was unnecessary. Thus, 53% of patients needed no additional therapy. The other 21 patients received bilateral adrenalectomy. There was no irradiation-induced hypopituitarism nor visual or neurologic deficit and, except for those with adrenalectomy, no required substitution therapy. Edmonds et al.,[29] using more lenient criteria, reported a 67% remission rate with an interval from radiotherapy to "complete remission" of one to six months. Eighteen months after irradiation, one patient showed evidence of recurrence, but this spontaneously disappeared and the patient was observed for an additional ten years without further indication of recurrence. There was no radiation complication.

Jennings et al.[30] treated 15 patients less than 16 years of age at onset of symptoms of Cushing's disease and less than 19 years of age at the time of radiotherapy. Some of these patients were included in the group reported earlier by Orth and Liddle. The criteria for cure were the same, namely the establishment of a mean plasma cortisol < 10 μg/100 ml, and a 24-hour urinary 17-hydroxycorticosteroid excretion of < 7 mg/gm of creatinine. Cure occurred in ten patients within nine months and in 12 (80%) within 18 months. There was no radiation-induced complication. Subsequent development, including secondary sexual characteristics, sexual function, and intellect, was said to be normal in all 15 patients. Four demonstrated fertility and growth resumed in 12. Three females, aged 16 years ± 5 months at the time of treatment, showed no further growth. One patient developed an abnormal GH response to hypoglycemia but in the other 11 so tested both basal and stimulated GH levels were normal.

The UCB experience with AP irradiation for Cushing's disease was updated by Linfoot[23] in 1979. Omissions in the data cited make interpretation of their results difficult. Length of follow-up and the number of patients serially studied are unclear. Pretreatment and post-treatment plasma cortisol levels were given as the mean for the patients studied without indicating numbers of patients with values outside the normal range. An average daily plasma cortisol of 16 μg/100 ml was accepted as normal. A total of 64 patients received AP irradiation by the technique described above for acromegaly. Fifty-nine of the 64 patients had small lesions with normal sellar volumes. The other five were of Grade 2, i.e., with sellar distortion but intact floor. Fifty-five patients (86%) were classified as "successfully treated"; this includes all five patients less than 20 years of age. Hypoadrenalism, hypothyroidism, and hypogonadism secondary to the AP irradiation and of sufficient degree to necessitate replacement therapy occurred in 20%, 27%, and 11%, respectively. The interval of risk for development of hypofunction extended up to ten years and many patients were followed for shorter periods of time. Thus the incidence of hypofunction will probably increase with further observation. There were two instances of injury to the third cranial nerve and one of chiasmal damage. Two thirds of the patients were treated between 1972 and 1978 and this data was presented in 1978. Thus, although AP irradiation appears promising, as yet a definitive evaluation cannot be made.

In summary, conventional pituitary irradiation controls Cushing's disease in 50% to 80% of patients with the apparent rate dependent on the endpoint chosen. Time to remission varies from a few months to a year or more, but appears shorter than that required for control of GH secretion in acromegaly. Reported complications are rare and recurrence virtually nonexistent. Childhood Cushing's disease responds better than that of adulthood. Adenomas producing Cushing's disease are generally very small, and limited volume-high dose AP irradiation may give a higher control rate, but final comparison is not yet possible. AP irradiation requires about the same time for response as does conventional radiotherapy and is associated with significant incidence of treatment-induced hypopituitarism.

## Nelson's Syndrome

The incidence of Nelson's syndrome in patients who have had adrenalectomy for Cushing's disease is probably around 10%. It may be higher in childhood Cushing's disease treated by bilateral adrenalectomy. Hopwood and Kenny [31] reported that eight of 30 children developed sellar enlargement and hyperpigmentation. Of the other 22, ten developed hyperpigmentation but did not have serial roentgenograms to investigate the possibility of sellar enlargement. According to these data, the incidence of Nelson's syndrome after adrenalectomy for childhood Cushing's disease is between 27% and 60%. In a series of 43 patients of all ages treated with pituitary irradiation for Cushing's disease, none developed Nelson's syndrome.[28] This in spite of the fact that 20 of the 43 patients had had bilateral adrenalectomies and were observed for a mean interval of eight years. Jennings et al.[30] reported no instance of Nelson's syndrome in 15 children who had received pituitary radiotherapy for Cushing's disease. Four of their children had been adrenalectomized and observed for a mean of 12 years. Failure to observe Nelson's syndrome in the irradiated patients of Orth and Liddle and of Jennings et al. has been used as suggestive evidence that pituitary irradiation might be effective as prophylactic therapy to prevent occurrence of this syndrome. Wild et al.,[32] however, described two isolated cases of Nelson's syndrome that occurred after pituitary irradiation. In adrenalectomized patients, Moore et al.[33] found two cases in 20 patients with pituitary irradiation and seven in 100 nonirradiated patients. Although the numbers are too small to permit definite conclusions, these data indicate that if pituitary irradiation does reduce the incidence of postadrenalectomy Nelson's syndrome, it is short of being 100% effective.

CFPRT with or without surgical resection also has been used in the therapy of Nelson's syndrome. Moore et al.[33] reported six of seven irradiated patients living and well and one dead of intercurrent disease an average of 9.4 years postirradiation. McKenzie and McIntosh[34] reported "apparent benefit" in two patients who received 4,800 rad, but follow-up time was not stated. Sheline and Wara[17] had two of three irradiated patients, two of whom also had subtotal resection, clinically controlled at two and five years. Linfoot[23] treated 15 patients with Nelson's syndrome; nine had only AP irradiation and six had a combination of surgical resection plus AP irradiation. He reported decreased pigmentation and adrenocorticotrophic hormone (ACTH) levels in all patients, but ACTH levels rarely returned to normal. One patient developed suprasellar extension and died. Six months postirradiation a second had either recurrence or radionecrosis. Although unsupportable from such meager data, it is the author's current preference that the pituitary tumor be surgically resected and, if excision is incomplete or the ACTH level remains elevated, to give postoperative radiotherapy.

## Prolactin-Secreting Tumors

Patients with hyperprolactinemia due to a pituitary adenoma often have small intrasellar adenomas, the majority of which can be dealt with quickly and effectively by transsphenoidal selective microresection. Hyperprolactinemia also may be associated with large tumors and varying degrees of sellar erosion and extrasellar extension. Prior to the prolactin assay, these tumors were usually classified as nonfunctional "chromophobe" or mixed adenomas. With the large tumors resection frequently fails to permanently control growth or to reduce prolactin levels to the normal range. The question of growth control will be dealt with in the following section. At this point, concern is regarding effectiveness of radiotherapy for control of excessive prolactin secretion. As will be seen, the published data relative to CFPRT are limited.

Samaan et al.[35] reported two patients with pituitary irradiation (4,900 to 5,400 rad) for hyperprolactinemia persistent after surgical resection. The plasma prolactin level was normal in one patient at three years but in the other remained elevated four years postirradiation. Kleinberg et al.,[36] Gomez et al.,[37] and Antunes et al.[38] reported on larger series of patients (Table 2), some treated surgically, some with radiotherapy, and others with both. Kleinberg et al. treated 15 patients with surgical resection (transsphenoidal in 13) and eight with radiotherapy for pituitary tumors associated with galactorrhea and hyperprolactinemia. All 23 patients had enlarged sellae and one fourth of them had visual field deficits. Transsphenoidal resection and radiotherapy appeared equally effective. Both groups had a similar reduction in mean prolactin level. Menses occasionally resumed. Irrespective of the method of therapy, galactorrhea was usually reduced but disappeared in only one third of patients. Gomez et al.[37] reported results for treatment of 19 patients with hyperprolactinemia; 18 tumors were microadenomas. Among 11 patients treated by transsphenoidal selective resection, prolactin level was normalized in seven patients with 3–8-mm diameter adenomas. Galactorrhea ceased and menses resumed in over one half of patients at risk. After irradiation there was a 62% decrease in mean prolactin concentration but only one of eight patients achieved a normal level. In four other patients, there was a gradual decline in serum prolactin over a period of three to four years.

Antunes et al.[38] used various combinations of surgery and radiotherapy (see Table 2). Sixteen patients had surgery alone for Grade

TABLE 2.—PROLACTINOMAS

| DATA | KLEINBERG ET AL.[36] | | GOMEZ ET AL.[37] | | | ANTUNES ET AL.[38] | |
|---|---|---|---|---|---|---|---|
| Treatment | S | CFPRT | S | CFPRT | S | S+CFPRT | CFPRT |
| Number of patients | 15 | 8 | 11 | 8 | 16 | 8 | 6 |
| Mean prolactin | | | | | | | |
| Pretreatment, ng/ml | 185 | 195 | 93 | 168 | 381 | 1204 | 2592 |
| | (4–3000) | (51–10,000) | (7–230) | (38–480) | (27–900) | (21–3600) | (110–10,000) |
| Posttreatment, ng/ml | 29 | 50 | — | 64 | 80 | 162 | 165 |
| | (0.5–170) | (32–1000) | | (12–200) | (6–361) | (3–490) | (32–560) |
| Decrease | 84% | 74% | | 62% | 79% | 87% | 93% |
| Prolactin normalized* | — | — | 7 | 1 | 7 | 2 | 0 |
| Galactorrhea ceased† | 5/15 | 3/8 | 5/9 | 2/8 | 4/12 | 1/3 | 2/3 |
| Menses resumed‡ | 2/12 | 2/6 | 4/6 | 4/? | 3/13 | 0/3 | 1/3 |
| Follow-up (mo) | 8–60 | | 8–60 | 6–57 | 1–28 | 3–39 | 13–72 |

S = surgical resection; CFPRT = conventional fractionated photon radiotherapy
*Number of patients with normal values after therapy.
†Number of patients controlled/number with pretreatment galactorrhea or amenorrhea.
‡Numbers in parentheses indicate range.

1 and 2 lesions. Radiotherapy was employed in 14 patients, eight of whom also had subtotal resection. Five of the irradiated tumors were Grade 3 or 4. The pretreatment serum prolactin level tended to be higher in those receiving radiotherapy; the mean pretreatment prolactin level for patients treated by transsphenoidal surgery was 381 ng/ml, whereas it was 1,204 for surgery plus radiotherapy and 2,592 for radiotherapy-only patients. Seven surgery-only and two surgery-plus-radiotherapy patients achieved normal serum prolactin levels after treatment. Normalization of serum prolactin was related to pretreatment prolactin level and tumor size. No patient with a pretreatment serum prolactin > 125 ng/ml, only one with a concentration of > 90 and none with a tumor larger than Grade 2 achieved a normal prolactin level regardless of the form of therapy. Cessation of galactorrhea and resumption of menses occurred at about the same rate in patients treated by resection and by radiotherapy.

Table 3 gives prolactin levels prior to and following CFPRT in 20 patients irradiated at UCSF. Patients #1–5 were treated with radiotherapy alone. Patients #16–20 had a subtotal resection prior to irradiation. In patients #8 and 20 surgery was transcranial; the remainder had transsphenoidal resections. Nineteen patients had tumors of grades 3 and 4, mostly accompanied by very large lateral and/or suprasellar extension. There was an inconsistent response to irradiation. In 5 patients (#1, 4, 5, 8, and 9) postirradiation prolactin concentrations were higher than preirradiation. Nine patients showed either a decrease after irradiation (#6, 7, 11, 12, 13, and 14) or progressive fall (#18, 19, and 20) suggesting an irradiation effect. Only patient 11 achieved a normal value that could be attributed to radiotherapy alone. Four patients were subsequently placed on bromocriptine with normalization of prolactin in only one case. Two patients (#2 and #3) were observed only one month and two others (#15 and 16) had normal prolactin postresection, hence the effect of irradiation could not be evaluated. Patient #7 is of particular interest as she was the only one treated for a microadenoma. She was 28 years old and had a five-year history of amenorrhea and galactorrhea. Six months following transsphenoidal selective adenectomy (at another medical center) her prolactin level ranged from 265 to 324 ng/ml. The levels decreased after irradiation, but did not return to normal range, and at 18 months the patient remained amenorrheic, although galactorrhea had ceased. Patient #4 also is of special interest. She was 27 years old and initially presented with a markedly enlarged sella, bitemporal hemianopia, and hypothyroidism, but with normal prolactin concentrations. Attempted surgical resection was

TABLE 3.—MACROPROLACTINOMAS: TRANSSPHENOIDAL
RESECTION AND/OR CONVENTIONAL RADIOTHERAPY AT UCSF

| | PROLACTIN, NG/ML | | |
|---|---|---|---|
| PATIENT | PRE-TS | PRE-RT | POST-RT (MO) |
| 1 | — | 88 | 180(20) |
| 2 | — | 33 | 39(1) |
| 3 | — | 200 | 160(1)* |
| 4 | — | 5.5; 4 | 35(31), 37(48), 41(72) |
| 5 | — | 32 | 17(6), 71(17), 62(24) |
| 6 | 380 | 90 | 89(3), 73(10), 50(17), 49(36)† |
| 7 | 96‡ | 300 | 76(11), 120(18) |
| 8 | 5,200§ | 160 | 634(19) |
| 9 | 1,070 | 101 | 1,380(27)* |
| 10 | 73 | 63 | 57(20) |
| 11 | 37 | 40 | 21(1), 14(2), 13(40) |
| 12 | 16,000 | 11,000 | 1,020(7), 634(13), 431(18), 335(24) |
| 13 | 6,500 | 2,700 | 2,070(5), 1,960(10), 1,320(18) |
| 14 | 115,000 | 33,000 | 17,000(1), 7,500(5) |
| 15 | 250 | 15 | 11(10), 7(28), 18(48) |
| 16 | 80 | 16 | 10(14) |
| 17 | 180 | — | 16(3) |
| 18 | 770 | — | 58(3), 23(50) |
| 19 | >200 | — | 111(1), 69*(7), 52(16), 57(25) |
| 20 | 800, 1300‡ | — | 1,150(4), 830(14), 250(16) |

TS = transsphenoidal resection.
RT = conventional radiotherapy.
*Placed on bromocriptine without normalization of prolactin level.
†Placed on bromocriptine with normalization of prolactin level.
‡Microadenoma.
§Surgery was by craniotomy.

aborted due to hemorrhage. Following CFPRT her visual fields improved but nine months later galactorrhea was noted and, subsequently, hyperprolactinemia documented. There was no evident exogenous cause for the prolactinemia, and the question arises as to whether or not this was secondary to hypothalamic irradiation with loss of prolactin-inhibiting factor. Shalet et al.[39] recently reported a patient irradiated for acromegaly who later developed hyperprolactinemia.

Final evaluation of the role of radiotherapy for control of hyperprolactinemia due to a pituitary adenoma awaits further data. Available information is based on too few patients, widely variable selection factors, and short or unstated period of observation. In patients with large tumors and very high prolactin levels, irradiation has produced a progressive decrease in prolactin levels but only occasionally to a normal value. Perhaps radiation reduces prolactin output from the adenoma, but this is partially offset by loss of prolactin-inhibiting factor acting on normal pituitary.

## Large Pituitary Tumors Treated For Growth Control

Many pituitary tumors attain clinical significance because of local invasion and/or expansion with pressure (mass) effects on surrounding structures. Moderately large tumors may be associated with acromegaly or Nelson's syndrome. The majority of large adenomas, however, either produce hyperprolactinemia or are without known endocrine function. The mass effects can cause headaches, visual field deficits, enlarged or eroded sellae, and/or secondary hypopituitarism. Depending upon growth pattern, such adenomas may extend superiorly to involve the optic chiasm, laterally into the cavernous sinus and oculomotor nerves, inferiorly into the sphenoid sinus and even into the substance of the brain. Occasionally, they extend into the ethmoid sinuses, orbit, and/or nasopharynx. As a general rule they are not completely resectable and after surgery alone, given sufficient time, they recur. Growth is slow and proof of "cure" necessitates prolonged observation. At UCSF[40] the mean time to recurrence for patients who failed after surgery alone was four years (range, one to 12 years) compared with nine years (range, two to 17 years) after a combination of surgery and postoperative radiotherapy. Erlichman et al.[41] found the median time to recurrence was 2.4 years for resection and 3.5 years for resection plus postoperative radiotherapy. Their latest recurrence was 15 years posttreatment.

The results of therapy for 140 consecutive patients treated for large pituitary tumors at UCSF prior to 1969 have been reported.[40] Prior to therapy, visual field deficits were present in 92%. Of the 11 patients with normal visual fields, nine had suprasellar extension demonstrated by pneumoencephalogram and the other two had biopsy-proved tumors extending into the nasopharynx. Although no attempt was made to grade these tumors, 96% had grossly enlarged sellae. Hypopituitarism was diagnosed in 53%; however, a number of patients had incomplete assessment of pituitary function and the real incidence of pretreatment hypopituitarism was undoubtedly higher. Twenty-three patients were treated with radiotherapy alone: five had refused surgery, seven were poor surgical risks, and seven had either normal visual fields or minimal visual field deficits. Of the 117 patients undergoing surgical resection, 80 were referred for postoperative irradiation. Although at present most patients at UCSF are operated via the transsphenoidal route, craniotomy was performed in 98% of this older series.

Most surgically related complications occurred in patients with huge locally invasive adenomas. There were eight operative or immediately postoperative deaths. Of the four surgical deaths subsequent to 1945, three were in patients with massively invasive tumors. Among the ten patients whose tumors were described at surgery as being invasive, there were three operative deaths and two instances of epilepsy with severe mental deterioration. Other authors have reported a similarly poor experience with invasive adenomas.[42-44] Surgery resulted in minor increases in visual deficit in ten patients with major loss occurring in 7; these were usually in situations where the optic nerve(s) and/or chiasm were enmeshed in tumor. Cerebrospinal fluid rhinorrhea developed in three patients in whom tumor extended through the floor of the sphenoid sinus into the nasopharynx.

Response to therapy was judged primarily on the basis of repeated visual field examinations. Each eye was evaluated separately and when surgical decompression was used, early responses were credited to the surgical procedure. With relatively minor visual field deficits involving one fourth or less of a visual field, irradiation alone or surgical decompression were equally effective: 65% and 67%, respectively, of the fields reverted to normal. When the pretreatment deficit involved two quadrants, radiotherapy gave a 60% improvement rate, but produced no normal fields. Surgical resection also gave a 60% improvement rate, but this included normalization of 32% of the abnormal visual fields. Thus, as measured by improvement of visual fields, patients with minimal deficits responded equally well to radiotherapy and surgical decompression, but the surgical decompression yielded better results for moderately advanced lesions.

Long-term recurrence-free survival rates were based largely on repeated visual field examinations, but roentgenograms of the sella turcica were also used. Repeated pneumoencephalograms and arteriograms were carried out only in those suspected of having recurrence. Patients treated with radiotherapy alone and those treated by partial resection plus postoperative irradiation experienced approximately equal recurrence-free survival rates. Five and ten years posttherapy the recurrence-free survival rates for radiotherapy were 93% and 71%, respectively. Several patients had died without recurrence of intercurrent disease before ten years. For resection plus postoperative radiotherapy recurrence-free survival rates were 90%, 79%, and 65% at five, ten, and 20 years, respectively. By contrast, only 25% of those treated by surgery alone were alive and recurrence-free at five years and no patient observed 15 years or longer was recurrence-free. Of the patients treated by radiotherapy only with a dose >2,000 rad, only one experienced a recurrence; however, the number so treated is small and there was a tendency to select patients with either relatively small tumors or limited life expectancy. When recently reviewed,[22] the five patients who at the time of the earlier report were without recurrence ten years following irradiation remained alive and disease-free 15 or more years after treatment. Since 14 patients irradiated during the earlier part of the study period received dosages less than 4,000 rad and response is dose-dependent, it is expected that modern radiotherapy techniques using doses of 4,500 to 5,000 rad will give better long-term control rates than those reported in this study. With improved surgery and radiotherapy, recurrences during the last 10–15 years have been exceedingly rare and a determinate control rate in the order of 95% is anticipated.

Other authors have had similar experiences with treatment of large adenomas. Kramer[14] reported 16 patients treated with radiotherapy alone. As in the UCSF series, these patients tended to be of advanced age and poor surgical risks. At the time of reporting, seven had died of intercurrent disease, two had had a recurrence, one was lost to follow-up, and six were alive and well. Thus, Kramer's absolute and determinate five-year survival rates with radiation alone were 38% and 75%, respectively. His determinate survival rate for patients treated by resection plus postoperative irradiation was 83%. Emmanuel[45] reported a 93% absolute four-year recurrence-free survival rate for combined surgery and radiotherapy, compared with 30% for resection alone. Pistenma et al.[44] had 86% and 82% absolute five-year control rates for irradiation alone and for surgery plus postoperative radiotherapy, respectively. Recently, Erlichman et al.[41] reported 87% disease-free survival rates for both radiotherapy alone and for surgery plus radiation. Thus, in these series, as in that from UCSF, irradiation alone and surgery followed by irradiation gave similar, long-term control rates and both were better than surgery alone. It would, however, be improper to conclude that radiotherapy was the equal of surgery plus radiotherapy. The patient populations were dissimilar: at UCSF, for example, there was a tendency to select patients who were poor surgical risks (hence, those who may not have lived long enough to develop a recurrence) and those with lesser visual deficits for treatment with irradiation alone. In the radiation-alone group, 16% had visual symptoms and 25% visual field deficits, whereas in those treated by combined surgery and irradiation, symptoms were present in 75% and field deficits in 89%.

It is concluded that postoperative conventional radiotherapy improves the control rate for large invasive pituitary tumors. Although the presently evaluable long-term experience is based on a mixture of prolactin-secreting and nonfunctioning pituitary adenomas, this is probably true for both tumor types. Radiotherapy alone also is effective, particularly with smaller tumors, but it is generally preferable to surgically debulk the tumor mass before administering radiation. This permits confirmation of diagnosis and gives the most rapid and reliable means of decompressing the optic apparatus. This is especially important with visual field deficits involving more than one quadrant.

## Radiation Complications of Conventional Radiotherapy

With modern CFPRT of pituitary adenomas, adverse effects appearing during or shortly after radiotherapy are negligible. Available techniques minimize skin and subcutaneous dose and, generally, even epilation is minimal and transient.

Possible late complications, those appearing several months to years after irradiation, include hypopituitarism, neoplasia, brain necrosis, and damage to optic apparatus. Radiation induction of hypopituitarism has been reported but data on incidence as a function of radiation dose and age of patient are not available. In our experience, GH production is particularly radiosensitive[46-48] but is of little concern in adult patients. Samaan et al.[49] reported a high incidence of hypopituitarism in patients treated for extracranial malignancies but many of their patients received higher doses than were used for pituitary adenomas, and little distinction was made between clinically significant and subclinical injury. Shalet et al.[50] emphasized the necessity of distinguishing between biochemically detectable and clinically significant (that requiring replacement therapy) hypofunction. As noted earlier, Eastman et al.[19] had an increase in hypothyroidism and hypopituitarism in patients irradiated for acromegaly.

Waltz and Brownell[51] reviewed the literature and found eight reported cases of fibrosarcoma and one osteosarcoma that arose in irradiated tissue subsequent to radiotherapy for a pituitary adenoma; nine fibrosarcomas were described but one case was duplicated. They added two fibrosarcomas and one osteosarcoma from their own experience. Subsequently, Powell et al[52] and Rubinstein[53] have reported two more fibrosarcomas. Of these 14 cases, seven had multiple courses of therapy usually with exceedingly high total dose, and in four others the dose was not stated. Thus, only three patients are known to have received a single course of irradiation with a dose within the currently advocated range. Since sarcoma can occur in unirradiated patients,[54] it is possible that one or more of these three cases was unrelated to irradiation.

With radiation doses currently advocated for pituitary adenomas, if radiation-induced brain necrosis does occur, it is exceedingly rare. Martins et al.[55] reported two cases in pituitary adenoma patients but the doses were 6,600 and 6,700 rad. Almquist et al.[56] and Aristizabal et al.[57] reported single cases after 5,000 rad, but none has been reported after irradiation of a pituitary tumor with a dose of 4,500 rad. Erlichman et al.[41] described one patient thought to have had a radiation-induced vasculitis that led to a fatal stroke. This patient received 4,000 rad in 18 fractions over three and a half weeks, but neither the age nor the blood pressure of the patient was stated and the actual cause of the vascular accident is unclear.

Injury to the optic apparatus although also rare, is more frequent than oncogenesis or necrosis. There are 13 reported instances of optic nerve or chiasm injury following irradiation of pituitary tumors. Of the four cases reported by Aristizabal et al.,[57] all received doses greater than 4,600 rad, and in two of the four, the daily fractions exceeded 220 rad. The daily dose was 250 rad or more in all five patients of Harris and Levene.[58] The patient reported by Sheline[22] received daily fractions of 225 rad. Kramer[59] had no injuries in 190 patients with "chromophobe" adenomas, but had three of 42 patients who received 5,000 rad in five weeks for acromegaly. Kramer suggested that small vessel disease associated with acromegaly may increase the risk of damage but has had no further injuries since reducing the dosage to 4,500 rad. There is evidence that for radiation injury of the nervous system, not only total dose but the number of fractions, conversely the size of each fraction, is of importance.[60] Aristizabal et al.[57] thought there was a disproportionately high incidence of optic injury reported in patients with Cushing's disease, but those patients generally had relatively high total doses or the daily fraction was in excess of 200 rad.

It may be concluded that with conventional radiotherapy given as a single course with a total dose of 4,500 rad and daily fractions ≤200 rad, the likelihood of radiation-induced sarcoma, brain necrosis, or injury to the optic apparatus (except possibly in acromegaly) is negligible.

## Radiotherapy Technique

While there will be no attempt to present a detailed discussion of radiation technique, consideration of general concepts seems appropriate. First, the tumor volume must be carefully defined by using all available information. Often this will include postoperative computerized tomographic scans with reconstruction in coronal and sagittal planes. Second, the treatment plan must be designed to give a uniform dose to the tumor volume with as little radiation as possible to surrounding structures. Third, a megavoltage radiation source with good beam characteristics is necessary. Depending upon the radiation equipment used, a variety of acceptable treatment plans can be generated. For very large tumor volumes where little can be gained by rotational or multiple fields, simple opposed bilateral coaxial fields occasionally are acceptable. However, this arrangement is rarely optimal for pituitary adenomas; it gives an unnecessarily high dose to the subcutaneous tissues and to the temporal lobes. Using a 4-meV linear accelerator, the author generally employs bicoronal 110-degree arc rotation with moving wedge filters.[22] Dose is calculated at the 95% isodose line designed to include the tumor mass. This technique provides a dose uniform to within ±2.5% throughout the tumor volume with a rapidly decreasing dose outside this volume. Arc angles and thickness of wedge filters are varied according to the site of residual tumor. Field size depends on the volume to be irradiated. A fairly similar dose distribution can be obtained with bilateral coaxial wedged fields used together with a coronal field. It is the author's opinion that with conventional fractionation, 180 to 200 rad per day and five treatments per week, a total dose of about 4,500 rad is optimal for most pituitary adenomas. The dose may be carried higher for very large invasive adenomas. When the dosage is calculated at the 95% isodose line, this gives a dose of 4,610 ± $2^{1}/2$% rad throughout the tumor volume. There is evidence that doses less than 3,500 or 4,000 rad yield a lower control rate,[17] and with doses above 5,000 rad complications begin to appear, particularly if the daily fraction is greater than 200 rad.

## REFERENCES

1. Frantz A.G.: Prolactin. *Physiol. Med.* 298:201, 1978.
2. Glick S.M., Roth J., Yalow R.S., et al.: Immunoassay of human growth in plasma. *Nature* 199:784, 1963.
3. Kovacs K., Horvath E., Ezrin C.: Pituitary adenomas, in Sommers, S.E. (ed): *Pathology Annals.* New York: Appleton-Century-Crofts, 1977.
4. Landolt A.M.: Progress in pituitary adenoma biology, in Krayenbuhl H.

(ed): *Advances and Technical Standards in Neurosurgery*. New York: Springer-Verlag New York, 1978, vol 5.

5. McCormick W.F., Halmi N.S.: Absence of chromophobe adenomas from a large series of pituitary tumors. *Arch. Pathol.* 92:231, 1971.

6. Pelletier G., Robert F., Hardy J.: Identification of human anterior pituitary cells by immunoelectron microscopy. *J. Clin. Endocrinol. Metab.* 46:534, 1978.

7. Hardy J., Vezina J.L.: Transsphenoidal neurosurgery of intracranial neoplasm, in Thompson R.A., et al. (eds): *Advances in Neurology: Neoplasia in the Central Nervous System*. New York: Raven Press, 1976, vol 15.

8. Wilson C.B.: Neurosurgical management of large and invasive pituitary tumors, in Tindall G.T., et al. (eds): *Clinical Management of Pituitary Disorders*. New York: Raven Press, 1979.

9. Sheline G.E.: Pituitary tumors: Radiation therapy, in Beardwell C.G., et al. (eds): *Butterworth International Medical Review-Clinical Endocrinology: The Pituitary*. London: Butterworth International, vol 1., 1981, pp 106–139.

10. Kernohan J.W., Sayre G.P.: Tumors of the pituitary gland and infundibulum, in *Atlas of Tumor Pathology*, section X, fascicle 36. Washington, D.C.: Armed Forces Institute of Pathology, 1956.

11. Sheline G.E., Goldberg M.B., Feldman R.: Pituitary irradiation for acromegaly. *Radiology* 76:70, 1961.

12. U H.S., Wilson C.B., Tyrrell J.B.: Transsphenoidal microhypophysectomy in acromegaly. *J. Neurosurg.* 47:840, 1977.

13. Pistenma D.A., Goffinet D.R., Bagshaw M.A., et al.: Treatment of acromegaly with megavoltage radiation therapy. *Int. J. Radiat. Oncol. Biol. Phys.* 1:885, 1976.

14. Kramer S.: Indications for, and results of, treatment of pituitary tumors by external radiation, in Kohler P.O., et al. (eds): *Diagnosis and Treatment of Pituitary Tumors*. New York: Elsevier North-Holland, 1973.

15. Glick S.M.: Acromegaly and other disorders of growth hormone secretion: Combined clinical staff conference at the National Institutes of Health, *Ann. Intern. Med.* 66:760, 1967.

16. Sheline G.E.: Treatment of chromophobe adenomas of the pituitary gland and acromegaly, in Kohler P.O., et al. (eds): *Diagnosis and Treatment of Pituitary Tumors*. New York: Elsevier North-Holland, 1973.

17. Sheline G.E., Wara W.M.: Radiation therapy of acromegaly and nonsecretory chromophobe adenomas of the pituitary, in Seydel H.G. (ed): *Tumors of the Nervous System*. New York: John Wiley & Sons, 1975.

18. Lawrence A.M., Pinsky S.M., Goldfine I.D.: Conventional radiation therapy in acromegaly. *Arch. Intern. Med.* 128:369, 1977.

19. Eastman R.C., Gorden P., Roth J.: Conventional supervoltage irradiation is an effective treatment for acromegaly. *J. Clin. Endocrinol. Metab.* 48:931, 1979.

20. Goldfine I.D., Lawrence A.M.: Hypopituitarism in acromegaly. *Arch. Intern. Med.* 130:720, 1972.

21. Williams R.A., Jacobs H.S., Kurtz A.B., et al.: The treatment of acromegaly with special reference to transsphenoidal hypophysectomy. *Q. J. Med.* 44:79, 1975.

22. Sheline G.E.: Conventional radiation therapy in the treatment of pitu-

itary tumors, in Tindall G.T., et al. (eds): *Clinical Management of Pituitary Disorders.* New York: Raven Press, 1979.

23. Linfoot J.A.: Heavy ion therapy: α-Particle therapy of pituitary tumors, in Linfoot J.A. (ed): *Recent Advances in the Diagnosis and Treatment of Pituitary Tumors.* New York: Raven Press, 1979.

24. Kjellberg R.N., Kliman B.: Lifetime effectiveness—a system of therapy for pituitary adenomas, emphasizing Bragg peak proton hypophysectomy, in Linfoot J.A. (ed): *Recent Advances in the Diagnosis and Treatment of Pituitary Tumors.* New York: Raven Press, 1979.

25. Cushing H.: The basophilic adenomas of the pituitary body and their clinical manifestations. *Bull. Johns Hopkins Hosp.* 50:137, 1932.

26. Dohan F.C., Raventos A., Boucot N., et al.: Roentgen therapy in Cushing's syndrome without adrenocortical tumor. *J. Clin. Endocrinol. Metab.* 17:8, 1957.

27. Heuschele R., Lampe I.: Pituitary irradiation for Cushing's syndrome. *Radiol. Clin. Biol.* 36:27, 1967.

28. Orth D.N., Liddle G.W.: Results of treatment in 108 patients with Cushing's syndrome. *N. Engl. J. Med.* 285:243, 1971.

29. Edmonds M.W., Simpson W.J.K., Meakin J.W.: External irradiation of the hypophysis for Cushing's disease. *Calif. Med. Assoc. J.* 107:860, 1972.

30. Jennings A.S., Liddle G.W., Orth D.: Results of treating childhood Cushing's disease with pituitary irradiation. *N. Engl. J. Med.* 297:957, 1977.

31. Hopwood N., Kenny F.: Increased incidence of postadrenalectomy Nelson's syndrome in pediatric versus adult Cushing's disease: A nationwide study, *Pediatr. Res.* 9:290, 1975.

32. Wild W., Nicolis G.L., Gabrilove J.L.: Appearance of Nelson's syndrome despite pituitary irradiation prior to bilateral adrenalectomy for Cushing's syndrome. *Mt. Sinai Med. J.* 40:68, 1973.

33. Moore T.J., Dluhy R.G., Williams G.H., Cain J.P.: Nelson's syndrome: Frequency, prognosis, and effect of prior pituitary irradiation. *Ann. Intern. Med.* 85:731, 1976.

34. McKenzie A.D., McIntosh H.W.: Hyperpigmentation and pituitary tumor as sequelae of the surgical treatment of Cushing's syndrome. *Am. J. Surg.* 110:135, 1965.

35. Samaan N.A., Leavens M.E., Jesse J.H. Jr.: Serum prolactin in patients with "functionless" chromophobe adenomas before and after therapy. *Acta Endocrinol.* 84:449, 1977.

36. Kleinberg D.L., Noel G.L., Frantz A.G.: Galactorrhea: A study of 235 cases, including 48 with pituitary tumors. *N. Engl. J. Med.* 296:589, 1977.

37. Gomez F., Reyes F.I., Faiman C.: Nonpuerperal galactorrhea and hyperprolactinemia: Clinical findings, endocrine features and therapeutic responses in 56 cases. *Am. J. Med.* 62:648, 1977.

38. Antunes J.L., Housepian E.M., Frantz A.G., et al.: Prolactin-secreting pituitary tumors. *Ann. Neurol.* 2:148, 1977.

39. Shalet S.M., MacFarlane I.A., Beardwell C.G.: Radiation-induced hyperprolactinemia in a treated acromegalic. *Clin. Endocrinol.* 11:169, 1979.

40. Sheline G.E.: Treatment of nonfunctioning chromophobe adenomas of the pituitary. *Am. J. Roentgenol.* 120:553, 1974.

41. Erlichman C., Meakin J.W., Simpson W.J.: Review of 154 patients with

non-functioning pituitary tumors. *Int. J. Radiat. Oncol. Biol. Phys.* 5:1981, 1979.

42. Martins A.N., Hayes G.J., Kampe L.G.: Invasive pituitary adenomas. *J. Neurosurg.* 22:268, 1965.

43. Ogilvy K.M., Jakubowski J.: Intracranial dissemination of pituitary adenomas. *J. Neurol. Neurosurg. Psychiatry* 36:199, 1973.

44. Pistenma D.A., Goffinet D.R., Bagshaw M.A., et al.: Treatment of chromophobe adenomas with megavoltage irradiation. *Cancer* 35:1574, 1975.

45. Emmanuel I.G.: Symposium on pituitary tumors: 3. Historical aspects of radiotherapy, present treatment, technique and results, *Clin. Radiol.* 17:154, 1966.

46. Richards G.E., Wara W.M., Grumbach M.M. et al.: Delayed onset of hypopituitarism: Sequelae of therapeutic irradiation of central nervous system, eye and middle ear tumors. *J. Pediatr.* 89:553, 1976.

47. Sheline G.E.: Radiation therapy of tumors of the central nervous system in children. *Cancer* 35:957, 1975.

48. Wara W.M.: Personal communication.

49. Samaan N.A., Maor M., Sampiere V.A., et al.: Hypopituitarism after external irradiation of nasopharyngeal cancer, in Linfoot J.A. (ed): *Recent Advances in the Diagnosis and Treatment of Pituitary Tumors*. New York: Raven Press, 1979.

50. Shalet S.M., Price D.A., Beardwell C.G., et al.: Normal growth despite abnormalities of growth hormone secretion in children treated for acute leukemia. *J. Pediatr.* 94:719, 1979.

51. Waltz T.A., Brownell B.: Sarcoma: A possible late result of effective radiation therapy for pituitary adenoma: Report of two cases. *J. Neurosurg.* 24:901, 1966.

52. Powell H.C., Marshall L.F., Ignelzi R.J.: Postirradiation pituitary sarcoma. *Acta Neuropathol. (Berl.)* 39:165, 1977.

53. Rubinstein L.J.: Tumors of the central nervous system, in *Atlas of Tumor Pathology*, 2nd series, fascicle 6. Washington, D.C.: Armed Forces Institute of Pathology, 1972.

54. Goldberg M.B., Sheline G.E., Malamud N.: Malignant intracranial neoplasms following radiation therapy for acromegaly. *Radiology* 80:465, 1963.

55. Martins A.N., Johnson J.S., Henry J.M., et al.: Delayed radiation necrosis of the brain. *J. Neurosurg.* 47:336, 1977.

56. Almquist S., Dahlgren S., Notter G., et al.: Brain necrosis after irradiation of the hypophysis in Cushing's disease: Report of a case. Acta Radiol. [Diagn.] (Stockh.) 2:179, 1964.

57. Aristizabal S., Caldwell W.L., Avila J.: The relationship of time-dose fractionation factors to complications in the treatment of pituitary tumors by irradiation. *Int. J. Radiat. Oncol. Biol. Phys.* 2:667, 1977.

58. Harris J.R., Levene M.B.: Visual complications following irradiation for pituitary adenomas and craniopharyngiomas. *Radiology* 120:167, 1976.

59. Kramer S.: Personal communication.

60. Sheline G.E., Wara W.M., Smith V.: Therapeutic irradiation and brain injury. *Int. J. Radiat. Oncol. Biol. Phys.* 6:1215, 1980.

# Panel II: The Pretreatment Pituitary Patient

*Moderator:* EDWARD R. LAWS, M.D.
*Panelists:* PETER KOHLER, M.D., JAMES ACKER, M.D., KALMAN T. KOVACS, M.D., GLENN SHELINE, M.D.

*I would like to invite people who presented papers this afternoon to come up to the stage. So many subjects were covered that I am sure that in the question period we can expand on a number of different areas, certainly from the radiotherapy standpoint. We need to see what the combination of bromocriptine and radiotherapy will do. And I think that in two or three years we will probably have some data that will be very impressive concerning the combination of both the medical and radiotherapeutic modalities, both as primary treatment and in salvaging the failures of surgery. That should be extremely useful data. Can we start with some questions from the audience?*

QUESTION FROM THE AUDIENCE: *Dr. Kovacs, what do you see in the way of pathologic changes after radiotherapy?*

KOVACS: It is a difficult question. We studied only a few cases and I can not give you any definite answer. There were a few cases in which there was no change; there were others in which there were binuclear cells, some nuclear pleomorphous and some fibrosis. But all these changes occurred without radiotherapy, so we cannot identify pathologic changes just by looking at the slides of a patient who is treated or not treated. Our material is really not sufficient to properly answer your question. As a matter of fact, it would be very smart to study this question in detail in the future.

QUESTION FROM THE AUDIENCE: *Have psychological studies been done at ten to 15 years after either whole brain or pituitary area radiation to determine its effect on intellect?*

SHELINE: There are a number of such studies. None is really very good. This is a very burning question and one that we wish we had

145

0-8151-3530-0/82/006-145-162-$03.75

a better answer to. Some of the problems are that we never have the preradiation assessment to compare with later on. Now I believe there are a few ongoing studies. I think there is one at Manchester. I believe that Anna Meadows and Audry Evans in Philadelphia are carrying out one where they are getting baseline studies and projecting these into the future. Looking at what is available, there is some penalty with large fields, certainly whole-brain radiation and certainly in very young patients. This is so particularly in patients under the age of two or three years. I would not anticipate a recognizable effect on intellect with appropriate therapy for pituitary tumors, using small volumes and not exceeding 4,500 rad and not exceeding 180 rad per day. I would be almost willing to wager we won't pick up any deficits there. But there are a couple of studies with the big fields. One from Jefferson that I have heard reported—it has not hit the literature yet—suggests that there may be a drop of about 10% in IQ as compared to various types of controls. I think there have been similar data from some of the acute leukemia studies. Dr. Raimondi, a neurosurgeon from Children's Memorial Hospital in Chicago, has reported suggestive evidence of reduced IQ and learning disabilities in children with medulloblastomas treated with high-dose, whole CNS radiation. Again, there seems to be a penalty, but that is whole brain and spinal cord radiation in children. I think it is a different ballgame that we are talking about here.

QUESTION FROM THE AUDIENCE: *How does the referring endocrinologist or neurosurgeon determine whether the radiotherapist, who is going to give the therapy, is doing it the right way? If the temporal lobes are fried, that is probably more important than whether radiotherapy is given or not. What matters is how well it is given. Are there any tips? Is there some author who says who is good and who is not?*

SHELINE: No, I'm afraid there isn't. I think that probably applies to all specialties.

QUESTION FROM THE AUDIENCE: *On those large tumors that you operated upon, how do you decide whether to utilize combined therapy or not?*

LAWS: I am persuaded that it depends on the size of the tumor and the extent to which it is removed and that it is part of the problem of individualization. We had a patient with a large tumor that has continued to cause a problem. The patient continued to have visual field defects and so forth. The data is pretty clear that that kind of patient is apt to continue to get into trouble, if he does not receive radiation, just with the simple mass effect. Now, if you have a smaller tumor that does not show any evidence of erosion or does not give you any visual field changes, or something like that, even without surgical therapy, that is a more controversial area. But I would think, and I will ask Dr. Sheline to comment, since this is his area, that large tumors that are incompletely removed should probably be irradiated.

SHELINE: This has been my thinking. If some of the smaller ones are not treated by one means or another, and are simply observed, then they must be observed for a long period of time, I think for the lifetime of the patient. We have a number of these in our files that I have pulled out and looked at serially. A good percentage of them develop visual field defects, although it may be five, ten or 15 years after therapy. So I think if they are left untreated they need to be followed. I think Dr. Wilson would like to comment on that last question, because for the last ten years he has been my chief source of material.

WILSON: Well, I think it has been fairly well stated by Ed Laws: when a tumor is incompletely removed, we don't need to relive history. Tumors grow and they should be irradiated because of the 95% probability of recurrence of growth. You are concerned about a life-stretching tumor. I think it is cavalier to say that probably there is not much left and let's just watch it. Because when you are dealing with a 95% cure rate, at least up to 20 years with radiotherapy, for tumors that have been treated surgically to reduce the bulk in radiotherapy, you have to be awfully optimistic, or have a patient who is unlikely to survive that period of time, to believe that something better will come along or to say that, because radiotherapy has a dangerous effect, the tumor should not be irradiated. Now, to answer that specific question, what to do for the incompletely removed tumor, I think you should fully inform the patient who elects to have the radiation for two months.

QUESTION FROM THE AUDIENCE: *A question for Dr. Acker. In St. Louis you have had the opportunity to follow two relatively young patients who had brain surgery and radiotherapy. You have followed them with CT scans over a period of three or three and a half years now. Both of them have developed a wavelike radiolucency through the area of the plane of therapy that has been ascribed to small cell vasculytes and wipeout brain tissue. Have you ever experienced postirradiation CT follow-up on these patients?*

ACKER: Yes, I am seeing more and more of them. Now describe again what you have seen.

A MEMBER OF THE AUDIENCE: Basically, what the CT pictures show is a loss of enhancing tissue right through the path of the beam.

ACKER: Oh, I see, with radiotherapy. Now I think that I have seen very many of the postradiotherapy patients. I cannot comment further.

QUESTION FROM THE AUDIENCE: *What were those patients and what do they have? What was their ages?*

DAUGHADAY: Most of them were relatively large, age between 32 and 45 and what we assumed at that point were adequate tumor doses in the range of 45 and under, treated at the university.

QUESTION FROM THE AUDIENCE: *Dr. Kovacs, not too many years ago, textbooks used to describe growth cell hormone hyperplasia as the cause of acromegaly. Have you seen that in your studies, macroplasia of GH cells only?*

KOVACS: We have seen hyperplasia of cortical tubes causing Cushing's disease, but up to now we have not seen hyperplasia of GH cells accounting for acromegaly. There is just one point that I would like to make and that is that the distribution of cells is uneven in the pituitary. The GH cells are located mainly in the lateral wings and very few in the central portion. So if we study only surgically removed fragments, and we don't know exactly from which part of the pituitary has the material been taken, then we can really not assess this question. So it is much easier to study autopsy material from a hemihypophysectomized patient. But this very small surgical tissue fragment, which usually we get, is just not suitable for diagnosis. Several patients referred to us were supposed to have GH cell hyperplasia, but we could never convince ourselves that they really had GH cell hyperplasia.

QUESTION FROM THE AUDIENCE: *Is there any reason why that entity should not exist?*

KOVACS: Theoretically it exists, but we have seen only one case.

QUESTION FROM THE AUDIENCE: Dr. Sheline, have you seen any patients treated with just radiation or whose tumor could not be completely removed at surgery, who had transient deterioration in the visual fields from swelling?

SHELINE: The answer to that is no. We have seen fields deteriorate before we have started, unfortunately, and then had them decompressed and patients had a bleed. We used to insist that the ones we treated with radiation, without decompression, get weekly visual field assessments, but this never paid off, and Bill Hoyt, who did these for us, won't even do them anymore.

LAWS: I have operated on two patients who had developed pituitary apoplexy during radiotherapy, so certainly it can occur. It is probably not very common.

SHELINE: I have not seen it, but the possibility is there.

LAWS: *Some neurosurgeons favor an intraoperative biopsy, during the course of removal of a microadenoma to determine if the microadenoma has been totally removed. Would you comment on the usefulness of that in your experience?*

KOVACS: Well, I am probably too conservative in this, but we think that from the fresh frozen section, very often, it is very difficult if not impossible to make the proper diagnosis. So we think that if the tissue is fixed properly and embedded properly, we have a much better chance to make the correct diagnosis than when frozen sections are made. I think many mistakes have been made when fresh frozen section has been diagnosed in the operating room.

QUESTION FROM THE AUDIENCE: *Does it bother anyone that until we had tomograms and prolactins and some of the recent tests, very few people died of pituitary tumors? Now, I happen to come from a small town in eastern Tennessee and in the last year or so have been personally responsible for the pituitary operations of eight or ten people. For 15 or 20 years before that, almost nobody had pituitary operations and nobody died of pituitary disease that I knew of. We are now finding these little things, and at every meeting all of the people on the front bench say take them out. And yet at autopsy we find that 15% to 20% of cadavers have microadenomas. It does bother me a bit that in past years not many people seemed to die of pituitary tumors. I would appreciate any comments that you gentlemen might have.*

KOHLER: What you are saying really is that we don't know the natural history very well, but we do know that death from a pituitary tumor is quite rare. We were interested in the same question. Thinking that maybe men had larger numbers of small prolactinomas that were being missed, we went to screen men at a geriatric facility. We were obviously taking a select population over 65 and we found an extraordinarily low incidence, in fact, there were only four men who had borderline prolactin elevation. I think that it really depends on the clinical situation. Whether the therapy would be surgical or not depends on what the goal is in the particular patient. I think that we are willing to tolerate some small prolactinomas that we are fairly confident are there and that presumably are what you would see at autopsy. If, in fact, the clinical situation is such, it does not seem to be causing any harm. I do think that the prolactin levels that Dr. Kovacs mentioned can be used to some degree to see whether an adenoma is expanding when radiologic studies are equivocal, which they frequently are.

KOVACS: It is very true that we do not know the natural history of pituitary adenomas sufficiently well. If one studies autopsy material, as Dr. Kohler has done, there is, depending on how many sections are taken, an incidence of about 10% to 20% of pituitary adenomas in autopsy material. But 50% of them contain prolactin by the amino staining; there is no sex difference. Males and females are probably the same. Males may have adenomas a little more frequently, but theirs are small. We think that maybe there are two types of pituitary adenomas, one that is growing and one that is just there and just doesn't grow anymore or has a very low potential to proliferate. It is very difficult to distinguish these two types. As a matter of fact, it is just not possible by morphology, to distinguish clearly these two types at all. But obviously, there is one pituitary adenoma that is there, does not cause any clean-cut symptoms, and is found by the pathologist at autopsy. But there is another type, which grows quite rapidly. In the last two or three years, we have seen two cases of patients with prolactin-producing adenomas who died. These cases are very interesting. If I may, I'd like to review them briefly. In the first case I got the tissue from Australia. This was a young patient who had a tumor at the base of the brain. It was rapidly growing. The neurosurgeon operated. The pathologist couldn't really tell what the tumor was because sometimes it is very difficult to tell. Then the patient died. Then I got the tissue for amino staining. It was fully loaded with prolactin, so obviously this was an invasive prolactin adenoma. In the second case the patient was diagnosed as having a nasal pharyngeal carcinoma, which invaded the brain. The patient died and we got the paraffin block, which turned out to contain a large amount of prolactin. Again, this was invasive prolactin adenoma. So I think that invasive adenomas are sometimes missed and unless we do amino staining, they will be not recognized, they are rare, but they occur.

KOHLER: May I add just one other point? I think there is a critical time at which you can watch a patient, but others at which you cannot, and there seems to be a relationship between them. Obviously, the smallest tumors are the ones most easily operated on. When a woman has been concerned about infertility, for instance, and has a small adenoma that is easily seen on x-ray and so forth, it has been a logical decision to go to surgery, because her goal is not survival, as it is with these large tumors, but fertility. I know this varies a great deal from place to place, but you can watch people who have prolactin in the elevated range; as they approach 100 or so, I think you are jeopardizing the chance of the surgeon to have a good success rate, particularly if this is associated with any x-ray changes. So although these very invasive tumors are rare, there are some that can be watched. Some patients really don't care about fertility and it doesn't matter. We would anticipate that their course would probably be benign. One final point that I should mention is the theory raised by Sherman and others, namely, that oral contraceptives have actually caused more prolactinomas and that is why we are seeing them now, where we did not see them a few years ago. I think others could comment on that. I personally doubt any cause and effect of oral contraceptives with prolactinomas, even though estrogens will raise prolactin levels.

LAWS: *I guess one of the questions is whether a bad invasive tumor starts as a small microadenoma and after a time evolves into a nasty tumor, or it is bad from the beginning. Do you have any insights into that?*

KOVACS: No.

LAWS: That would obviously be pertinent to when you treat.

SHELINE: I have seen a few, of course. I recall one that had a depressed sellar floor and it was thought to be a nonfunctioning small chromophobe adenoma. It was in a boy about 15. This patient, for reasons I am not sure of, was followed for the next five years and you can look at his films year after year and watch that tumor go right down; it finally presented as a tumor in the nasal pharynx. As far as we know, it is nonfunctional. I suppose it was a prolactin-secreting one, but we have seen this sort of thing enough to worry about it.

DAUGHADAY: I think another comment ought to be made, and that is, as mentioned before, people do die of pituitary apoplexy. That is one of the complications of untreated tumors. People have acromegaly, despite some writings to the contrary, and, I believe have a high risk of cardiovascular renal disease. And there are complications related to that. There are also people who have tumors associated with Cushing's disease, where the tumors become malignant and invasive and kill the patients. And the fourth thing is that all of us who are a little bit older and who have been around before the surgeons became so aggressive and we turned over so many patients so early to the surgeons, did see patients who would die of brain stem pressure from a tumor that had not been treated early enough and had got out of hand. So I don't by any means think that pituitary tumors are innocuous.

KOHLER: Yes, I think that is an oversimplification to justify therapy, yes or no, on the basis of life or death, because acromegaly cuts at least 20 years out of your life expectancy. With Cushing's disease, few patients live five years beyond their initial clinical manifestation. I would look at that as justification for therapy. I think that you can argue about the quality of life, desire for pregnancy and so forth, and whether that is an issue more than complications. I would hate to think we would judge a pituitary therapy fairly based upon mortality alone.

KOHLER: *May I ask a question? This comes up all the time. Does prior irradiation of the pituitary gland influence the surgical outcome? We are often faced with the issue of trying to decide on primary radiation therapy. The neurosurgeons tell us that we better be careful because if that patient gets into trouble, I am going to have a much harder time taking the tumor out.*

LAWS: No, I don't think it does. I have operated on a number that have had previous x-ray therapy and I have not found it to be very difficult at all, not in the immediate phase. I think if you operate several years later, you can run into difficulty with wound healing or cysts. But not immediately.

KOHLER: I think it can, Ed. I don't think it should be used as a reason not to radiate as initial therapy, but I actually think that many cases may not be tumors. The incidence of hyperplasia and tumors is the problem.

KOVACS: It is difficult to assess the presence of hyperplasia on surgical material, especially when we receive small fragments. In addition, the area very close to the adenoma is compressed and very difficult to evaluate. Despite these reservations, I think that in Cushing's disease there is not infrequently hyperplasia also outside the adenoma. I have seen cases where there was no tumor, there was hyperplasia. Prolactin has proved more difficult. I am quite sure that there are some cases in which there is hyperplasia outside the tumor. There is usually no regression. As a matter of fact, it is quite evident that there is no regression of prolactin cells outside the tumor. In some cases, there might be hyperplasia. As far as GH cell adenomas are concerned, we have never seen hyperplasia outside the adenoma.

GIVENS: Have you seen suppression of the normal cells in the surrounding normal gland?

KOVACS: You mean in GH? I don't think that I can answer this.

QUESTION FROM THE AUDIENCE: *Dr. Kovacs, have you seen at postmortem sections, when you can look at the whole pituitary, any evidence of multicentric adenomas?*

KOVACS: We have seen some, but obviously you have to do serial sections, because sometimes you see two independent adenomas. If you do serial sections, there is only one adenoma. So this really needs a very, very careful study. I don't think that our study in this regard was so careful that I could answer your question really conclusively, but we have seen a few patients in whom there were definitely two adenomas present. In some of these patients, the adenoma was the same histologically and immunocytologically. But I have seen also patients in whom there was a GH cell adenoma and a fallopian cell adenoma with a prolactin cell adenoma, and they were nonfunctioning. So there are variations. But this has to be done, really, on a much larger scale, because if you don't do serial sections, in most patients you cannot exclude the possibility that this is just not one adenoma.

QUESTION FROM THE AUDIENCE: *Dr. Laws, how do you treat prolactin cell microadenomas that cause impotence in males?*

LAWS: Well, the question, as I gather, is what are the indications for surgery on prolactin-secreting microadenomas in the male?

A MEMBER OF THE AUDIENCE: *I'd like to know your views.*

LAWS: Of course, one would assume that you have discovered the lesion, because the patient has a specific complaint, and if he has a specific complaint that is mass related, like headache or visual loss, microadenoma should not produce visual loss, and I think we would probably recommend surgical therapy. If his complaint is impotence or infertility or azoospermia, and the endocrinologic workup seems to indicate prolactin as the cause of that, we would probably give him a trial of bromocriptine and see what happens and then discuss the pros and cons of maintaining bromocriptine therapy before trying for a surgical excision. If the prolactin level as measured in the serum was over 200, we would tend, I think, much more toward operating early, because I think that tumor would have the potential for growth. So there is no good evidence for that. I assume my colleague in endocrinology would agree.

BESSER: *Are there any data on postoperative recurrences of prolactinomas? Do you have a good initial response and so forth, in terms of hyperprolactinemia? Is surgery a proved cure for prolactinomas?*

LAWS: I think it depends on what the initial prolactin is. I think if the preoperative prolactin is under 200, surgery can provide a cure.

BESSER: I think it is a question of recurrence, though. How many patients have you had who initially looked as if they were cured and then developed a recurrent hyperprolactinemia?

TINDALL: There are probably about six or seven with recurrences that I can identify out of about 120 and most of those had prolactin levels over 200 to start with. I think you have to be careful, though, because if you have a development of prolactin postoperatively, it does not necessarily mean that you have persistent or recurrent tumors. You could have the stalks syndrome or the stalk section syndrome.

LAWS: I think our results have been even a little less than that, with a follow-up that ranges about every two years. I think we probably had three recurrences out of 200 and some odd cases.

BESSER: You would be very disappointed if I did not ask you.

ROBERTSON: I would like to comment on that recurrence thing. I have just reviewed the entire literature that I can find on it and if a recurrence is defined as someone who had an operation and then had a perfectly normal prolactin level, and who then seemed perfectly normal and then, in x number of months or years later, had a recurrence of the syndrome, that is a recurrence to me. What George is saying is that one of the mechanisms can be the stalk syndrome. But as far as I am concerned, if the prolactin level does not return to normal fairly soon, you have to be concerned that you left the tumor there. So I call that a surgical failure, regardless of what the cause is. Now, true recurrences are hard to come by and in my series, which approaches 75, I can only find one true recurrence using that definition, and you said three. Mine occurred three years later.

LAWS: We had these one, two and three years afterwards, but we will talk more about that tomorrow.

QUESTION FROM THE AUDIENCE: *My question is to Dr. Acker and Dr. Sheline regarding the radiologic follow-up in terms of how much radiation is given to the patients, the periodicity of repeating tests, especially CT scans, sella tomograms, and just getting a lateral telemetry with cone down view of the sella. What do you recommend and how often would you do it for patients who had postoperative or primary radiotherapy? What would you recommend for someone without hormone elevation, and who, on CT scan and other tests, shows no empty cells, or someone whom you felt had an enlarged sella with a tumor that was hormonal inactive and not progressive, whose tumors have been operated on and irradiated and just been followed? How frequently do you follow them?*

ACKER: The nice thing about the CT scan and especially the coronal technique is that you are directing the beam away from the critical organ of the lens. Certainly you would not like to repeat axial scans on these patients. The way we do it currently is to do the coronal scan with a thin columella at 1.5, and you can usually cover that area very nicely in five or six slices. So you have directed your beams away from the lens, so the falloff is tremendous. You are not putting very much radiation into that category. Certainly, if you are going to follow them with polytomography, you probably are going to require putting the lens over the eyes. Certainly, the radiation is quite high, so I am not so concerned with the coronal technique or use of thin columella as far as any significant radiation to any of the critical organs is concerned.

QUESTION FROM THE AUDIENCE: *How does a coronal scan with CT compare with an annual chest x-ray and would you do it annually without worrying about it?*

ACKER: Oh, I think we could do it annually without worrying about it.

QUESTION FROM THE AUDIENCE: *Could I ask what the cost might be?*

ACKER: The single contrast scan in various places from Alabama to Memphis ranges from $250 to $400 or so for a single scan.

QUESTION FROM THE AUDIENCE: *Do you do this every year on patients who have received primary radiation?*

ACKER: First of all, I am not sure how good the CT is going to be as far as following these people. It has been very difficult with the ones that I have seen to obtain serial scans. These may help because you would be able to detect a change. I don't even recommend it as far as following these patients postoperatively. I don't think there is any good evidence that I know of at the current time that is going to be that helpful. We will just have to wait and see. Some of the people in California or somewhere else may have more experience.

SHELINE: This is an issue that I have been struggling with and I don't really have a good answer, a firm answer. My tendency at present is to get one six months or so after the therapy is over with. Of course, these are the ones that are radiated, or I would not have seen them. Looking at this pretty much as a baseline scan for future comparison, I am not at all surprised if I see some residual tumor setting there, under the circumstances that you described, if it is doing no harm and will sit there and not grow and radiation has prevented cell replication in the future. I am not very concerned about that. Sometimes, in fact, I think you would be better not to know it, because it gets people itchy to do something. But then, beyond that period of time, and we have got two or three of these, that one I showed you, the special short arcs and what-not Dr. Wilson operated on that one, it had failed, I think it had two previous surgeries, or three, had been radiated once prior to that, that patient—Dr. Wilson removed part of it. We radiated it and he has been out now about three or four years and he does have something sitting there, but as long as it does not change, I don't think we should do anything about it. Now, what we are worried about, something that we are concerned about, is whether he is getting an annual CT scan. I don't know if it is worthwhile on every patient or not.

KOHLER: *How about the patients that are treated with bromocriptine? How often?*

SHELINE: That is not for me.

BESSER: We x-ray them at six months, 12 months, and then yearly, but that is because we like to see the fossa getting smaller.

ACKER: You are talking about x-ray rather than CT.

SHELINE: With sellar tomograms, or just by x-ray?

BESSER: Oh no, we get a right lateral skull film, always the same side. It doesn't matter if it is right or left, as long as it is the same side and frontal view. We will only do tomograms if we think there may have been a change that we can't make out. We use the CT scan after the initial investigation period if it is clinically evident.

QUESTION FROM THE AUDIENCE: *What is the dosage of radiation with a properly done hypocycloidal polytome? AP and lateral? How much dosage do you need to damage the lens and when does the damage appear?*

ACKER: That is a very good question and I don't know the answer. We looked at this in Alabama. I even had a couple of twins. A neuro-ophthalmologist and I studied the problem and I do not know the answer to that question. How much radiation does it take on different fractionated examinations? How much does it take to cause cataract formation?

SHELINE: There isn't a good solid answer, but I can get you into the ballpark. A few hundred rad, depending on the size of the dose and how fast it is given. If you gave 600 or so in a single crack to the lens, you would probably get a cataract, although that exact number is debated a good deal. If you fractionated it into 200-rad fractions, it would take a bit more to do it. The more you gave and the bigger the fractions, the earlier it would appear. But again, if you are talking 600 to 800 rad fractionated over a period of a week or so, you might look for the cataract 6, 12, 18 months down the line. With smaller doses, the latent interval becomes longer and I would think that with the doses we are talking about, the latent interval would be so long that the patient is not going to survive to see it.

QUESTION FROM THE AUDIENCE: *What was the dose to the lens? I did not hear the answer.*

ACKER: In Alabama, we took the detector chips and put them over the eyes, and with axial scans we got doses anywhere from 5 rad up to 7 rad. I have not done it with the coronal scan since the beam is directed so far away from the lens of the eye.

SAME QUESTIONER: That is on CT. Now with the polytome, it is much higher than that.

ACKER: With the polytome, it is much, much higher. You are getting up over ten rad. The statistics that have come out on CT scans show a high variability in the amount of radiation that is given.

ROBERTSON: I want to get this straight. If you operate on a chromophobe nonsecreting tumor and you really feel that you have removed all of the tumor, should the patient receive postoperative x-rays? I have no quarrel if you know that you have left the tumor, but I wasn't trying to be cavalier. Five years ago, I thought I had removed the tumor very carefully in five people and this year they all came back with their tumors. Now I wish I had given them all x-rays. In the chromophobe you don't have any kind of biologic marker to know whether or not it is a recurrence or whether you did or didn't get it all out, like GH secretion, etc. So I am wondering whether they should all receive postoperative x-rays.

SHELINE: I think if there is doubt in the surgeon's mind that he removed it all, that it is probably appropriate. The larger tumors are the ones with the higher recurrence rate, if observed long enough.

LAWS: Philip Atkinson, who is a neurosurgeon in New Zealand, did a very nice study of half a dozen autopsies of patients who had large chromophobe adenomas that were big enough to fill the sella turcica but were not invasive. Between the two layers that make up the dura mater of the cavernous sinus in each of those cases there were viable tumor cells. So it is my feeling, and I think that my colleagues in endocrinology agree, that if the patient has a tumor that is large enough to fill the sella turcica and to stretch the dura mater and that tumor is probably not surgically curable, we would tend to recommend radiotherapy.

SHELINE: I want to add a little bit to that question of surgery following radiotherapy. I think part of the answer is how the therapy is given again. If we use those lateral, opposed fields and then go into the surgery, goes into those fields, 5 years or so later, you may have some wound complications. I would not anticipate that if you use a different technique. You might have a little fibrosis or something down around the region of the sella turcica itself, but I certainly would not expect wound problems.

ROGOL: Do you feel that pituitary tumors are basically regular tumors from the pituitary gland, or do they represent some abnormal tonic influence from the hypothalamus causing these things in the first place?

REICHLIN: Alan, that is a very good question and some of the questions directed to Dr. Kovacs were designed to try to bring that out. That is, what is the character of the noneffective pituitary tissue? Is there hyperplasia? If there were and the disease lay in the adenoma intrinsically, you would expect, in prolactinomas, corticotropin-producing tumors, and acromegalics, that the surrounding tissue would be suppressed. That is the point that you addressed. I was very interested in his answers. Now, we have just completed a detailed analysis of 37 prolactinoma patients with very extensive physiologic testing before and after surgery. In that group, there were 24 patients who we were absolutely certain were cured according to our criteria, namely, that their prolactin levels came down to normal and they resumed menses. Several patients got pregnant. When those patients were studied baseline prolactin levels were all in the normal range. They had normal reserve responses to TRH as judged by delta increase in prolactin level. They had slightly impaired hypoglycemia responses, but were in the normal range. Now, depending on how you interpret the mild impairment that persists, is this what you would expect in a patient who has had an adenoma removed and has surgical manipulation in the region of the pituitary gland or is this a reduction of residual dysfunction? My own interpretation is that you can find a lot of patients in whom, after removal of the adenoma, there is absolutely normal pituitary regulation and it comes right back to normal range and very quickly. From my point of view, then, that group must be primary intrinsic autonomous adenoma similar to the solitary adenoma of the thyroid gland. On the other hand, in the same series, there were about 12 patients who were not cured, and we were left with the question that cannot be resolved. Were they not cured because the surgeon failed to remove all the tumor, or is the residual abnormality due to hypothalamic dysfunction? But even if we did remove all the tumor, it still wouldn't prove that it is in the hypothalamus, because it could be a primary abnormality of the pituitary gland in responding to normal hypothalamic influences. So to summarize the answer, I think that most prolactinomas start out as intrinsic disease of the pituitary gland, and there is a certain number, I don't know how many, that may not be, and that is the group where detailed histologic studies may give us the answer.

BESSER: Could I ask Dr. Reichlin if he doesn't think there is an alternative explanation possible which would put the microprolactinoma genesis in the hypothalamus? The explanation may lie in our latex studies of the whole capillary system. Do you think that it is at least possible that there is delivery of hypophysiotrophic substances, very specifically from point A in the immediate eminence to point B in the pituitary? After all, the prolactin cells are the natural wings. Now if you had a microvascular block, so that dopamine was not delivered to one wing of the pituitary, you could get the hyperplasia that is characteristic of the initial stages of these microadenomas. After all, they don't have a fibrous capsule, they have depressed normal pituitary gland. You could then produce precisely the situation that you described when the area of tissue involved in that microvascular block and dopamine deficiency were removed, the rest of the pituitary would be normal. There is, after all, a low function of beta, which suggests that the rest of the pituitary gland is exposed to excessive dopamine, like Scanlon's results using dopa and receptor blockers and the excessive response of TSH.

REICHLIN: I can't answer that, but I would like to make a couple other arguments for the intrinsic pituitary origin of these tumors. One is the finding that many of these tumors are mixed. Dr. Kovacs described this data and there are other studies that indicate that what appears to be a prolactinoma may also secrete GH, TSH, and even ACTH. I can't think of any singular hypothalamic deficit that would cause an abnormality in multiple pituitary secretions. Again, that speaks to me of instability of the pituitary. That is one argument. The second argument is that there are two circumstances in which one sees chronic neurogenic, that is brain-induced hypoprolactinemia. One is chronic administration of tranquilizer drugs. There has been at least one survey of prolactin regulation in chronically psychotic hospitalized patients who have been on chlorpromazine or similar drugs for decades, and in every one of those patients, as soon as the phenothiazine is stopped, prolactin levels start down, and then, after a week or two, they come into the normal range. This suggests to me that simple abolition of dopamine input is not sufficient to bring about tumor. I would say that issue is not resolved. It is a challenge to all of us here. I don't think the instances of prolactinoma in hospitalized or chronically treated schizophrenics are any higher than those in the general population. I wonder if anyone has any other information on this, because that is really the essential neurogenic hypoprolactinemia.

BESSER: Not really, because in chronic neuroleptic therapy, the blood levels that are drawn get into the levels where they act as partial agonists, but on chronic neuroleptic therapy, the prolactin levels are nowhere near as high as the normal person acutely given it.

REICHLIN: But they do run high though. You do agree that even a person who has been on phenothiazine for ten years will still run two or three times the normal level of prolactin? They may not go up to 80, 90, or 100, but they do run in the 20s anyway.

GIVENS: Would you alter your thinking if you took a prolactinoma out of one wing and went to the other side and biopsied it and found hyperplasia?

REICHLIN: Well, that would be a terrific experiment. That is the kind of experiment one needs to do—to really get the material from both sides and let Dr. Kovacs examine it.

KOVACS: I think this is an open question. There is really no good evidence about whether the hypothalamus plays a role in the development of prolactinomas or not. I just would like to mention one animal experiment. Namely, there is a great strain the longer one sweats, which is a very interesting great strain. They develop prolactinomas, quite frequently when these animals become old. This aging is really a gold mine for endocrine studies, because many of these rats have medullary carcinoma of the thyroid, islet cell, and also of the pancreas, pheochromocytoma, and very interestingly they have prolactinomas quite frequently. Now, we have studied these rats, but obviously from the rats it is very difficult to extrapolate to the human pituitary gland. In these rats, the hyperplasia with the prolactin precede the development of the tumor. So you see, you can fool all of these rats into becoming older with high prolactin level and more prolactin access, and when they become old they develop prolactin cell adenomas. But this is a rat module and I just don't think that it is justified to make any comment in the human being. But I think this is a very important question for man.

GIVENS: I think that it is important to follow the reports of recovery of the hormone situation postoperatively. We had a patient of Dr. Laws' here, whom Dr. Roberts operated on. She had Cushing's disease. A 2-mm tumor was taken out. Postoperatively the cortisol level was 1 or 2 μg/100 ml. We elected not to treat her and it took her nine months to recover. Now she is fully recovered and has a normal pituitary test. We think that the prolactinoma took so long for her to recover is again the increased pituitary driving force talked about a little earlier.

KOHLER: I think that generally has been the experience with successfully treated patients with Cushing's disease.

QUESTION FROM THE AUDIENCE: *Dr. Kovacs, why is it that prolactin-secreting adenomas are so much more frequent?*

KOVACS: I don't know. Probably prolactins are more susceptible to carcinogenic stimuli, or they cannot metabolize oncogenic agent in a different way, or they have different receptors or hyperthalamic factors. There are a lot of explanations. But that proves that prolactinomas are much more frequent than, for example, tumors arising from TSH.

QUESTION FROM THE AUDIENCE: *What is the normal distribution? What is the distribution of prolactin cells in the healthy person?*

KOVACS: In the human being, prolactin cells were previously assumed to represent 5% of the adenohypophyseal cell population. Studies were performed using nonspecific staining techniques. We have recently completed a study, and found that there is quite a significant range in the number of prolactin cells in autopsy pituitaries. But again, you can argue that autopsy pituitaries cannot be regarded as normal.

KOHLER: You have to look at the patients who come to autopsy after an auto accident or similar occurrence, or after a stroke.

KOVACS: Yes, we are very fortunate, because we collected about 20 of these pituitary glands from people who died after suicide, auto accidents, shootings, or something and in these patients there is still quite a significant variation between 15 and 35 persons there is a number of prolactin cells, but again they are obviously the age factor, the sex factor, then the time of menstruation and all these things which make it more difficult to assess this patient. But there is one interesting thing: there is a definite prolactin cell hyperplasia in pregnancy and in lactation. We can confirm this in the human pituitary gland. It is also true that if you do cell counts of a pregnant patient you can see significant increase in the number of prolactin cells in the pituitary gland. Very interestingly, the D cells regress, but they do not regress entirely, whereas there are no prolactin cells in multiparas and they are 70 years of age, than those who are nulliparous. So physically, just looking at the prolactin cell number, you can more or less tell which patient had many pregnancies and which did not. So this is a very complicated question and the autopsy material is just not suited for it. We have to study many more cases than we have. There is a wide range of variation in the normal number of prolactin cells. This makes it very difficult to discuss the hyperplasia because hyperplasia is really the increase in the number of cells and we don't know exactly what is the normal number. It is very difficult to talk about prolactin cell hyperplasia.

QUESTION FROM THE AUDIENCE: *Do you go through by lumbar puncture or intrasternally?*

ACKER: Since I follow it with the CT scan, and I am using a hanging head technique and my biggest problem seems to be the patient's motion, I would rather stick them in the back than in the neck and then have them complain. So yes, I am using a little more stick. Now I am not using Metrizamide very often at all with that last technique. I do not use that very frequently.

QUESTION FROM THE AUDIENCE: *Are you able to rule out empty sella to identify an empty sella syndrome without the use of it, just with your coronal*

ACKER: Yes, you can be fairly adequate and accurate in doing that, especially if you can follow the pituitary stalk down into the sella turcica. Then you can be sure that the low density that you are looking at is not a cystic tumor.

# The Role of the Pituitary Foundation

## LOIS DAVIDSON, M.B.A.

*President, Pituitary Foundation of America, Inc.*

THE PITUITARY FOUNDATION OF AMERICA, INC. (PFA) is a nonprofit organization that services patients with pituitary and endocrine disorders. It was founded in August of 1979 by James T. Robertson, M.D., and myself. Chapters are being formed in Memphis, Atlanta, Augusta, Philadelphia, and San Francisco; there are plans to establish others in Los Angeles, Houston, and Phoenix.

Because of my personal involvement with pituitary disease, I began a campaign with local doctors to convince them that pituitary patients and their families need more than surgical expertise and qualified endocrine management. Objectives for the organization were planned. Basically the objectives include nationwide chapter development, development of research programs, establishment of fellowships, programs of medical education designed to increase appreciation to bring about more expedient diagnosis and thus increase the chances of complete recovery with the least possible physical and emotional damage, and promotion of a program of general education designed to increase public appreciation and understanding of the extent of the social and human costs imposed by endocrine disorders and what can be done to assist in the alleviation, control, and prevention of these diseases and their effects.

The objectives of the Foundation can easily be attained by citizens and competent physicians working together in a voluntary movement.

Chapter development, perhaps first in order of priority, requires the support of physicians, more than does any other objective. Without patient participation, it would be virtually impossible to make PFA

0-8151-3530-0/82/006-163-165-$03.75

a success. I am convinced it would be in the best interest of all patients to be referred to the Foundation as well as in the best interest of all of you that practice medicine. By having others take on the task of educating your patients and families, it will tend to ease frustrations of your patients and thus take quite a load off the physician.

The purpose and duties of individual committees will evolve as the chapter becomes more involved in the foundation's objectives. The following types of committees are suggested:

1. A visitation committee to visit patients and/or their families in the hospital or in their homes to share experiences and lend the necessary emphathetic support to patients who are undergoing the anxiety, depression, fear, and confusion accompanying these disorders. In order to accomplish this, the local chapter of PFA must set up a visitor registry, a list of volunteers willing to donate their time and provide emotional support to patients undergoing prediagnostic, preoperative, and postoperative care for endocrine disorders.

2. A training committee to train volunteers to become visitors so they may competently visit patients and their families in their local hospitals and communities.

3. A planning committee to develop, implement, and schedule new chapter activities and directions.

4. A community outreach committee to develop ways in which volunteers can contact community organizations who would be interested in learning about and supporting PFA. This may involve volunteers' delivering informal talks to organizations desiring information about the Foundation, such as nursing societies, parent groups, local medical societies, and social groups.

5. A program committee to enlist services of knowledgeable people for continuing patient education.

At the outset, divulging personal histories and donating time to lend emotional support to those in need will be the primary function of the local chapters. Unquestionably, as the group develops other directions will evolve.

Special services within the community structure should be identified and made available to all patients. There are many community services that could be of benefit to your patients that are provided by your state and county human services department. I cannot state emphatically enough the needs of your patients. We all know that they need the best medical care available, but as I have previously stated they need much more.

Most patients, by the time they reach the neurosurgeon or endocrinologist, have already been made to feel like hypochondriacs, have developed acute visual problems, have had their sexuality challenged, and in the many cases have been denied the right to have children because of poor diagnosis on the part of the original attending physician. Most of the symptoms are so easily recognized that I stand in amazement that patients are so often misdiagnosed and therefore mismanaged.

I am convinced that more compassion and understanding should be demonstrated with the preoperative and postoperative pituitary patient than any other patient you will encounter. Be aware, be sensitive, and most importantly, be a good and understanding listener.

A local chapter can be a tremendous asset to the busy physician. Trained visitors will take a lot of pressure off the doctor and promote better understanding for the patient and the family.

Ideally, when a patient is diagnosed and scheduled for surgery but must wait a week or two for space on the surgery schedule, the visitation committee should be notified so the patient does not experience the anxiety that will take place without proper knowledge of the disease and procedures to treat it.

Within the realm of the Foundation I have traveled to medical centers across the country. I have been able to observe various treatments and gather statistical information on the treatments currently being used in the United States. Some of the methods you may be familiar with and some you may not. I would not presume to recommend any specific treatment, but if you are in question, I think statistical information should be available to patients.

The patient registry, a project of our medical committee, is becoming a reality. A registry of patients with documented pituitary disease will be an invaluable asset for researchers as well as physicians. Most neurosurgeons and endocrinologists cannot readily identify all the cases they have treated. By participating in the registry, a physician could not only have an instant overview of his/her own patients but could also have statistical information on all patients in the registry or an overview of a select group or age. Besides the medical information input, we are also doing a sociology study on all patients. This is done basically to find out how the patient views recovery and determine social costs of the disease. Forms are available for your review. With the forms you will also find an extensive release form, but it is stressed that the registry is designed so that the patient's personal confidentiality is rigorously maintained.

Again, I solicit the help of physicians actively involved in treatment of pituitary patients. Without accurate reporting procedures, the registry would not have creditability as a scientific instrument.

# Cushing's Disease: Medical Therapy

## DOROTHY T. KRIEGER, M.D.

*Director, Division of Endocrinology Mount Sinai
Medical Center, New York, New York*

## Definition and Pathophysiology

HYPERCORTISOLISM is seen with a variety of pituitary, adrenal, and
ACTH-producing tumors. The term Cushing's disease is reserved for
those patients with adrenal hyperfunction or hyperplasia with or
without demonstrable pituitary adenomata, small or large, while hypercortisolism secondary to other etiologies is termed Cushing's syndrome. In patients with adrenal or ectopic ACTH-producing tumors,
the pathogenesis of the hormonal abnormalities is clear. There are
questions as to whether Cushing's disease is a primary pituitary or
hypothalamic disorder, or whether there are subgroups in which the
primary site of pathology is localized to one or the other tissue. Hypothalamic dysfunction could be secondary either to excessive production of the still-elusive "corticotropin-releasing factor,"* or to a decrease in concentrations of a substance inhibitory to corticotropin
release. (Whether this is a specific corticotropin inhibitory factor or
another CNS peptide, such as somatostatin, which has been reported
to decrease ACTH release in some conditions characterized by ACTH
hypersecretion, but not in normal people, is purely speculative.) Either situation could result in prolonged stimulation of pituitary corticotrophs and lead either to hyperplasia with subsequent adenoma-

---

*The sequence of a corticotropin-releasing factor was reported in September 1981
(Vale W., Speiss J., Rivier C., Rivier J.: Characterization of a 41-residue ovine hypothalamic peptide that stimulates secretion of corticotropin and β-endorphin. *Science*
213:1394, 1981.)

0-8151-3530-0/82/006-167-198-$03.75

© 1982, Year Book Medical Publishers, Inc.

tous transformation (as is seen in the case of experimentally induced tumors) or to stimulation and adenomatous transformation of a uniquely sensitive subset of corticotrophic cells. If one postulates a pituitary etiology, this would be via in situ adenomatous transformation, as occurs in many endocrine glands, a transformation the basis for which is unknown.

Table 1 summarizes the pathologic findings encountered at autopsy or surgery in patients with Cushing's disease. Although autopsy studies of normal people with no apparent evidence of endocrine disease may reveal a maximum 10% incidence of basophilic adenomas (some of which have been found immunocytochemically to stain for ACTH), the incidence of such adenomas is much greater in patients with Cushing's disease. The reported incidence of 70% to 80% remission following microadenomectomy in this condition would also favor a pituitary etiology.

There is evidence, however, that may support a hypothalamic etiology in certain instances of Cushing's disease. There have been reports of degranulation and swelling in the paraventricular and supraoptic nuclei of some patients with Cushing's disease,[1] as well as of ventricular dilatation. These findings, however, are of questionable significance, since they might be secondary to the existing hypercorticism. A case report[2] of a patient presenting with episodic emotional disturbance, fever, obesity, hypertension, and elevated plasma ACTH levels was felt to be suggestive of a CNS etiology, although neurologic examination revealed a normal EEG and evidence on pneumoencephalography of only slight ventricular dilatation. More recently, we have reported evidence of altered circadian periodicity of plasma GH and prolactin concentrations as well as of ACTH concentrations and absence of Stage 3 and 4 slow-wave sleep in patients with Cushing's disease.[3] Since these reflect CNS dysfunction, the persistence of such

TABLE 1.—PITUITARY HISTOLOGY (LIGHT MICROSCOPY)

| Cushing's Disease 171 patients | Surgical or Autopsy |
|---|---|
| 52% to 81% | Incidence of pituitary tumors; 80% to 85% of these are basophilic adenomata |
| 8% to 26% | Incidence of basophilic hyperplasia |
| ? | Incidence of combined adenoma, hyperplasia |
| Normal persons 1260 patients | Autopsy |
| 8% to 20% | Incidence of pituitary tumors; 20% to 50% of these are basophilic adenomata |

abnormalities in these patients when in laboratory and clinical remission was felt to support a CNS etiology.[4] This might be effected by means of increased activity of a neurotransmitter involved in stimulation of corticotropin-releasing factor (CRF), although obviously other possibilities involving factors potentiating CRF action or factors directly inhibiting pituitary ACTH are possible.

A variety of neurotransmitters have been implicated in the regulation of CRF release. There is general consensus that cholinergic and serotoninergic inputs are stimulatory, and contradictory evidence with regard to adrenergic effects.[5-7] In view of the considerable body of evidence from in vivo and in vitro animal and human studies of serotoninergic stimulation of ACTH release, cyproheptadine, a putative serotonin antagonist, has been used in the treatment of Cushing's disease (see below), with remission occurring in approximately 50% of such patients. Although the high incidence of basophilic adenomata in patients with Cushing's disease was alluded to previously, it should be noted that there have been several reports of the occurrence of basophilic hyperplasia alone or in association with basophilic adenoma in such patients, an occurrence that suggests exogeneous stimulation. There has also been one case report demonstrating transition from hyperplasia to a mucoid adenoma.[8-10] Lastly (see below), reports of recurrences following clinical and laboratory remissions produced by microadenomectomy have raised the question as to whether these cases represent the continued effect of excessive hypothalamic stimulation.

## Clinical Presentation

Most of the clinical manifestations can be directly ascribed to either physiologic or pharmacologic effects of glucocorticoids (Table 2), together with additive effects of the adrenal androgens that are hypersecreted in some cases. Table 3 indicates the percentage incidence of clinical manifestations in Cushing's disease. Table 4 indicates some of the clinical features that help to establish a differential diagnosis between Cushing's disease (bilateral hyperplasia) and other etiologies of hypercortisolism.

There is a higher incidence of this disease in females of reproductive age. The characteristic presenting signs and symptoms in adult patients with Cushing's disease are weight gain, facial puffiness and plethora, easy bruisability, weakness, fatigue, insomnia, depression or irritability, back pain, amenorrhea or oligomenorrhea, and occasionally hirsutism in females, and decreased body hair and libido in

TABLE 2.—EFFECTS OF GLUCOCORTICOIDS*

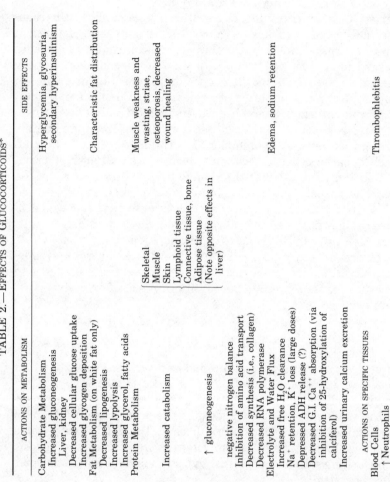

| ACTIONS ON METABOLISM | SIDE EFFECTS |
|---|---|
| Carbohydrate Metabolism<br>Increased gluconeogenesis<br>Liver, kidney<br>Decreased cellular glucose uptake<br>Increased glycogen deposition | Hyperglycemia, glycosuria, secondary hyperinsulinism |
| Fat Metabolism (on white fat only)<br>Decreased lipogenesis<br>Increased lipolysis<br>Increased glycerol, fatty acids | Characteristic fat distribution |
| Protein Metabolism<br><br>Increased catabolism   ⎰ Skeletal<br>  Muscle<br>  Skin<br>  Lymphoid tissue<br>  Connective tissue, bone<br>  Adipose tissue<br>  (Note opposite effects in liver)<br><br>↑ gluconeogenesis<br>negative nitrogen balance<br>Inhibition of amino acid transport<br>Decreased synthesis (i.e., collagen)<br>Decreased RNA polymerase | Muscle weakness and wasting, striae, osteoporosis, decreased wound healing |
| Electrolyte and Water Flux<br>Increased free $H_2O$ clearance<br>$Na^+$ retention, $K^+$ loss (large doses)<br>Depressed ADH release (?)<br>Decreased G.I. $Ca^+$ absorption (via inhibition of 25-hydroxylation of calciferol)<br>Increased urinary calcium excretion | Edema, sodium retention |
| Blood Cells<br>← Neutrophils<br>← Platelets<br>← → Erythrocytes<br>← → Lymphocytes<br>← → Eosinophils<br>→ Basophils | Thrombophlebitis |

| | SIDE EFFECTS |
|---|---|
| ACTIONS ON SPECIFIC TISSUES | |
| Peripheral Vascular | |
| Potentiate pressor effects of catecholamines | Hypertension |
| Increased hepatic production of angiotensinogen | |
| Central Nervous System | |
| Possible effects on enzymes involved in neurotransmitter synthesis (i.e., serotonin) | Sleeplessness, mood changes, psychosis |
| Alteration in thresholds of electrical excitability and of sensory perception | |
| Stomach | |
| Increase in stimulated gastric secretion | Peptic ulcer (?) |
| High doses inhibit cell growth | |
| Lung | |
| Induction of surfactant production in fetal lung | |
| ACTIONS ON BODY PROCESSES | |
| Immune System | |
| High doses suppress certain antibody responses | Increase susceptibility to infection (?) |
| Lymphocyte cytolysis or growth inhibition | |
| Suppresses cell-mediated immune response | |
| Thymus regression | |
| Inflammatory Response | |
| Inhibit phagocytic mechanisms | |
| Inhibit kinin release | |
| ACTIONS ON OTHER HORMONES | |
| ↔ Prolactin | Galactorrhea |
| ↓ Growth hormone release | Growth retardation |
| ↑ TSH release | |
| ↓ Gonadotropin release | |
| ↓ ACTH release | |

*From Krieger D.T.: *Cushing's Syndrome.* New York: Springer-Verlag New York, 1982. Used by permission.

TABLE 3.—PERCENTAGE INCIDENCE OF SIGNS
AND SYMPTOMS IN 450 PATIENTS WITH
CUSHING'S SYNDROME*

| SIGN OR SYMPTOM | INCIDENCE (%)† |
|---|---|
| Moon facies | 88 (0)‡ |
| Obesity | 86 (0)‡ |
| Buffalo hump | 54 |
| Weakness | 67 |
| Fatigue | 74 |
| Hypertension | 85 |
| Plethora | 77 |
| Violaceous striae | 60 |
| Easy bruisability | 59 |
| Ecchymoses | 52 |
| Mild polycythemia | 20 |
| Poor wound healing and leg ulcers | 35 |
| Ankle edema | 57 |
| Puffiness of eyes | 26 |
| Osteoporosis | 58 |
| Back pain and bone pain | 54 |
| Pathologic fractures | 38 |
| Kyphosis | 25 |
| Renal calculi | 20 |
| Urinary frequency and nocturia | 32 |
| Polydipsia | 28 |
| Mental changes | 46 |
| Headache | 40 |
| Neurologic symptoms | 34 |
| Menstrual disorders | 77 (0)‡ |
| Hirsutism (in females) | 73 (0)‡ |
| Acne | 54 |
| Exophthalmos | 14 |

*From Krieger D.T.: *Cushing's Syndrome.* New
York: Springer-Verlag New York, 1982. Used by permission.
†Data of Dr. L.J. Soffer.
‡(0)—Present at onset of disease.

male patients. The weight gain is usually truncal, with sparing of the
extremities, and is usually moderate; massive obesity is usually not
seen in patients with Cushing's disease.

Special mention should be made of the mental changes that have
been described in patients with Cushing's syndrome. Depression is
the most common symptom, although the other classic psychoses may
be simulated, as well as anxiety or a chronic confusional state. Similar mental changes have been noted in patients on exogenous steroid
therapy. Patients with depression may also manifest evidence of increased cortisol secretion, which may sometimes pose diagnostic difficulties. Since psychiatric manifestations are present in patients

TABLE 4.—CLINICAL FEATURES OF DIFFERENTIAL DIAGNOSIS

| | ADRENAL ADENOMA | ADRENAL CARCINOMA | BILATERAL HYPERPLASIA | ECTOPIC TUMOR | PRIMARY PITUITARY TUMOR* |
|---|---|---|---|---|---|
| Clinical course | Slow | Rapid | Slow | Rapid | Slow |
| Clinical manifestations | Mild to moderate | Florid, severe | Mild to moderate | Atypical (i.e., myopathy) | Mild to severe |
| Virilization ♀ or feminization ♂ | Rare | Frequent | Rare | 0 | Rare |
| Palpable suprarenal mass | 0 | + | 0 | 0 | 0 |
| Visual, CNS Sx | 0 | 0 | 0 | 0 | + |
| Sex of patient | 80% 20% ♀ > ♂ | | 80% 20%† ♀ > ♂ | ♂ > ♀ | |
| Age of patient (majority of cases) | All ages | Comprise 60% of cases in children | 20–40 yr | 40–60 yr. | 20–70 yr |
| Pigmentation | 0 | 0 | Rare | Present | Present |

*Primary pituitary tumor refers to patients with Cushing's disease in whom *gross* sellar enlargement is seen at the time of initial presentation.
†Ninety percent of men with Cushing's disease, however, have hyperplasia.

with Cushing's syndrome as well as those with Cushing's disease, it is felt that such symptoms are secondary to the hypercortisolism present (and not to ACTH). Cortisone may exert direct effects on thresholds of neural excitability and sensory perception by acting on cerebral enzymes or altering brain serotonin concentrations. It has also been suggested that hypercorticism merely accentuates a previous personality disturbance. There have been reports of both persistence[12] and alleviation[13] of psychiatric symptomatology following normalization of plasma cortisol concentrations.

In some patients with Cushing's disease, the clinical manifestations may be cyclic and may appear to be manifestations of periodic hormonogenesis. In some instances such periodic hormonogenesis may be present with no fluctuation or remission of the clinical syndrome and may be detected only in consecutive laboratory tests, while in others cyclic manifestations of disease may also be evident. Such periods of hormonal and/or clinical activity may persist two weeks to two months; there may be symptom-free intervals of several weeks to a year, although the usual course is one of increasingly shorter periods of remission. This should be contrasted with the cases of patients reported to have spontaneous remission of hypercorticism.

As noted above, many of the characteristic features (Fig 1) noted on physical examination may be related to the effects of glucocorticoids. The buffalo hump and increase in the fat pads of the cheek may be secondary to cortisone stimulation of accumulation of "brown fat" (the decreased lipogenetic effect of cortisol noted in Table 2 refers only to its effects on white fat), whereas the insulin hypersecretion present in these patients may well account for the generalized lipogenesis. The apparent sparing of the limbs is secondary to muscle atrophy. Such atrophy, together with the associated hypokalemia, accounts for much of the muscular weakness noted in these patients. The characteristic plethora, ecchymoses, and striae are manifestations of thinning of skin and of capillaries secondary to decreased collagen synthesis. Such thinning of skin and the stretching caused by fat accumulation are responsible for the striae. Plethora may in part also be due to the presence of polycythemia, which may occur especially in patients with increased androgen secretion. The poor wound healing and leg ulcers observed in these patients may also be ascribed to thinning of skin with superimposed infection, due to decreased resistance. Decreased circulation due to atherosclerotic vascular changes (see below) may also account for the ankle edema and puffiness of the eyes sometimes seen, although enhanced mineralocorticoid activity has also been postulated to be etiologic. (It should be

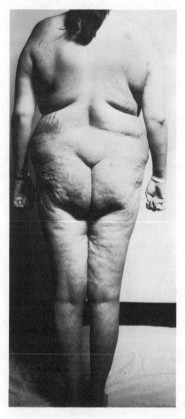

**Fig 1.**—Patient with Cushing's disease showing the characteristic truncal obesity.

noted, however, that detectable elevations of mineralocorticoids are only occasionally reported in patients with Cushing's disease.)

In female patients, varying degrees of hirsutism are present, usually confined to moderate body and facial hirsutism, although occasionally some degree of alopecia is observed. Clitoromegaly may also be present. Male patients may exhibit some decrease in body hair. These manifestations in the female are attributable to increased adrenal androgen secretion, while in the male they may be secondary to decreased testosterone levels, which may be due to inhibitory effects of corticosteroids on gonadotropin secretion.

Hypertension is usually moderate, with increases in both systolic and diastolic pressure, the extent of which do not appear to be related to the severity or duration of disease. It should be noted that approximately half of these patients with hypertension have evidence of cardiac enlargement and ECG evidence of myocardial involvement. It is postulated that the hypertension is secondary to hyperresponsiveness to pressor agents and to increased formation of angiotensin secondary to corticoid induction of increased plasma renin substrate, rather than to excessive mineralocorticoid production. Evidence of bone pain on physical examination may be evidence of osteoporosis; rarely, kyphosis is present. This is seen more frequently in cases of long duration.

Less common manifestations of Cushing's disease are hyperpigmentation and galactorrhea. Hyperpigmentation is more common in the ectopic ACTH syndrome and in patients with Cushing's disease who present with gross evidence of sellar enlargement, in whom it is more likely that plasma ACTH levels will be elevated. Thus far, no increase in circulating concentrations of melanocyte stimulating hormone has been documented in patients with Cushing's disease; β-lipotropin, concentrations of which are also elevated in these patients, has only minor pigmentary effects. At present, therefore, the increased levels of ACTH in these patients provide the most likely explanation for the hyperpigmentation due to some inherent melanotropic activity of ACTH itself, although there is no correlation between extent of pigmentation and concentrations of ACTH present. The galactorrhea may be secondary to the moderate increase in serum prolactin concentrations present in patients with Cushing's disease. This may occur in the absence of a grossly visible pituitary tumor on polytomography of the sella turcica. It is of interest that galactorrhea has been described as an initial manifestation of Cushing's disease, with other signs and symptoms appearing as long as several years afterwards.[11]

Cushing's disease in children is an infrequent cause of hypercortisolism, as noted in Table 4. However, in children over seven years of age, hyperplasia may equal or exceed adrenal tumor in frequency. Clinical manifestations are similar to those reported for the adult, save that obesity is present in all patients and may be more massive,[14] and shortness of stature is present in 84% of such children. Although the latter is postulated to be secondary to glucocorticoid suppression of GH secretion, it should be noted that children appear to be less susceptible to such suppression than are adults. Another form of Cushing's disease that has been reported in younger subjects is micronodular hyperplasia. This occurs mostly in females between the ages of two and 21.[15] Usually, only mild manifestations of hypercortisolism are present, and such hypercortisolism may only be detected in the course of workup of the marked osteopenia that is present in these patients. There may be presenting symptoms of fracture or back pain. Unlike the adrenal glands of patients with Cushing's disease, which are either normal or enlarged, the adrenal glands of those with micronodular hyperplasia are normal or decreased in weight and are characterized by the presence of many small nodules throughout the gland that contain black or brownish pigment (melanin or lipofuscin), with atrophy of internodular adrenal tissue. In many instances, plasma ACTH concentrations are low or undetectable, in contrast to what is found in Cushing's disease (see below). It has been hypothesized that this entity is primarily adrenal in origin.

## Laboratory Diagnosis of Cushing's Disease

The purpose of laboratory testing is, first, to distinguish those patients who may have suggestive signs and symptoms of hypercortisolism, but who are actually eucorticoid, from those with increased corticosteroid production. The most common categories in which the first type of distinction has to be made involve patients with obesity or depression. Once hypercortisolism is documented it becomes necessary to distinguish patients with Cushing's disease from those with other etiologies of corticoid excess.

Interpretation of laboratory tests requires some familiarity with the physiology of the hypothalamic-pituitary-adrenal system, as well as some knowledge of the circulating forms of corticosteroid hormones, their metabolism, and their excretory products. A large number of tests are available to make the requisite distinctions; in many instances no single test offers the specificity and precision necessary to make an unequivocal diagnosis, so that assessing the results of a combination of tests may be necessary. Prior to discussing a scheme for laboratory testing, it is first necessary to consider the available tests that are in current use and that in some instances have replaced older tests of pituitary-adrenal function. In most instances, such tests consist of measurement of blood and urinary cortisol and of plasma ACTH and their response to suppression and stimulation.

### PLASMA CORTISOL

Cortisol in plasma exists in bound and free forms. The major binding proteins are corticosteroid-binding globulin (CBG), which accounts for binding of approximately 75% of plasma cortisol, and albumin, which has a much lower affinity binding constant and accounts for 15% of binding. Thus 10% of circulating cortisol is free under conditions of normal secretion. CBG is saturated by plasma cortisol concentrations greater than 25 μg/dl, so that when cortisol production is increased, a greater proportion will be free.[16] Most available methods for measuring plasma cortisol concentrations measure the total amount that is both bound and free. In the presence of elevated CBG concentrations (i.e., estrogen administration), plasma cortisol concentrations appear to be elevated in eucorticoid patients, whereas in patients with CBG insufficiency (liver disease, nephrosis, or hereditary defects in CBG synthesis), plasma cortisol levels will be low in eucorticoid patients. A discrepancy between total plasma cortisol and urinary free cortisol may therefore give a clue as to a possible abnormality in CBG concentrations in these instances. Liver disease and hypothyroidism may also cause apparent increases in plasma cortisol concentrations in eucorticoid patients secondary to decreased cortisol clearance, whereas the converse may be seen in hyperthyroidism. Usually, the presence of normal feedback mechanisms will minimize such changes.

The major methodology for measuring plasma cortisol at present is either that of competitive protein-binding assay (based on the ability of endogenous plasma cortisol to compete with radiolabeled cortisol for binding sites on corticosteroid-binding globulin) or radioimmunoassay employing a specific cortisol antibody. In healthy persons there are no significant changes in plasma concentrations in the 15 to 90 age range, nor are there significant sex differences in plasma concentrations of single specimens.

From inspection of Table 5, it is apparent that there is a circadian variation in plasma cortisol concentrations in normal people, whereas in patients with Cushing's disease and syndrome such variations are absent. Hypercorticism is a strong possibility in the presence of A.M. plasma cortisol concentrations exceeding 23 μg/dl and 15 μg/dl between noon and midnight. Normal 8:00 A.M. levels may be seen in approximately one third to one fifth of patients with Cushing's disease or syndrome, whereas less than 17% of such patients have levels in the normal range at 8:00 P.M., and should sampling be performed at 11:00 P.M. an insignificant number of patients with hypercorticism will have normal levels. The overlap of such concentrations in normal people and patients with disease may be explained by the episodic secretion of plasma cortisol. This occurs (in normal people) in rapid, irregular bursts over the 24-hour period, superimposed on the curve describing the circadian rhythmicity of plasma cortisol concentrations, leading to the occurrence of rapid and wide fluctuations in plasma cortisol concentrations within relatively short periods. Such

TABLE 5.—NORMAL BASAL PLASMA AND
URINARY CORTICOSTEROID
CONCENTRATIONS*

| ITEM | CONCENTRATION |
| --- | --- |
| Plasma Cortisol† | |
| 0800 | 10.0 ± 4.0 µg/dL |
| 2000 | 4.5 ± 2.5 µg/dL |
| Urine cortisol | 20–100 µg/24 hr |
| Urine 17-OHCS | 3–10 mg/24 hr (♂) |
| | 2–8 mg/24 hr (♀) |
| Cortisol production rate | 6–30 mg/day‡ |

*From Krieger D.T.: *Cushing's Syndrome.*
Heidelberg: Springer-Verlag, 1982. Used by permission.
†Competitive protein binding assay; see reference 17 for review.
‡See reference 25 for review.

episodic secretion is also present in patients with hypercortisolism who, however, do not exhibit circadian secretion. If sampling is performed only at two time points in the 24-hour cycle, by chance one may obtain separate specimens either at the peak of or at the beginning of a secretory episode, the former falsely conveying the impression of elevated P.M. cortisol concentrations in normal people, while the latter may falsely convey the impression of a lower plasma cortisol concentration than actually exists in patients with hypercorticism.

## URINARY CORTICOSTEROID CONCENTRATIONS

Three methods of measurement are currently used: (1) 17-OH corticosteroids (Porter-Silber chromogens, 17-OHCS; (2) 17-ketogenic steroids; and (3) urinary free cortisol, which is the current preferred method. The Porter-Silber method measures the tetrahydrometabolites of cortisol and cortisone, which account for approximately 50% of the cortisol produced. Positive reactions may be given by naturally occurring ketones, as well as by drugs such as spironolactone, tranquilizers (such as Atarax and Librium) and antidepressants (such as Monase). 17-Ketogenic steroid determinations measure a larger fraction of urinary metabolites, since in addition to the tetrahydrometabolites, cortols and cortolones, which are reduced forms of the tetrahydro derivatives, are also determined. However, other steroids, such as pregnanetriol, and several drugs (such as penicillin, meprobamate, and radiopaque dyes), as well as glucose, may falsely elevate levels obtained with this method. Free cortisol is most commonly measured with a competitive protein-binding assay. From what has previously been noted with regard to binding of plasma cortisol to CBG, it is apparent that in states in which excessive amounts of cortisol are produced (since CBG does not increase concomitantly), a larger fraction of plasma cortisol would be free and available for glomerular filtration. Therefore, a change in total plasma cortisol level is greatly amplified by determination of urinary free cortisol. For example, a threefold increase in urinary 17-OHCS excretion is reflected in an eightfold to tenfold increase in urinary free cortisol excretion.[16]

## Plasma ACTH

This is measured most commonly by radioimmunoassay. Determination by bioassay is important only in those instances in which there appears to be a dissociation between endogenous immunoreactive ACTH concentrations and measurable cortisol concentrations. Unfortunately, because of methodological difficulties, immunoassay determinations are not available at all medical centers, although they are currently being offered by some commercial laboratories. Table 6 depicts the range of plasma ACTH concentrations. The wide range noted in normal people is in part secondary to the episodic fluctuations of plasma ACTH concentrations. This, in view of the shorter half-life of ACTH, makes such concentrations subject to even more rapid fluctuations than those of plasma cortisol. Hence, a single ACTH determination, unless markedly below the lower limits of the normal range or above the upper limits of the normal range, is of little help in establishing a diagnosis of the presence and etiology of hypercorticism. An afternoon concentration greater than 100 pg/ml is highly suggestive of Cushing's disease, whereas morning levels may be within the normal range, indicative again of the abnormal circadian periodicity present in patients with Cushing's disease. Plasma ACTH concentrations greater than 300 pg/ml are infrequently seen in patients with Cushing's disease. Morning concentrations less than 20 to 30 pg/ml, together with evidence of hypercorticism, would suggest adrenal tumor.

With the demonstration of the existence of a common precursor molecule for ACTH, β-lipotropin, γ-lipotropin, and endorphin, it would be expected that there would be concomitant secretion of these peptides, as well as of ACTH, in conditions characterized by ACTH hypersecretion. This has been borne out,[18, 19] but such tests are not necessary for the diagnosis of hypercortisolism.

TABLE 6.—PLASMA ACTH AND CORTISOL CONCENTRATIONS IN CUSHING'S DISEASE OR SYNDROME*

| CLINICAL CONDITION | 8:00 A.M.–9:00 A.M. | | 5:00 P.M.–6:00 P.M. | |
| | PLASMA CORTISOL (CBG METHOD) | PLASMA ACTH (IMMUNOASSAY) | PLASMA CORTISOL | PLASMA ACTH |
|---|---|---|---|---|
| Normal | 8–20 µg/100 ml | 20–140 pg/ml† | 4.4–11 µg/100 ml | 10–88 pg/ml† |
| Nontumorous adrenocortical hyperfunction | Normal or ↑ | Usually moderately ↑ | | |
| Adrenal adenoma | Normal or ↑ | → | ↑ | → |
| Adrenal carcinoma | ↑ | → | ← | → |
| 1° pituitary tumor | Normal or ↑ | ↑ | ← | ← |
| "Ectopic" ACTH | ↑ | ← | ← | ← |

*From Krieger D.T.: Plasma ACTH and corticosteroids, in DeGroot et al. (eds): *Textbook of Endocrinology.* New York: Grune & Stratton, 1979, pp 1139–1156. Used by permission.
†Mean.

### Tests Involving Pituitary-Adrenal Suppression and Stimulation

ACTH STIMULATION TESTS.—At present, the most common test employed is one in which 0.25 mg synthetic ACTH[1-24] is administered intravenously. A normal response consists of doubling of plasma corticosteroid concentrations within the hour following such administration. The majority of patients with Cushing's disease manifest hyperresponsiveness to ACTH administration, whereas patients with adenomas will have a normal or an absent response; response is usually absent in patients with adrenal carcinoma, and in those with ectopic ACTH secretion.

VASOPRESSIN TEST.—Vasopressin is employed as a prototype of corticotropin-releasing factor, since there is no available preparation of the latter for clinical testing. In normal people, parenteral administration of either lysine vasopressin or aqueous Pitressin is followed by an increase in plasma cortisol and ACTH concentrations.[20] In patients with Cushing's disease, a normal or an enhanced response is seen, since pituitary stores of ACTH are increased. In other etiologies of hypercorticism, suppression of pituitary ACTH stores leads to an absent or diminished response, although responses have been reported in some patients with ectopic ACTH-producing tumors.

METYRAPONE TEST.—This test is based on the rationale that inhibition of cortisol synthesis (which occurs via 11-β-hydroxylase blockade by metyrapone) leads to a rise in plasma ACTH concentrations. In view of the difficulty in obtaining plasma ACTH determinations, plasma 11-deoxycortisol (compound S) concentrations are frequently measured. (These would be elevated in response to increased ACTH secretion because of the metyrapone-induced enzymatic blockade.) Two forms of testing are available. The first is that originally proposed by Liddle et al.,[21] in which 750 mg metyrapone are administered every four hours for six doses. Usually, urinary 17-OHCS levels (which will reflect the increased 11-deoxycortisol present) are measured. A normal response is a twofold increase in urinary 17-OHCS concentrations or greater than a 5 mg/24-hr increment over baseline levels. Another method of testing is a single-dose test[22] in which 30 mg/kg of body weight of oral metyrapone are administered at midnight; levels of either plasma 11-deoxycortisol or plasma ACTH are determined at 8:00 A.M. the following morning. To be certain that adequate suppression of 11-hydroxylation has been obtained, determination of both plasma cortisol and 11-deoxycortisol or ACTH levels is performed. An 8:00 A.M. plasma cortisol level less than 7.5 μg/dl is considered to indicate adequate suppression. A normal response is an increase in plasma deoxycortisol concentrations from their usual value of less than 1 μg/dl to 16.4 ± 0.6 μg/dl, or a fourfold to eightfold increase in plasma ACTH concentrations. Patients with Cushing's disease manifest normal or increased responsiveness to metyrapone with either type of testing, whereas patients with adrenal tumor usually show an absent responsiveness. False negative tests are seen in patients receiving drugs enhancing metyrapone metabolism, such as dilantin. In patients receiving drugs that influence metabolic pathways of tetrahydrodeoxycortisol (such as patients on estrogen therapy), subnormal urinary responses may be present, whereas plasma deoxycortisol responses may be normal. Other conditions that interfere with steroid metabolism or excretion, such as hypothyroidism, liver disease, malnutrition, and renal disease, will also falsely influence results based on urine 17-OHCS, but not those based on plasma deoxycortisol determination. Lastly, the administration of progestational agents, which may also bind to glucocorticoid receptors, will suppress pituitary ACTH release, and false negative responses to metyrapone may be seen.

DEXAMETHASONE SUPPRESSION TEST.—Two types of tests are available: the standard dexamethasone test introduced by Liddle[23] and the overnight test first suggested by Nugent et al.[24] The presence of a suppressed response to the overnight test negates the need for the more prolonged dexamethasone test. In the overnight test, 1 mg dexamethasone is administered orally at 11 P.M. or midnight and plasma cortisol concentrations are determined on a sample obtained at 8:00 A.M. the following day. The accepted criterion of normal suppression is a plasma cortisol level below 6 μg/100 ml. Patients with Cushing's disease do not suppress to this level. However, studies have shown that 28% of obese control subjects fail to exhibit normal suppression, as do 20% of hospitalized or chronically ill patients.[25] Drugs such as phenobarbital and dilantin, which increase dexamethasone metabolism, thereby lowering effective plasma concentrations, will result in false negative suppression tests (i.e., failure of suppression in a eucorticoid patient). Estrogen administration will also result in false negative tests as the result of decreased cortisol disposal rates and increased binding to CBG. Stressed patients may also fail to show suppression, since in stress there is an increase in steroid requirements to produce suppressibility.

Where ambiguous results are obtained in the overnight suppression tests, greater discrimination may be obtained with the use of the 2 mg low-dose dexamethasone suppression test, in which 0.5 mg dexamethasone is administered orally every 6 hours for 2 consecutive days. Urinary 17-OHCS concentrations less than 4 mg/24 hours or urine free cortisol of less than 20 μg/24 hours on 24-hour samples collected on the second day of such dexamethasone administration represent a normal response. A review of the literature reveals that patients with hypercorticism do not suppress with this dose in approximately 90% of such instances. Occasional normal responses in patients with proven Cushing's disease can be explained by the existence in these patients of a decreased metabolic clearance rate of dexamethasone, leading to higher dexamethasone concentrations than would normally be seen. Plasma cortisol concentrations at 8:00 A.M. following two days of dexamethasone administration should be less than 5 μg/dl.

The high-dose dexamethasone suppression test is used to distinguish various etiologies of hypercorticism. In this test, 2 mg is administered orally every six hours for eight doses. A normal response is suppression of urinary 17-OHCS to less than 50% of the initial value on the second day of such dexamethasone administration and of urinary free cortisol to less than 20% of the initial value. Patients with Cushing's disease exhibit suppression in the high-dose test, whereas those with adrenal tumors or ectopic ACTH syndromes usually do not (see below). Plasma cortisol levels are reported to be undetectable following high-dose administration in patients with Cushing's disease, but there has been no reported series on such patients using either plasma cortisol or plasma ACTH concentrations as criteria. In patients with bilateral nodular adrenocortical hyperplasia, it may be necessary to use 16 to 32 mg dexamethasone daily for two days to achieve normal suppression.

Patients receiving drugs such as dilantin, which may induce enzymes that enhance metabolism of dexamethasone, may fail to suppress on the 8-mg dose. In some patients with Cushing's disease, a paradoxical increase is seen in both plasma ACTH concentrations and those of urinary 17-OHCS following dexamethasone administration.[26] The concept of periodic hormonogenesis has been used to explain this, with the "paradoxical" response coinciding with the phase of increased secretion. There have been reports in which suppression has been obtained in the case of adrenal tumors, but repeat testing to see if such suppressibility was reproducible was not performed in either of the two reported patients. Ectopic tumors may suppress with high-dose administration in approximately 25% of such cases, such suppression being most common in instances of bronchial carcinoids, thymomas, and hepatomas.

OTHER HORMONAL CONCENTRATIONS AND RESPONSES

Such tests are not commonly employed in routine clinical testing, but may be of interest with regard to understanding of pathophysiology. The administration of TRH to patients with Nelson's syndrome and Cushing's disease is associated with an increase in plasma concentrations of ACTH and of lipotropin, in contrast to the absence of such a response in normal people,[27] while TSH responses are blunted and prolactin responses are normal. Inhibition of spontaneous ACTH secretion following somatostatin administration has been reported in a patient with active Cushing's disease and in two patients with Nelson's syndrome,[28] although it has not been confirmed by our unpublished observations or those of others.[29] There is a tendency for basal prolactin concentrations to be elevated in patients with Cushing's disease (unpublished observations,[30]) and $T_4$ concentrations are mildly suppressed (secondary to a reduction in thyroxin binding globulin).[31] Serum $T_3$ and free $T_3$ levels are both reduced, while the free $T_4$ level is normal. Decreased plasma testosterone concentrations have also been reported in male patients with Cushing's disease and syndrome, even in the presence of normal plasma gonadotropin concentrations. Other nonspecific diagnostic considerations are indicated in Table 7.

USEFULNESS OF TESTING IN DIFFERENTIAL DIAGNOSIS
(TABLES 8 AND 9)

In choosing tests, the factors of utility (i.e., their discriminant function for either distinguishing hypercortisolism vs eucorticism and for distinguishing among the various courses of hypercortisolism) and practicality should be considered. The availability of assays, ease of testing, and risk or discomfort of a given test procedure are all factors to be considered. Much of the testing described in this chapter can be performed on an outpatient basis. For the initial discrimination between patients with hypercortisolism from those who may have suggestive clinical manifestations but who are actually eucorticoid, there are two readily available procedures. These are the determination of early morning plasma cortisol concentrations following the administration of 1 mg dexamethasone at midnight, and on a separate occasion, determination of 24-hour urinary free cortisol excretion. Hypercortisolism can be ruled out if the plasma cortisol level at 8:00 A.M. following the overnight dexamethasone test is

TABLE 7.—Nonspecific Diagnostic Determinations

Electrolyte and acid-base balance
   Serum sodium—usually normal; may be increased
   Serum potassium—usually normal; may be decreased
      Hypokalemia most prominent in Cushing's syndrome due to nonendocrine tumor
   Serum chlorides—Usually normal; may be decreased
   Venous $CO_2$ content—usually elevated (with high blood pH)
Blood volume—usually normal
Carbohydrate metabolism
   Diabetic glucose tolerance curve usually present
Lipid metabolism
   Serum cholesterol—normal or elevated
   Serum triglycerides—normal or elevated
   Serum phospholipids—normal or elevated
Calcium and phosphorous metabolism
   Urinary calcium—normal or increased
   Serum calcium—normal
   Serum phosphorus—normal
   Serum alkaline phosphatase—normal or increased
Blood cells
   Total leukocytes—usually increased up to 20,000
   Neutrophils—usually increased
   Lymphocytes—usually decreased to less than 15% of the total leukocyte count, due
     to involution of lymphoid tissue
   Eosinophils—usually decreased to less than 50/cu mm due to sequestration in
     lungs and spleen and increased destruction in the bloodstream
   Basophils, plasma cells—usually decreased, as with eosinophils; associated with a
     fall in circulating antibodies
   Erythrocytes—usually increased, but rarely above 6,000,000/cu mm. Hematocrit
     often above 50%
   Platelets—often increased
Other nonspecific manifestations
   Increased gastric acid and pepsin
   Increased urinary excretion of uropensin
   Occasional decrease in plasma albumin and γ-globulin
   An increase in angiotensinogen production may occur

equal to or less than 6 µg/dl and if the urinary cortisol level is equal to or less than 100 µg/24 hours. In the latter case, if hypercortisolism is strongly suspected, several repeat determinations should be performed, in view of the above-noted intermittency of cortisol production in some cases. In instances where the plasma cortisol level at 8:00 A.M. in the overnight suppression test is greater than 6 but equal to or less than 10 µg/dl, performance of the low-dose 2-mg dexamethasone test should provide discrimination between normal people and those with hypercortisolism. If there are facilities for determination of late afternoon and evening plasma cortisol levels, then screening with determination of plasma cortisol concentrations at 8:00 A.M. and 8:00 P.M. may indicate in a limited way whether or not normal circadian variation is present. Cortisol concentrations greater

TABLE 8.—Plasma Corticosteroid Responses to Diagnostic Maneuvers Designed to Demonstrate Nonautonomy* or Autonomy† of Adrenal Function

| CONDITION | BASAL (8:00 A.M.) | CIRCADIAN VARIATION | PLASMA 11-HYDROXYCORTICOSTEROIDS‡ | | | BASAL PLASMA ACTH |
|---|---|---|---|---|---|---|
| | | | RESPONSE TO DEXAMETHASONE (1 MG AT MIDNIGHT) | RESPONSE TO AQUEOUS PITRESSIN, 10 UNITS INTRAMUSCULARY | RESPONSE TO ACTH | |
| Normal | 10–20 µg/dl | A.M. > P.M. 10 P.M.: 2–10 µg/dl | >6 µg/dl | Increment ≧ 8 µg/dl above baseline | Doubling of baseline value | 20–100 pg/ml 8:00 A.M. |
| Adrenal hyperplasia | Normal or increased | Absent | >6 µg/dl | Normal or increased | Increased | Normal or increased |
| Adrenal adenoma | Normal or increased | Absent | >6 µg/dl | Absent§ | No or normal response | Decreased |
| Adrenal carcinoma | Increased | Absent | >6 µg/dl | Absent§ | No response | Decreased (rare exceptions) |
| Pituitary tumor | Increased | Absent | >6 µg/dl | Absent§ | No to slight response | Moderately or markedly increased |
| Ectopic ACTH | Increased | Absent | >6 µg/dl | Usually absent§ (occ. exceptions) | Usually no response | Moderately or markedly increased |

*Nonautonomy of adrenal function, as would be seen in adrenal hyperplasia.
†Autonomy of adrenal function, as would be seen in adrenal, pituitary, or "ectopic" tumors.
‡From Krieger D.T.: *Cushing's Syndrome.* Heidelberg: Springer-Verlag New York, 1982.
§Response of plasma ACTH must be determined if adrenal response to ACTH is absent.

TABLE 9.—URINARY CORTICOSTEROID RESPONSES TO DIAGNOSTIC MANEUVERS DESIGNED TO DEMONSTRATE NONAUTONOMY* OR AUTONOMY† OF ADRENAL FUNCTION

| CONDITION | URINARY 17-HYDROXYCORTICOSTEROIDS§ | | | ACTH STIMULATION | METYRAPONE | URINARY 17-KETOSTEROIDS BASAL |
|---|---|---|---|---|---|---|
| | BASAL | SUPPRESSION WITH 2 MG | DEXAMETHASONE 8 MG | | | |
| Normal | 3–10 mg/24 hr | <4 mg/24 hr | <50% to 60% initial value | Twofold to threefold increase over baseline | Twofold increase over baseline (or >5 mg increment/24 hr) | Female: 5–15 mg/24 hr Male: 8–20 mg/24 hr |
| Adrenal hyperplasia | Increased | Not suppressed | <50–60% initial value, occasional "paradoxical response" | Hyperresponsive | Hyperresponsive | Normal or increased |
| Nodular hyperplasia | Increased | Not suppressed | May not suppress | Normal response or none | Variable | Normal or increased |
| Adrenal adenoma | Increased | Not suppressed | Not suppressed | Normal response or none | Decreased response or none | Normal or decreased |
| Adrenal carcinoma | Markedly increased | Not suppressed | Not suppressed (rare exceptions) | No response (rare exceptions) | No response | Markedly increased |
| Pituitary tumor | Increased-markedly increased | Not suppressed | Not suppressed | No to slight response | No response | Increased |
| Ectopic ACTH | Markedly increased | Not suppressed | Usually not suppressed | Usually no response | No response | Increased |

*Nonautonomy of adrenal function, as would be seen in adrenal hyperplasia.
†Autonomy of adrenal function, as would be seen in adrenal, pituitary, or "ectopic" tumors.
‡From Krieger D.T.: *Cushing's Syndrome.* New York: Springer-Verlag New York, 1982.
§Same considerations apply for the most part to urinary cortisol. Normal basal levels, 20 to 100 μg/24 hours; <20 μg/24 hours; p 2 mg dex, <100 μg/24 hours; p 8 mg dex, <20% of basal level; quantification of response in pathologic situations may show greater variability than seen in urinary 17-OHCS response. Basal levels are not affected by liver disease or drugs affecting hepatic metabolism; they are affected only by severe renal disease.

than 15 μg/dl at 8:00 P.M. are highly suggestive of hypercortisolism. Frequently, such determinations are combined with a subsequent overnight dexamethasone suppression test, providing two criteria for differentiation.

These tests usually exclude the diagnosis of simple obesity in contradistinction to hypercortisolism, which is one of the clinical situations most confused with Cushing's disease. Such tests, however, may not exclude patients with depression who present with some stigmata suggestive of Cushing's disease. In these patients, abnormal dexamethasone suppressibility and a suggestion of normal circadian periodicity may be present if this is assessed by determination at only two time points in the circadian cycle. (When repeated frequent plasma cortisol determinations over 24 hours are obtained in patients with depression, a normal circadian periodicity is evident.)

To differentiate between various forms of hypercortisolism, the most direct approach is determination of plasma ACTH concentrations. Morning levels less than 30 pg/ml are not present in patients with Cushing's disease or with ectopic ACTH-producing tumors, whereas levels above this are not seen in patients with adrenal adenoma or carcinoma (save in very rare instances where there may possibly be ectopic production of ACTH by an adrenal carcinoma). Plasma ACTH levels greater than 300 pg/ml are rarely seen in patients with Cushing's disease (although there may be some exceptions in patients who present with gross sellar enlargement at the time of initial diagnosis), whereas levels above this are common in patients with ectopic tumor production. The high-dose (8-mg) dexamethasone suppression test is also a good means of discriminating between Cushing's disease and other etiologies. Exceptions have been noted above; in these instances, the plasma ACTH concentration will be of further aid.

Vasopressin or metyrapone testing are infrequently required; with either of these tests, the absence of normal responsiveness is suggestive of adrenal tumor or ectopic ACTH production. The simplicity of the vasopressin test (which, however, is contraindicated in patients with significant hypertension and with which occasional unpleasant side effects such as pallor, abdominal cramps, and/or defecation may be present) has much to recommend it over the standard metyrapone test—there are no comparative data with the overnight metyrapone test.

In such testing, a major source of confusion may arise in the differentiation of Cushing's disease from ectopic ACTH production, especially in patients whose plasma ACTH concentrations are in the intermediate range between 250 and 400 pg/ml and from whom evidence of suppression with 8 mg of dexamethasone may be obtained. Although in clinically obvious cases of carcinoma the clinical manifestations may give a clue as to the correct diagnosis, the difficulty arises in cases of relatively slow-growing tumors, such as bronchial carcinoids, thymomas, medullary thyroid carcinomas, and occasional pancreatic neoplasms, where the underlying neoplasm may not be readily visible on routine x-ray studies and where the clinical symptomatology may be more suggestive of hypercortisolism than of malignancy. Screening of patients with suspected Cushing's disease with determinations of urinary 5-hydroxyindoleacetic acid levels is helpful in diagnosing the presence of asymptomatic bronchial carcinoid, and, if followed by additional tomographic and/or bronchoscopic procedures, may help to visualize these small neoplasms.

## Other Diagnostic Procedures

### Venous Catheterization for Tumor Localization

In theory, in patients with pituitary-dependent Cushing's disease, there should be a significant gradient in ACTH concentrations in blood obtained from the jugular vein or inferior petrosal sinus and that simultaneously obtained from a peripheral vein, whereas in ectopic production there would be no such gradient but there would be a step-up in ACTH concentrations of samples obtained from the immediate vicinity of the tumor. There is, however, little information as to normal jugular-peripheral vein gradients, and there have been reports of such gradients in patients with documented ectopic ACTH secretion. If an ectopic tumor is also secreting CRF-like material, a condition that has been reported in some instances, a jugular-peripheral gradient may still be present. When such venous catheterization is done, it is important, in view of the phenomenon of pulsatile secretion, to perform simultaneous sampling from a peripheral vein to compare concentrations with those derived from internal vessels.

### X-ray Studies

Pituitary.—Conventional lateral sellar x-rays may reveal evidence of enlargement in as many as 20% of patients presenting with Cushing's disease. With the advent of hypocycloidal polytomography for the detection of microadenomas, it appears that 60% of patients may show some abnormalities.[32, 33] The significance of such findings may be somewhat questionable, however, for some abnormalities may be present in 20% to 30% of endocrinologically normal people.[34] X-ray studies may also reveal the presence of osteoporosis, which in these patients is most evident in the skull, extremities, and spine. The role of computerized tomography is still unclear.

ADRENAL TUMORS.—Such studies are not really germane to the diagnosis of Cushing's disease, but may occasionally come up for consideration where tests suggest the presence of an adrenal tumor, as in bilateral adrenal nodular hyperplasia. Briefly, there are four available methods: radioscanning, ultrasonography, computerized tomography, and angiography. Radioscanning[35] is limited by problems of radiochemical availability, which at present is restricted to very few centers. Laterality of localization is the hallmark of adrenal tumor with all methods of visualization, although in some patients with adrenal carcinoma radiocholesterol scanning fails to show visualization of either adrenal. In obesity, which is usually present in patients with hypercortisolism, the quality of the sonogram may be poor due to excessive fat, in which case computerized tomography may be more useful.

## Medical Therapy of Cushing's Disease

Without any form of treatment, approximately 50% of patients with Cushing's disease die within five years of diagnosis. The major causes of death are infection, complications from generalized arteriosclerosis, and suicide. As noted, there are rare patients with Cushing's disease in whom spontaneous remissions have been described, and there are reports of patients with prolonged, relatively nonincapacitating clinical courses in the absence of any therapeutic intervention. These latter instances are rare, and the appreciable mortality in untreated patients is attested to by the number of therapeutic procedures that have been devised. In the past, therapy has been directed at correction of the enhanced cortisol secretion by either surgical or medical adrenalectomy. Such therapy, while effective in correcting the hypercortisolism, produces endocrine deficiencies that in themselves constitute medical hazards. Ideal therapy would be one which corrects ACTH hypersecretion without the introduction of associated pituitary insufficiency. In view of the present concepts of either a pituitary or a hypothalamic etiology, current approaches are directed at one or the other of these loci.

Figure 2 indicates the hierarchy of CNS-pituitary adrenocortical regulation and the points at which medical therapeutic measures are postulated to act. Surgical therapy is considered here only for comparison, since it is the subject of a later chapter. Besides their differ-

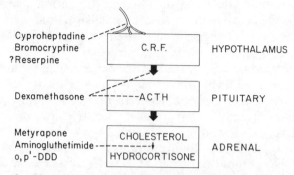

**Fig 2.**—Levels of hypothalamic-pituitary-adrenal axis at which medical therapy is postulated to act. Dotted line indicates points of blockade. Pituitary irradiation may possibly act via a hypothalamic as well as a pituitary locus. (From Krieger D.T.: *Cushing's Syndrome*. Heidelberg: Springer-Verlag. In press. Used by permission.)

ent mechanisms of action, the various approaches differ in the rapidity with which therapeutic control is achieved. Choice of a given therapy, in addition to its inherent efficacy, may be influenced by need for rapid control of the hypercortisolemic state (as in instances of progressive severe hypertension, severe and progressive osteoporosis, and psychiatric disturbances). In these instances, approaches that require a moderately long time before a maximum therapeutic effect is observed would be less desirable, although such approaches would be effective for treatment of patients with mild or moderate disease.

## MEDICAL ADRENALECTOMY

Four drugs that act by inhibition of steroidogenesis are available. Most experience has been obtained with the use of o,p'DDD (Mitotane, Lysodren), a drug that blocks steroidogenesis at a number of steps. Orth and Liddle[36] reported cure in all eight patients treated with three to six gm daily over a four-month to six-month period, with subsequent smaller maintenance doses. In a more recent report, Luton et al.[37] reported a 50% relapse rate on patients treated for an eight-month period with doses ranging from six to 12 gm daily. Subsequent additional courses of therapy, combined with pituitary irradiation, resulted in an overall remission rate of 60%. Most of Orth and Liddle's patients experienced sufficient loss of adrenocortical reserve to require maintenance corticosteroid therapy. This may be a necessary concomitant of effective therapy, since in Luton's series there was a greater tendency to relapse when adrenal insufficiency was not obtained. It should be noted that effective lowering of corticosteroid concentrations to the normal range may take as long as four to six months following initiation of o,p'DDD therapy.

The other three drugs available are more suitable for short-term use; two of these (aminoglutethimide and trilostane) are only available for investigative use in Cushing's disease. Aminoglutethimide acts by interfering with the conversion of cholesterol to pregnenolone, as well as by blocking various steroid hydroxylations. Adrenal insufficiency may appear within five days following onset of aminoglutethimide therapy. However, drug escape with resumption of enhanced steroidogenesis usually occurs in Cushing's disease as the result of compensatory increases of ACTH secretion, which is sufficient to overcome the initially effective enzymatic blockade. Side effects, such as goiter, somnolence, and skin rashes, have been reported with the usual therapeutic doses of 0.75–1.5 gm/day. Concomitant use of metyrapone has been advocated, with reduced toxicity as the result of employment of lower doses of each drug. Trilostane has been employed in one investigational study in which clinical and laboratory improvement (without significant side effects) were reported in all of seven treated patients,[38] although therapy was only continued for one month in five of these patients. The drug acts as an inhibitor of the 3-β-HSDH $\Delta^4$–5 isomerase enzyme system. Escape may also occur because of associated secondary rises in ACTH secretion.

Metyrapone is believed to act by its inhibition both of 11-β hydroxylation and of cholesterol cleavage to pregnenolone, although a direct action to suppress pituitary ACTH release was also suggested when it was noted that some patients receiving such treatment exhibited a decrease in plasma ACTH concentrations.[39] Corticosteroid concentrations usually fall to the normal range within a week following onset of therapy. Hirsutism may be noted in some patients. The drug may be contraindicated in patients with marked hypertension because of the concomitant increases in deoxycorticosterone concentrations secondary to 11β hydroxylase block.

It is felt that metyrapone and aminoglutethimide, singly or in combination, are best used, not as primary therapy for normalizing adrenocortical function, but either to prepare patients for surgery or while awaiting achievement of a therapeutic response to pituitary irradiation. Since adrenal insufficiency may be seen with the use of these agents, concomitant dexamethasone administration is usually indicated.

## PITUITARY IRRADIATION

This is usually accomplished by conventional cobalt radiotherapy (about 4,500 rad) and less frequently by proton-beam irradiation or by pituitary implantation of radioactive material. A survey of the literature over the past 20 years indicates that with conventional radiotherapy, 46% to 83% of the patients are improved within each reported series. Two thirds of such therapeutic responses are classified as cures; the remainder represents significant improvement with only modest residual elevation of corticosteroid concentrations and minimal disability. Laboratory and clinical improvement may not be fully apparent for a period as long as 18 months following completion of radiotherapy, so that, should more rapid control be required, interim treatment with metyrapone or aminoglutethimide might be indicated; o,p'DDD would be less preferable, since this might occasion permanent adrenal atrophy. To date, there is no evidence of production of any other endocrine deficits following such irradiation. Irradiation has been reported to be even more efficacious in children than in adults,[40] with resumption of normal growth and sexual development following such treatment-induced remission. A group of English investigators has used pituitary implantation of radioactive gold or yttrium.[41] This form of therapy requires a short period of hospitalization. It appears to be most effective in patients with no evidence of pituitary tumor on routine sellar x-ray, in whom an 81% improvement rate is reported, while only 50% of patients showed improvement if there were minor abnormalities of size or shape on routine sellar x-ray. The median interval between implantation and demonstration of complete remission is approximately four months. Two groups have used heavy-particle irradiation.[42, 43] As much as 15,000 rad may be delivered to the center of the pituitary with this technique by means of the Bragg peak effect. A cure rate of approximately 90% to 95% has been reported, with, however, an incidence of partial or panhypopituitarism of 7% to 10%. Although with other methods of pituitary irradiation there is a small percentage of patients in whom relapse may occur after apparent remission, there have been no such instances reported following heavy-particle irradiation.

## NEUROPHARMACOLOGIC TREATMENT

Cyproheptadine therapy was introduced for Cushing's disease in view of the above-cited experimental evidence implicating serotonin as an excitatory neurotransmitter in the regulation of ACTH secretion and the experimental evidence of CNS pathophysiology in Cushing's disease.[44] It is believed that cyproheptadine acts via antiserotoninergic mechanisms, although effects on other neurotransmitters are reported. Studies to date indicate that in adult patients this drug appears to be effective in approximately 50% of patients. In responsive cases, administration of 24 mg daily is associated with evidence of clinical and laboratory remission within a two-month to three-month period, such remission usually being maintained with continued drug medication. In addition to normalization of cortisol secretion, there is also return of normal dexamethasone suppressibility and of normal corticosteroid and ACTH circadian periodicity. In a small number of patients, relapse may occur (while on medication) after a successful treatment period of up to 15 months. The longest treatment period to date has been 18 months; relapses almost always occur after discontinuance of treatment. Initial side effects of hyperphagia and of somnolence usually disappear spontaneously with continuation of medication. Negative reports on the efficacy of cyproheptadine therapy have in most instances concerned treatment with less than the suggested dose and for a short duration. It is reported that the drug is less effective in children; there is, however, a report of complete clinical remission in a 14-year-old boy, a remission maintained after discontinuance of cyproheptadine therapy after 18 months of treatment.[45] This author has also observed a case of remission in a patient with Cushing's disease that has persisted for two years following discontinuance of cyproheptadine therapy; the patient subsequently became pregnant and delivered a normal infant. Remission for a similar length of time following discontinuance of therapy has also been reported in a patient with Nelson's syndrome.[46]

Metergoline, which may be a more specific antiserotoninergic agent than cyproheptadine, has also been tried; there are two reports of its efficacy in the treatment of childhood Cushing's disease.[47, 48] Another agent that has been employed is bromocriptine. Although dopamine does not affect release of corticotropin-releasing factor in vitro, studies showing an inhibitory role of catecholamines in the central regulation of corticotropin-releasing factor, however, implicate norepinephrine as the neurotransmitter involved. Acute administration of bromocriptine may suppress ACTH and cortisol levels in some patients with Cushing's disease and Nelson's syndrome. However, the most detailed study involving chronic treatment[49] indicates escape in two of five responsive patients after two to six weeks of therapy.

At present, there is still some question as to the role of neuropharmacologic therapy in the treatment of Cushing's disease, which may be better resolved with further followup and comparison of surgically and medically treated patients and when other neuropharmacologic agents are developed. If such neuropharmacologic treatment is effective, and if the rationale for its use is correct, such therapy should prevent the development of Nelson's syndrome. The problems of need for continued therapy and the occasional relapses noted in some patients while on therapy might indicate a use for cyproheptadine, if not for definitive therapy, as adjunct therapy, together with pituitary irradiation or in preparation for pituitary surgery, should long-term studies for this latter modality indicate a lack of significant recurrence of disease.

## REFERENCES

1. Heinbecker P.: Pathogenesis of Cushing's syndrome. *Medicine* 23:225, 1944.
2. Wolff S.M., Adler R.C., Buskirk E.R., et al.: A syndrome of periodic hypothalamic discharge. *Am. J. Med.* 36:956, 1964.
3. Krieger D.T.: The central nervous system and Cushing's disease. *Med. Clin. North Am.* 62:261, 1978.
4. Krieger D. T., Glick S.M.: Sleep EEG stages and plasma growth hormone concentration in states of endogenous and exogenous hypercortisolemia or ACTH elevation. *J. Clin. Endocrinol. Metab.* 39:986, 1974.
5. Krieger H.P., Krieger D.T.: Chemical stimulation of the brain: Effect on adrenal corticoid release. *Am. J. Physiol.* 218:1632, 1970.
6. Jones M.T., Gillham B., Mahmoud S.: Hypothalamus and ACTH secretion, in James V.H.T., et al. (eds): *The Endocrine Function of the Human Adrenal Cortex*. New York: Academic Press, 1978, pp 55–85.
7. Ganong W.F.: Neurotransmitters involved in ACTH secretion: Catecholamines, in Krieger D.T., et al. (eds): *ACTH and Related Peptides: Structure, Regulation, and Action*. New York: New York Academy of Sciences, 1977, pp 509–517.
8. Ludecke D., Kautzky R., Seager W., et al.: Selective removal of hypersecreting pituitary adenomas. *Acta Neurochir. (Wien)* 35:27, 1976.
9. Carmalt M.H.B., Dalton G.A., Fletcher R.F., et al.: The treatment of Cushing's disease by transsphenoidal hypophysectomy. *Q. J. Med.* 46:119, 1977.
10. Saeger W.: Die morphologie der paraadenomatosen adenohypophyse. *Virchows Arch. [Pathol. Anat.]* 372:299, 1977.
11. Young R.L., Bradley E.M., Goldzieher J.W., et al.: Spectrum of nonpuerperal galactorrhea: Report of two cases evolving through the various syndromes. *J. Clin. Endocrinol. Metab.* 27:461, 1967.
12. Gifford S., Gunderson J.G.: Cushing's disease as a psychosomatic disorder. *Medicine* 49:397, 1970.
13. Jeffcoate W.J., Silverstone J.T., Edwards C.R.W., et al.: Psychiatric manifestations of Cushing's syndrome: Response to lowering of plasma cortisol. *Q. J. Med.* 191:465, 1979.

14. McArthur R.G., Cloutier M.D., Hayles A.D., et al.: Cushing's disease in children. *Mayo Clin. Proc.* 47:318, 1972.
15. Ruder J.H., Loriaux D.L., Lipsett M.B.: Severe osteopenia in young adults associated with Cushing's syndrome due to micronodular adrenal disease. *J. Clin. Endocrinol. Metab.* 39:1138, 1974.
16. Beisel W.R., Coss J.J., Horton R., et al.: Physiology of urinary cortisol excretion. *J. Clin. Endocrinol. Metab.* 24:887, 1964.
17. Krieger D.T.: Plasma ACTH and corticosteroids, in DeGroot L., et al. (eds): *Textbook of Endocrinology*. New York: Grune & Stratton, 1979, pp 1139–1156.
18. Krieger D.T., Liotta A.S., Li C.H.: Human plasma immunoreactive β-lipotropin: Correlation with basal and stimulated plasma ACTH concentrations. *Life Sci.* 21:1771, 1977.
19. Suda T., Liotta A.S., Krieger D.T.: β-endorphin is not detectable in plasma from normal subjects. *Science* 202:221, 1978.
20. Krieger D.T., Liotta A.S., Suda T., et al.: Human plasma immunoreactive lipotropin and ACTH in normal subjects and in patients with pituitary-adrenal disease. *J. Clin. Endocrinol. Metab.* 48:566, 1979.
21. Liddle G.W., Estep H.L., Kendall J.W. Jr., et al.: Clinical application of a new test of pituitary reserve. *J. Clin. Endocrinol. Metab.* 19:875, 1959.
22. Jubiz W., Meikle S.W., West C.D., et al.: Single-dose metyrapone test. *Arch. Intern. Med.* 125:472, 1970.
23. Liddle G.W.: Tests of pituitary-adrenal suppressibility in the diagnosis of Cushing's syndrome. *J. Clin. Endocrinol. Metab.* 20:1539, 1960.
24. Nugent C.A., Nichols T., Tyler F.H.: Diagnosis of Cushing's syndrome: Single dose dexamethasone suppression test. *Arch. Intern. Med.* 116:172, 1965.
25. Crapo L.: Cushing's syndrome: A review of diagnostic tests. *Metabolism* 28:955, 1979.
26. Brown R.D., Van Loon G.R., Orth D.N., et al.: Cushing's disease with periodic hormonogenesis: One explanation for paradoxical response to dexamethasone. *J. Clin. Endocrinol. Metab.* 36:445, 1973.
27. Krieger D.T., Luria M.: Plasma ACTH and cortisol responses to TRF, vasopressin of hypoglycemia in Cushing's disease and Nelson's syndrome. *J. Clin. Endocrinol. Metab.* 44:361, 1977.
28. Tyrrell J.B., Lorenzi M., Forsham P.H., et al.: The effect of somatostatin on secretion of adrenocorticotropin in normal subjects and in patients with Nelson's syndrome and Cushing's disease. *57th Meeting Endocrine Society*, 1975, p 350.
29. Hall R., Besser G.M., Schally A.V., et al.: Action of growth-hormone-release inhibitory hormone in healthy men and in acromegaly. *Lancet* 2:581, 1973.
30. Hashimoto K.: The pituitary ACTH, GH, LH, FSH, TSH and prolactin reserves in patients with Cushing's syndrome. *Endocrinol. Jpn.* 22:67, 1975.
31. Duick D.S., Wahner H.W.: Thyroid axis in patients with Cushing's syndrome. *Arch. Intern. Med.* 139:767, 1979.
32. Tyrrell J.B., Brooks R.M., Fitzgerald P.A., et al.: Cushing's disease: Selective transsphenoidal resection of pituitary microadenomas. *N. Engl. J. Med.* 298:753, 1978.

33. Salassa R.M., Laws E.R. Jr., Carpenter P.C., et al.: Transsphenoidal removal of pituitary microadenoma in Cushing's disease. *Mayo Clin. Proc.* 53:24, 1978.
34. Swanson H.A., du Boulay G.: Borderline variants of the normal pituitary fossa. *Br. J. Radiol.* 48:366, 1975.
35. Sakar S.D., Cohen E.L., Beierwaltes W.H., et al.: A new and superior adrenal imaging agent $^{131}$I-6β-iodomethyl-19-nor-cholesterol (NP-59): Evaluation in humans. *J. Clin. Endocrinol. Metab.* 45:353, 1977.
36. Orth D.N., Liddle G.W.: Results of treatment in 108 patients with Cushing's syndrome. *N. Engl. J. Med.* 285:243, 1971.
37. Luton J.P., Mahoudeau J.A., Bouchard P., et al.: Treatment of Cushing's disease by o,p'DDD: Survey of 62 cases. *N. Engl. J. Med.* 300:459, 1979.
38. Komanicky P., Spark R.F., Melby J.C.: Treatment of Cushing's syndrome with trilostane (WIN 24,540), an inhibitor of adrenal steroid biosynthesis. *J. Clin. Endocrinol. Metab.* 47:1042, 1978.
39. Jeffcoate W.J., Rees L.H., Tomlin S., et al.: Metyrapone in long-term management of Cushing's disease. *Br. Med. J.* 2:215, 1977.
40. Jennings A.S., Liddle G.W., Orth D.N.: Results of treating childhood Cushing's disease with pituitary irradiation. *N. Engl. J. Med.* 297:957, 1977.
41. Burke C.W., Doyle F.H., Joplin G.F., et al.: Cushing's disease: Treatment by pituitary implantation of radioactive gold or yttrium seeds. *Q. J. Med.* 42:693, 1973.
42. Linfoot J.A.: Heavy ion therapy: Alpha particle therapy of pituitary tumors, in Linfoot J.A. (ed): *Recent Advances in the Diagnosis and Treatment of Pituitary Tumors.* New York: Raven Press, 1975, pp 254–267.
43. Kjellberg R.N., Kliman B.: A system for therapy of pituitary tumors, in Kohler P.O., et al. (eds): *Diagnosis and Treatment of Pituitary Tumors.* New York: Elsevier North-Holland, 1973, pp 234–252.
44. Krieger D.T., Amorosa L., Linick F.: Cyproheptadine induced remission of Cushing's disease. *N. Engl. J. Med.* 293:893, 1975.
45. Grant D.B., Atherden S.M.: Cushing's disease presenting with growth failure: Clinical remission during cyproheptadine therapy. *Arch. Dis. Child.* 54:466, 1979.
46. Aronin N., Krieger D.T.: Persistent remission of Nelson's syndrome following discontinuance of cyproheptadine treatment. *N. Engl. J. Med.* 302:453, 1980.
47. Soyka L.: Successful trial of metergoline in juvenile Cushing's disease. *Pediatr. Res.* 13:385, 1979.
48. Ferrari C., Bertazzoni A., Ghezzi M.: Letter to the editor. *N. Engl. J. Med.* 296:576, 1977.
49. Lamberts S.W.J., Stefanko S.Z., Delange S.A., et al.: Failure of clinical remission after transsphenoidal removal of a microadenoma in a patient with Cushing's disease: Multiple hyperplastic and adenomatous cell rests in surrounding pituitary tissue. *J. Clin. Endocrinol. Metab.* 50:793, 1980.
50. Krieger D.T.: Cushing's Syndrome. Heidelberg: Springer-Verlag, 1982.

# Cushing's Disease: Surgical Management

CHARLES B. WILSON, M.D., J. BLAKE TYRRELL, M.D., PAUL A. FITZGERALD, M.D., AND PETER H. FORSHAM, M.D.

*The Departments of Neurological Surgery and Medicine, and the Metabolic Research Unit, University of California, San Francisco*

ALMOST FIFTY YEARS AGO, Harvey Cushing[1] reported 12 patients who during their lives had clinical manifestations of hypercortisolism. He found basophilic adenomas in a postmortem study of six of these patients and implicated a pituitary disorder in the disease that now bears his name. Emphasizing the small size of these occult pituitary adenomas, he warned that without serial sections of the gland the tumor might escape detection.

In December, 1933, Howard C. Naffziger performed a craniotomy on a young woman with Cushing's disease. This was, to our knowledge, the first operation for removal of a corticotropic adenoma. Incomplete removal of the tumor produced a dramatic remission lasting one year, but despite irradiation of the sella, and later of the adrenal glands, the disease recurred and the patient died in 1940. Lisser's account of the case was published in 1944, on the occasion of Dr. Naffziger's sixtieth birthday.[2]

The introduction of cortisone promoted bilateral adrenalectomy as the accepted treatment of Cushing's disease, in the face of undisputed evidence that the anterior pituitary was linked to the condition in some, if not most, cases. With few exceptions, intrasellar pathology could not be defined by radiographic methods available at the time, and uncertainty regarding the pathogenesis of the process argued against the then radical treatment by total hypophysectomy.

199

0-8151-3530-0/82/006-199-208-$03.75

Selective removal of pituitary microadenomas emerged as a therapeutic alternative with Hardy's report in 1969.[3] Using a surgical microscope and making a transsphenoidal approach to the sella turcica, Hardy proved that an endocrine-active pituitary adenoma could be removed selectively, an operation that would result in restoration of normal pituitary function. This pivotal achievement inaugurated an immediate redirection of the therapeutic approach to pituitary adenomas. Subsequent refinements in the biochemical definition of pituitary-based hypercortisolism and the evolution of neuroradiologic techniques capable of detecting minor abnormalities of the sella turcica and its contents have afforded additional precision and certainty in the diagnosis of pituitary disorders, but the therapeutic reorientation of the past decade undoubtedly began with Hardy's report that microadenomas could be removed—selectively, completely, and safely.

In 1978 we published our report of a group of 20 patients who underwent transsphenoidal operations for Cushing's disease.[4] This chapter concerns the follow-up of this initial group, and the results of transsphenoidal exploration in an additional 57 patients.

## Patients and Methods

### PATIENTS

Between February, 1974, and October, 1980, 77 patients, diagnosed as having Cushing's disease on the basis of laboratory findings, underwent transsphenoidal exploration of the sella turcica. The majority of these patients were women; seven were children. Three of the patients had undergone unsuccessful pituitary irradiation, and three had recurrent Cushing's disease after a presumed total bilateral adrenalectomy. The only death occurred six weeks after operation in a patient whose postoperative course was benign; her death was attributed to myocardial infarction, although postmortem verification was not obtained. The period of follow-up ranged from three months to six and a half years. Included in this series are all patients whose preoperative and postoperative evaluations were performed in the Metabolic Research Center at the University of California, San Francisco.

### PREOPERATIVE AND POSTOPERATIVE EVALUATION

The methods for the preoperative and postoperative endocrinologic evaluations described in our earlier report[4] have undergone no change. The preoperative radiologic evaluation now includes thin-section computerized tomographic (CT) scans of the sella and body CT scans of the adrenal glands, as well as thin-section polytomograms of the sella. Although in this series the manner of performing sellar exploration was influenced by any abnormality detected by polytomography and CT scanning, the decision to explore the sella was based entirely on the endocrinologic diagnosis. Radiographic studies served only to direct the operative procedure to an observed abnormality of the sella or its contents. In the first few patients, carotid angiography provided no useful information, and it was abandoned as a preoperative study.

## OPERATIVE PROCEDURE

The patients (or in the case of children, their parents) were informed that a microadenoma, even if not identified during the course of intrasellar exploration, was the probable cause of their disorder. After the three alternatives—pituitary irradiation, bilateral adrenalectomy, and total hypophysectomy—were described, adult patients were advised to have a total hypophysectomy if the exploration proved negative. The same alternatives were described to the parents of children and to young adults, but irradiation rather than hypophysectomy was recommended if no adenoma was identified.

If hypophysectomy was a possibility in a particular case, a lumbar subarachnoid catheter was introduced after the induction of general anesthesia and before the patient was positioned for the transsphenoidal approach. At the surgeon's request, the anesthesiologist was prepared to inject normal saline (without preservative) through the catheter to prevent intracranial aspiration of blood and to check the adequacy of sellar closure at the end of the procedure.

The transsphenoidal procedure was used, with no major deviation from the technique described by Hardy.[5] Exposure of the dura is wide, from the tuberculum sellae to the horizontal plane of the sellar floor and to the medial edge of both cavernous sinuses. The dura is coagulated with a bipolar forceps along a line adjacent to the bone edges, and is excised. If the preoperative tomograms and CT scans indicate a focal abnormality, or if the appearance of the exposed anterior lobe suggests the tumor's location, the suspect region is explored initially. In the absence of a clue to the location of the tumor, the initial exploratory incision is made vertically in the midline, and the incision is extended from the upper surface of the anterior lobe to the sellar floor, and to the surface of the posterior lobe. The importance of fully exposing the posterior lobe relates to the occasional adenoma occupying the pars intermedia and, as illustrated in one of Cushing's original cases,[1] invading the posterior lobe.

The second and third vertical incisions are made into the lateral wings. Because the adenoma may arise on the surface of the anterior lobe, the next maneuver is the separation of the gland from the cavernous sinus and the sellar floor and inspection of the upper surface beneath the arachnoid and sellar diaphragm for tumor. The last step is a horizontal incision to the plane of the posterior lobe, literally bisecting the anterior lobe, which at this point has been divided into eight sections. Any disproportionately large section can be divided, but the four initial incisions—three vertical and one horizontal—approach the limitations of technical practicality.

If the exploration failed to disclose a tumor, and if the patient had consented to hypophysectomy, a total hypophysectomy was performed with removal of all intrasellar tissues. Subcutaneous fat has become the preferred graft for packing the sella, and a carved piece of nasal septal cartilage was used to reconstitute the anterior wall of the sella.

Since complete removal of an identified adenoma requires direct visualization of adjacent normal structures, it was necessary in some cases to excise a wedge of uninvolved anterior lobe. After all abnormal tissue had been removed (including a portion of the posterior lobe if it had been in contact with the adenoma), the cavity was irrigated with absolute alcohol, and was then filled with gelatin foam saturated with absolute alcohol. After being exposed to alcohol for ten minutes, the cavity was packed either with alcohol-saturated gelatin foam or with this foam plus fat, and the sella was closed with cartilage. Depending on the surgeon's concern about the potential for a postoperative cerebrospinal fluid leak, the sphenoid sinus was filled with fat.

## Results

A total of 77 patients underwent transsphenoidal exploration; the overall results are given in Table 1. Selective adenomectomy cured 51 patients (66%), and an additional eight patients (10%) were cured by total hypophysectomy.

Five patients (two in the initial series of 20 reported, and three in the subsequent 57 patients) are designated technical failures. In each case, the exposed dura contained formidable venous sinuses. Because identification and removal of a microadenoma requires wide exposure of the sella and a bloodless surgical field, the procedure was aban-

TABLE 1.—CUSHING'S DISEASE: RESULTS OF
PITUITARY MICROSURGERY

| RESULT | NO. OF PATIENTS | PERCENT |
|---|---|---|
| Selective microsurgery | | |
| Correction of hypercortisolism | 51 | 66 |
| Persistence | | |
| Adenoma proved (8) | 9 | 12 |
| Adenoma not proved (1) | | |
| Recurrence | 4 | 5 |
| Total hypophysectomy | | |
| Adenoma proved (6) | 8 | 10 |
| Adenoma not proved (2) | | |
| Technical Failure | | |
| Dural venous sinus | 5 | 7 |
| Total | 77 | 100 |

doned in these cases without opening the dura. More than one half of microadenomas have a diameter of 5 mm or less, and with suboptimal exposure and operating conditions, an anatomically compromised operation exposes the patient to the risks of entering the sella with a greatly reduced likelihood of performing a curative selective adenomectomy. Consequently, to abandon the operation in the face of technical obstacles seemed preferable to a compromised intrasellar exploration. After additional experience, and with the availability of newly designed forceps that have 45-degree and 90-degree angled tips, however, two cases identical to these five were later managed successfully, with curative selective adenomectomy in both instances.

Except for the five cases in which the sella was not entered, 13 adenomas extended beyond the sella. Of these, four had suprasellar extension, three extended laterally, four extended into the sphenoid sinus, and two had both suprasellar and sphenoid-sinus extension. Whereas age, sex, clinical manifestations of the disease, and laboratory values failed to predict the outcome of operation, extrasellar extension, observed in 18% of cases, proved to be an unfavorable predictor of outcome (Table 2). The small numbers in each category preclude any distinction among the different types of extrasellar extensions according to curability, except in the case of tumors that extend laterally, either into or beneath the cavernous sinus, and by definition cannot be completely removed.

Tumors that are designated microadenomas (see Table 2) were entirely intrasellar and had a diameter of less than 10 mm. Two tumors that met the volumetric criterion of a microadenoma extended beyond

TABLE 2.—CUSHING'S DISEASE: RESULTS OF
PITUITARY MICROSURGERY*

| RESULT | NO. | PERCENT |
|---|---|---|
| Microadenomas | | |
| Corrected with selective removal | 48 | 81 |
| Corrected with total hypophysectomy | 7 | 12 |
| Persistence | 3 | 5 |
| Recurrence | 1 | 2 |
| Total | 59 | 100 |
| Extrasellar extension | | |
| Corrected with selective removal | 3 | 23 |
| Corrected with total hypophysectomy | 1 | 8 |
| Persistence | 6 | 46 |
| Recurrence | 3 | 23 |
| Total | 13 | 100 |

*Patients with dural venous sinus excluded.

the sella; one was suprasellar and one lateral. Both of these tumors were assigned to the extrasellar category despite their small size.

Among the 59 patients with microadenomas, 55 were cured by operation. In seven, an adenoma was not identified during exploration and a total hypophysectomy was performed; these patients were cured, but at the expense of panhypopituitarism. Selective removal of an adenoma with preservation of anterior pituitary function was successful in 48 patients.

Of the four patients who were failures in the group with microadenomas, three had persistent hypercortisolism and one had a recurrence after initial correction. One of the patients with persisting disease has normal cortisol values and is clinically well four years after removal of the microadenoma, but dynamic testing has shown that the patient does not have normal diurnal cycles.

The results in the group of 13 patients with extrasellar adenomas were decidedly inferior to the outcome for the patients with microadenomas. Only three patients were cured by selective adenomectomy, and one additional patient was cured by total hypophysectomy. The overall cure rate of 31% for extrasellar tumors contrasts sharply with the 93% successful outcome for patients with microadenomas.

Postoperative follow-up has identified four patients who had recurrent Cushing's disease after initial correction (Table 3). None of the eight patients treated by total hypophysectomy suffered a recurrence. Among the 49 patients considered cured after selective removal of a microadenoma, only one had recurrent disease. Stated differently, 48 of 49 patients whose early postoperative endocrine evaluation indi-

TABLE 3.—CUSHING'S DISEASE:
POSTOPERATIVE FOLLOW-UP OF TUMORS
WITH INITIAL CORRECTION OF
HYPERCORTISOLISM

| FOLLOW-UP PERIOD (YEARS) | NO. OF PATIENTS | RECURRENCE |
|---|---|---|
| Microadenomas | | |
| <1 | 15 | 0 |
| 1–2 | 8 | 0 |
| 2–3 | 8 | 0 |
| 3–7 | 18 | 1 |
| Total | 49 | 1 |
| Extrasellar tumors | | |
| <1 | 1 | 0 |
| 1 | 2 | 2 |
| 2 | 2 | 1 |
| 4 | 1 | 0 |
| Total | 6 | 3 |

cated cure of the disease have remained well. The excellent prognosis for patients whose disease is initially corrected by selective microadenomectomy is reinforced by the follow-up observation of 26 patients for two to seven years. After an initially successful removal of extrasellar adenomas, three recurrences were evident within two years after operation.

## PATHOLOGY

The tumors were examined by both conventional and immunofluorescent staining techniques and by electron microscopy. When stainable granules were observed by light microscopy, the tumors were designated basophilic, but the majority contained no identifiable secretory granules and were designated "chromophobe," an imprecise term meaning, roughly, "devoid of observable granules." In recent years immunofluorescent staining has shown ACTH-secreting granules in the cytoplasm of the adenomas removed from patients with Cushing's disease. We can add nothing to the excellent pathologic study reported by Robert et al.[6]

Of particular interest in our series are the three patients in whom an adenoma was not proved by pathologic examination (see Table 1). The typical adenoma responsible for Cushing's disease is white or gray-white, and is soft to the point of being gelatinous or even semiliquid in some instances. These adenomas can be minute: the smallest accurately measured tumor, detected by serially sectioning an excised pituitary gland, has a diameter of 1.5 mm. Because of the small size and semiliquid consistency of many adenomas, insufficient material was obtained for microscopic examination from several patients cured by selective adenomectomy, but with clinical justification, an adenoma can be assumed in these cases.

The failure to find an adenoma after serially sectioning an excised pituitary gland does not exclude the possibility that a microadenoma was present, but the specimen "lost," i.e., went undiscovered. Cushing recognized that the adenoma could occupy the pars intermedia and invade the posterior lobe; in our series, three tumors were confined to the pars intermedia and adjacent posterior lobe.[1] During total hypophysectomy, the anterior lobe is more easily removed than the posterior lobe because of its firmer consistency and smoother surface. The posterior lobe often excavates the base of the dorsum sellae, and small lobules may be either overlooked or aspirated while the surgeon clears the field of blood coming from the frequently opened basal dural venous sinuses. Both the adenoma and the posterior lobe are soft and white, adding another possible source of error in identifying and obtaining a specimen. Although none of our adenomas involved the pituitary stalk, a small adenoma originating in the pars tuberalis could theoretically be overlooked in dividing the pituitary stalk.

In a recent case not included in this series, we failed to identify an adenoma initially; the pituitary gland was being mobilized in preparation for a total hypophysectomy, when a 2-mm adenoma was found on the surface of the anterior lobe lying against the cavernous sinus near the dorsum sellae. We suspect that the adenoma was similarly overlooked in the two cases of "adenoma not proved" after total hypophysectomy (see Table 1). Schnall et al.[7] recently reported a case of Cushing's disease with diffuse hyperplasia of corticotrophs and no adenoma in the removed pituitary gland; but because both of our patients were cured by hypophysectomy, and because hyperplasia of corticotrophs was not present in either patient, our presumption of an overlooked adenoma is reasonable in these instances. We are not surprised by a well-documented case of Cushing's disease caused by corticotroph hyperplasia, but the exceptional nature of the case reported by Schnall et al. should be apparent.

The third "adenoma not proved" in Table 1 would have been considered proved had the patient's hypercortisolism been corrected, because a tumor was seen grossly even though an adequate specimen was not obtained. It seems reasonable to accept this as a case of incomplete removal rather than one of negative exploration.

# Discussion

This series of 77 cases extends our initial observations[4] and supports the conclusions we reached three years ago. The diagnosis of Cushing's disease accurately predicts the presence of a corticotrophic adenoma. The responsible adenoma may be minute and elusive, and in our experience, a successful selective adenomectomy requires the utmost surgical skill.

The initial treatment of Cushing's disease should be transsphenoidal exploration, regardless of the patient's age. Although, in children, the operation presents the technical obstacle of frequently limited pneumatization of the sphenoid sinus, our results in children have been excellent; we have achieved correction without recurrence in all seven children.

In comparison with alternative modes of therapy—pituitary irradiation and bilateral adrenalectomy—transsphenoidal adenomectomy has a superior record of success. Adenomectomy provides immediate correction of hypercortisolism in the great majority of patients. The operative risk is low: in a series of 600 endocrine-active adenomas at our institution there were no deaths related to the operation. The probability of achieving and maintaining normal pituitary function is high, although it may be necessary to accept panhypopituitarism in an adult if hypercortisolism is corrected. Furthermore, the potential complication of Nelson's syndrome is averted, an important consideration in view of our poor results in the treatment of postadrenalectomy adenomas.

Medical treatment of Cushing's disease, the most recent trials involving the use of bromocriptine, has had disappointing results.[8] Medical therapy may eventually supercede present forms of surgery and irradiation, but the prospects now are no brighter than they were three years ago.

We can add nothing to the discussion contained in our earlier report. Cushing was correct, and the direct form of treatment that he conceived has been applied with salutary results.

## REFERENCES

1. Cushing H.: The basophil adenomas of the pituitary body and their clinical manifestations (pituitary basophilism). *Bull. Johns Hopkins Hosp.* 50:137, 1932.
2. Lisser H.: Hypophysectomy in Cushing's disease. *J. Nerv. Ment. Dis.* 99:727, 1944.

3. Hardy J.: Transsphenoidal microsurgery of the normal and pathological pituitary. *Clin. Neurosurg.* 16:185, 1969.
4. Tyrrell J.B., et al.: Cushing's disease: Selective transsphenoidal resection of pituitary microadenomas. *N. Engl. J. Med.* 298:753, 1978.
5. Hardy J.: Transsphenoidal surgery of hypersecreting pituitary tumors, in Kohler P.O., et al. (eds): *Diagnosis and Treatment of Pituitary Tumors.* New York: Elsevier North-Holland, 1973, pp 179–194.
6. Robert F., Pelletier G., Hardy J.: Pituitary adenomas in Cushing's disease. *Arch. Pathol. Lab. Med.* 102:448, 1978.
7. Schnall A.M., et al.: Pituitary Cushing's disease without adenoma. *Acta Endocrinol. (Copenh.)* 94:297, 1980.
8. Lamberts S.W.J., et al.: The mechanism of the suppressive action of bromocriptine on adrenocorticotropin secretion in patients with Cushing's disease and Nelson's syndrome. *J. Clin. Endocrinol. Metab.* 51:307, 1980.

# Pathophysiology of Acromegaly

## WILLIAM H. DAUGHADAY, M.D.

*Metabolism Division, Washington University School of*
*Medicine, St. Louis, Missouri*

IN THIS BRIEF REVIEW I will describe some aspects of the endocrine pathophysiology of acromegaly. Focusing primarily on the differences between the normal secretion of GH and the secretion in acromegaly, I will also consider the possible ectopic secretion of GH and GH-releasing hormone by tumors. Lastly, I will discuss the changes that occur in the somatomedin peptides during acromegaly and the clinical usefulness of somatomedin C/IGF-I measurements.

### GH Circadian Secretory Pattern

Normal individuals secrete GH in discrete bursts that interrupt extremely low levels of basal secretion (Fig 1). The most regularly occurring burst occurs on the average of 90 minutes following the onset of nocturnal sleep.[1] Lesser secondary and tertiary periods of GH secretion can occur in sleep. During the day GH secretory bursts occur every four to six hours. These may occur spontaneously or be provoked by moderate physical activity.

This normal pattern of GH secretion makes it clear that it cannot be characterized by one or two isolated measurements. This has led investigators to measure the integrated GH level over a 24-hour period either by continuous or intermittent sampling. The results of such measurements have provided evidence of a substantial increase in mean GH levels during puberty and a progressive decrease in GH secretion as a function of age.[2] The same pattern has been observed

This study was supported by Research Grants AMO 1526 and AMO 5105, National Institute of Arthritis, Metabolism and Digestive Diseases, Bethesda, Maryland.

209

0-8151-3530-0/82/006-209-223-$03.75
© 1982, Year Book Medical Publishers, Inc.

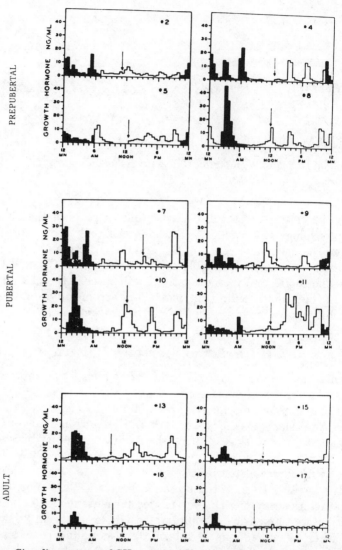

**Fig 1.**—Circadian pattern of GH secretion. *Upper panels,* studies in four prepubertal individuals. *Middle panels,* studies in four pubertal individuals. *Lower panels,*
results of studies in four older individuals. Solid columns represent blood samples obtained during sleep. (From Plotnick L.P., et al.: *J. Clin. Endocrinol. Metab.* 40:240,
1975. Used by permission.)

with measurements limited to the sleep-entrained GH secretory surge.

The circadian pattern of GH secretion in acromegaly is variable[3] (Fig 2). In some patients serum GH varies very little from hour to hour, whereas in others a fourfold to fivefold difference may occur. In nearly all patients studied, the peaks and valleys appear to lack any predictable pattern and are unassociated with the onset of sleep.

The pattern of GH secretion in normal and acromegalic persons limits the usefulness of single testing GH measurements in acromegalic patients. Some normal individuals, particularly young women who are physically active or anxious before blood sampling, can have serum GH levels above the "normal" range. This can be largely prevented by obtaining blood an hour or two after the ingestion of 75 gm of glucose. Under those conditions the vast majority of normal individuals will have serum GH below 5 ng/ml, while acromegalic patients almost always have serum GH levels above this value. Even with glucose loading, the diagnosis of acromegalic activity on the basis of GH levels alone may be difficult and has led to the proposed use of serum somatomedin as a more sensitive index of GH excess (see "Serum Somatomedin Levels in Acromegaly" below).

## Effect of Major Nutrients on GH Secretion

Ingestion of glucose has a twofold effect on GH secretion. As mentioned above, glucose can suppress mild elevations of GH secretion due to anxiety or mild exertion. Insulin induced hypoglycemia and

**Fig 2.**—Diurnal pattern of GH secretion in a patient with acromegaly showing extreme variability of GH secretion. (From Cryer P.E., Daughaday W.H.: *J. Clin. Endocrinol. Metab.* 29:386, 1969. Used by permission.)

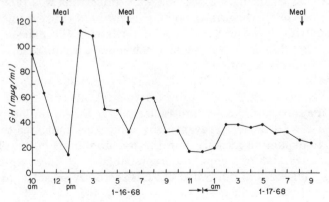

the falling blood sugar in the three to four hours after glucose ingestion can also increase GH secretion. Experiments with animals have indicated that these effects of glucose are mediated by a hypothalamic glucose receptor.

Arginine infusion also acts on a hypothalamic site to stimulate GH secretion in most normal individuals and like insulin induced hypoglycemia is extensively used to stimulate GH secretion in patients with suspected hypopituitarism. Increased plasma fatty acids, induced experimentally by heparin activation of lipoprotein lipase after a fatty meal, inhibit GH secretion

The effect of acute alteration of blood sugar on GH secretion in acromegaly has been extensively studied in acromegaly.[3] Glucose ingestion rarely lowers serum GH to normal levels and in 14% of patients may actually increase GH secretion. The normal serum GH rise after hypoglycemia is observed in about 60% of acromegalic patients. Similarly, arginine infusion can lead to GH secretion in 45% of acromegalic patients.

The response to glucose and arginine in acromegaly is evidence of partial hypothalamic secretory dependence, as there is no evidence that in the concentrations achieved these nutrients act directly on the pituitary gland.

## GH Regulation by Biogenic Amines

There is much evidence that hypothalamic catecholamines are important in the normal regulation of GH secretion. Blackard and Heidingsfelder[4] first demonstrated that the GH response to insulin-induced hypoglycemia was augmented by prior β-blockade with propranolol and inhibited by phentolamine pretreatment. Further evidence that α-adrenergic pathways are important was provided by Toivola and Gale[5] who stimulated GH secretion by direct injection of norepinephrine into the ventromedial nucleus of the baboon. In human beings, clonidine, a central α-adrenergic agonist, is a potent stimulator of GH secretion.[6]

L-Dopa ingestion stimulates GH secretion in most normal individuals and so provides a useful provocative stimulus of GH secretion in clinical diagnosis of hyposomatotropism. That this stimulatory effect of L-dopa can be largely prevented by α-blockers indicates that it is due not to dopamine formation in the hypothalamus but to the subsequent conversion of L-dopa to norepinephrine.[7] α-Adrenergic blockade is also effective in inhibiting the GH secretory effects of arginine, hypoglycemia, exercise, and glucagon, a fact that indicates a role for norepinephrine in mediating the response to these secretagogues. α-Adrenergic pathways are not important in controlling sleep-related GH secretion.

In acromegaly, some adrenergic modification of GH secretion persists. α-Blockade induced by phentolamine infusion partially suppressed GH levels in acromegalic patients; addition of a β-agonist, isoproterenol, led to further fall in GH levels (Fig 3).[8]

Dopaminergic modification of GH secretion in acromegaly is more potent than adrenergic modification. Oral ingestion of L-dopa will lower GH secretion in most acromegalic patients. This effect is due to pituitary conversion of L-dopa to dopamine. Subsequent conversion to norepinephrine is not required because α-blockade does not modify the effect of L-dopa.[7] When pituitary conversion to dopamine is prevented by carbidopa, the effect is abolished.[9] Evidence that dopaminergic agents act directly on the pituitary has been provided by the lowering of serum GH in acromegaly by dopamine infusions.[10] It is known that dopamine cannot traverse the blood brain barrier to a significant degree. The direct inhibitory effect of dopamine on GH secretion by GH-secreting tumors has also been demonstrated in vitro.[11]

Bromocriptine, a dopaminergic agent, has been used extensively in the medical treatment of acromegaly in Great Britain and Europe. Substantial lowering of GH levels can be achieved in most patients (Fig 4).[12] This form of treatment has had limited acceptance in the United States. In the first place, GH levels are seldom restored completely to normal and the dose of bromocriptine required for maxi-

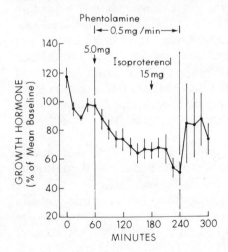

**Fig 3.**—Effect of phentolamine infusion and sublingual isoproterenol on serum GH concentration in ten acromegalic patients. (From Cryer P.E., Daughaday W.H.: *J. Clin. Endocrinol. Metab.* 39:658, 1974. Used by permission.)

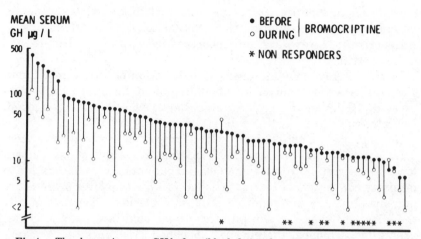

**Fig 4.**—The change in mean GH before *(black dot)* and on *(circle)* bromocriptine in 73 patients with acromegaly. Note serum GH has been plotted on a logarithmic scale. (From Besser G.M., et al.: *Acta Endocrinol. [Suppl. 216] (Copenh.)* 88:187, 1978.)

mum benefit is much higher than that used in the treatment of prolactinomas. The medication is expensive and may induce gastrointestinal or circulatory side effects.

## Control of GH by Hypothalamic Peptides

The normal secretion of GH is under dual control. There is clear biologic evidence that the hypothalamus contains a GH-releasing factor (GHRF) that is secreted into the portal sinusoids in the median eminence. Until recently, the isolation of GHRF has frustrated several groups of investigators. The interference from large amounts of somatostatin has recently been eliminated and elucidation of the primary structure of the molecule will not be long in the offing.

The second hypothalamic peptide that regulates GH secretion is somatostatin. While the familiar 14 amino acid peptide has been extensively studied, larger fully active somatostatin peptides exist in hypothalamus.

While a number of other hypothalamic peptides have been shown to release GH under various experimental conditions, their importance in physiologic GH release is questionable.[7]

From what has already been said about the normal control of GH secretion, it is clear that many neurogenic mediators impinge on the ventromedial nucleus and median eminence to alter the secretion of GHRH and somatostatin. Particularly relevent to this discussion is the negative feedback exerted by GH and somatomedin on GH secretion. GH administration of normal and hypophysectomized rats increases median eminence somatostatin concentration.[13] Intraventricular injection of GH markedly decreased the amplitude of the periodic bursts of GH secretion in the rat.[14] Lastly, when GH and somatomedin C (IGF-I), the GH-dependent mediators of some of GH's action, are added to rat hypothalamic explants in vitro they increase somatostatin release.[15, 16]

It has long been speculated that acromegaly might be the result of prolonged stimulation of somatotroph cells and the eventual development of nodular hyperplasia and ultimately of adenoma (Fig 5). Plasma from acromegalic patients has been reported to stimulate GH release by monkey hemipituitaries in vitro,[17] but the significance of this finding is in doubt. There is much evidence against such a stimulation. First, diffuse or nodular somatotroph hyperplasia is rarely found in acromegalic patients. Almost without exception the condi-

**Fig 5.**—Possible pathogenesis of acromegaly. Normal hypothalamus and pituitary shown above with normal regulation of GH secretion by somatostatin and GH-releasing hormone *(GHRH)*. *Right,* a postulated phase of GH hypersecretion resulting from increased secretion of GHRH. *Left,* GH hypersecretion resulting from development of an autonomous GH-secreting tumor. The possible conversion of somatotroph diffuse proliferation to autonomous focal neoplasm is shown. The existence of a preceding phase of diffuse somatotroph hyperplasia has seldom been established. (From Daughaday W.H., Cryer P.E.: *Hosp. Pract.* 13:75, 1978. Drawing by Nancy Lou Gahan.)

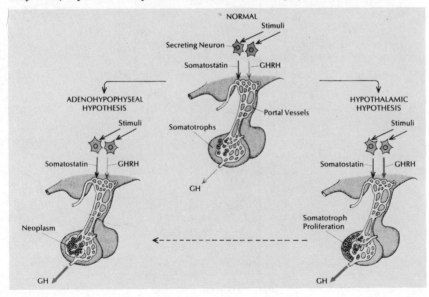

tion is associated with discrete somatotroph adenomas. The somatotrophs in the uninvolved pituitary appear normal or suppressed. Second, selective removal of a somatotroph adenoma has led to normal or suppressed GH secretion. This observation would suggest that the initial hypersomatotropism is due to a primary autonomous adenoma rather than the result of prolonged hypothalamic stimulation.

As has been mentioned above, GH and somatomedins can stimulate somatostatin secretion in vivo and in vitro in various experimental studies, but is somatostatin secretion activated in acromegaly? Somatostatin infusion will lower GH secretion in acromegalics (Fig 6).[18] The dose of somatostatin required to suppress GH secretion in acromegalics does not appear to be greatly different than that required to block GH responses in normal individuals.[19] This observation would suggest that marked somatostatin resistance is not present. A more subtle partial resistance of adenomatous somatotrophs as compared to normal somatotrophs may have been missed by past, rather crude, dose response studies. Somatostatin has not proven to be of practical therapeutic benefit because of a requirement for parenteral adminis-

**Fig 6.**—Lowering of serum GH in eight acromegalic patients during 75-minute infusions of somatostatin. (*Black square*, 100 μg; *black dot*, 250 μg; *black triangle*, 500 μg; *circle*, 1000 μg). (From Besser G.M. et al.: *Br. Med. J.* 1:352, 1974. Used by permission.)

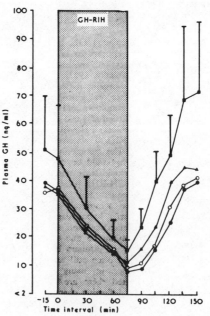

tration and the simultaneous suppression of insulin and other hormonal secretion.

As yet there is no way to determine hypothalamic secretion of somatostatin in man. Plasma somatostatin is derived from pancreatic and other extraneural sites as well as the median eminence. Plasma measurements are of little avail in reflecting median eminence secretion.

An interesting property of somatotroph adenomas is their ability to respond in vivo and in vitro to thyrotropin releasing hormone (TRH) and gonadotropin-releasing hormone (LRH) (Fig 7).[20, 21] The frequency of these aberrant GH responses has varied from series to series but has averaged from 40% to 60% of the cases.

The effects of TRH and LRH are believed to be directly exerted on the pituitary tumor. Ishibashi and Yamaji[22] have shown that TRH can stimulate GH release by somatotroph adenomatous tissue in vitro. The unmasking of TRH and LRH receptors by the neoplastic process may be related to the unmasking of dopamine receptors in the tumor.

The TRH test in acromegaly is of clinical usefulness. A rise in serum GH preoperatively supports the diagnosis. Persistence of a positive TRH response postoperatively strongly suggests incomplete tumor removal and probable eventual clinical relapse.[23]

## Ectopic Production of GH and GHRH

Ectopic production of GH has been suspected in certain patients with cancer, particularly small cell carcinoma of the lung and carcinoid tumors. In some cases increased GH content of the tumor and release of GH from tissue culture have been demonstrated.[24] Generally the secretion of GH by these tumors is modest and does not contribute significantly to the clinical course of the patients.

Evidence is accumulating that carcinoid tumors (including bronchial adenomas) can produce significant hypersomatotropism and clinically evident acromegaly by secretion of a GH-releasing factor. Even when the sella turcica is enlarged, suggesting a pituitary tumor, successful removal of the carcinoid has led to clinical and hormonal remission. Uz Zafar et al.[25] reported that extracts of such a tumor were devoid of GH but stimulated release of GH by primary pituitary cell culture. Similarly, Shalet et al.[26] were able to maintain such a tumor in cell culture and show that the conditioned medium could stimulate GH release by isolated rat pituitary cultures.

We have described a young man with gigantism and a metastatic

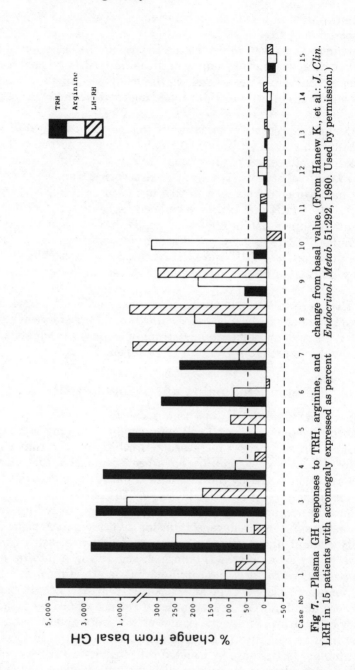

**Fig 7.**—Plasma GH responses to TRH, arginine, and LRH in 15 patients with acromegaly expressed as percent change from basal value. (From Hanew K., et al.: *J. Clin. Endocrinol. Metab.* 51:292, 1980. Used by permission.)

duodenal carcinoid.[27] Extracts of plasma from this patient contained a GH-releasing factor. Although the tumor itself contained little GH, GH-containing cells identified by immunofluorescent staining were scattered throughout the tumor. The pituitary contained a large adenoma composed of sheets of mature-appearing somatotroph cells. This case is an example of a carcinoid tumor that contained some GH-producing cells but that also stimulated the pituitary to adenomatous change by secreting a potent releasing hormone.

Frohman et al.[28] have partially characterized the GH-releasing factor from our patient's tumor and from three other similar tumors. The factor is a peptide that appears to be somewhat larger than previously reported.

## Serum Somatomedin Levels in Acromegaly

Somatomedins are components of serum that mediate some but not all effects of GH on target tissues. They may be most important in regulating skeletal growth. There are two main types of somatomedin whose structure is known.[29] IGF-I is a 70 amino acid peptide with a striking structural homology to insulin. This peptide appears to be identical or nearly identical to somatomedin C, isolated by Svoboda and his colleagues.[30] IGF-I/ (Sm C), which is now measured by radioimmune assay (RIA), virtually disappears in hypopituitarism and is restored by GH administration.[31]

A second related peptide, IGF-II, has been isolated from human plasma proteins.[32] This peptide can now be measured by a specific radioreceptor assay in our laboratory and an RIA is under development in Dr. Froesch's laboratory. IGF-II has slightly different biologic properties than IGF. It is less GH-dependent than IGF-I, however, and levels of it only fall partially in pituitary dwarfism.

In acromegaly there is a marked rise in IGF-I (Sm C) by RIA to values that are two to 20 times normal. The clinical usefulness of the Sm C RIA in acromegaly has been investigated by Clemmons and his co-workers.[33] They found that somatomedin measurements were an extremely sensitive method in establishing hypersomatotropism in acromegalic patients with serum GH levels in the normal range (Fig 8). Moreover, a number of clinical parameters of the severity of acromegaly correlated better with somatomedin elevations than they did with GH elevations. Treatment of acromegalic patients with large doses of estrogens reduces somatomedin concentration without affecting GH concentration. Our experience with an improved IGF-I RIA confirms the conclusions of Clemmons et al. In view of the expense of

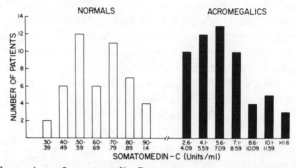

**Fig 8.**—Comparison of somatomedin C serum concentrations in 48 normal persons *(open columns)* and 57 patients with acromegaly *(solid columns)*. (From Clemmons D.R., et al.: *N. Engl. J. Med.* 301:1138, 1979.)

the current commercial Sm C RIA determination, it is only needed in a minority of patients whose GH levels are indeterminant.

In contrast to the elevations of Sm C/IGF-I that occur in acromegaly, measurements of IGF-II by a specific radioreceptor assay[34] fail to show a consistent rise above normal. It is clear that this insulin-like peptide is less affected by GH and must have a separate role to play in cellular regulation.

## Summary

In acromegaly, GH secretion may be variable and does not show the sleep-related bursts characteristic of normal persons. Serum GH of some acromegalic patients is acutely altered by changes in glucose and arginine concentrations. As these stimuli appear to act on the hypothalamus, some residual hypothalamic control exists.

In acromegaly, hypothalamic adrenergic pathways of regulating GH secretion are generally interrupted. Most somatotroph tumors acquire potent dopaminergic receptors, which, when activated by dopamine or the synthetic agent bromocriptine, inhibit GH secretion.

Most of the evidence suggests that somatotroph tumors generally arise without preceding somatotroph hyperplasia. Complete selective adenomectomy usually results in restoration of normal pituitary function. These observations argue against a hypothalamic etiology for the disease. GH and somatomedin excess stimulate somatostatin secretion in laboratory animals. The failure of this negative feedback in acromegaly remains unexplained. Perhaps somatotroph tumors possess only a relative resistance to somatostatin that has escaped recognition.

Certain tumors, particularly carcinoid tumors, can secrete GH in low amounts. Well-recognized cases of clinical acromegaly have been associated with the ectopic secretion of GH releasing factor(s).

GH acts on certain target tissues by stimulating release of somatomedins. IGF-I (Sm C) is highly GH dependent. Marked elevations in serum IGF-I (Sm C) occur in acromegaly. This measurement is of great usefulness in evaluating the significance of borderline GH measurements. Another somatomedin, IGF-II, is not elevated in acromegaly.

## REFERENCES
1. Takahashi Y., Kipnis D.M., Daughaday W.H.: Growth hormone secretion during sleep. *J. Clin. Invest.* 47:2079, 1968.
2. Plotnick L.P., Thompson R.C., Kowarski A., et al.: Circadian variation of integrated concentration of growth hormone in children and adults. *J. Clin. Endocrinol. Metab.* 40:240, 1975.
3. Cryer P.E., Jacobs L.S., Daughaday W.H.: Regulation of growth hormone and prolactin secretion in patients with acromegaly and/or excessive prolactin secretion. *Mt. Sinai J. Med.* 40:402, 1973.
4. Blackard W.G., Heidingsfelder S.A.: Adrenergic receptor control mechanisms for growth hormone secretion. *J. Clin. Invest.* 47:1407, 1968.
5. Toivola P.T., Gale C.C.: Stimulation of growth hormone release by microinjection of norepinephrine into hypothalamus of baboons. *Endocrinology* 90:895, 1972.
6. Gil-Ad I., Topper E., Laron Z.: Oral clonidine as a growth hormone stimulation test. *Lancet* 2:278, 1979.
7. Martin J.B.: Functions of central nervous system neurotransmitters in regulation of growth hormone secretion. *Fed. Proc.* 39:2902, 1980.
8. Cryer P.E., Daughaday W.H.: Adrenergic modulation of growth hormone secretion in acromegaly: α- and β-adrenergic blockade produce qualitatively normal responses but no effect on L-dopa suppression. *J. Clin. Endocrinol. Metab.* 44:977, 1977.
9. Camanni F., Picotti G.B., Massara F., et al.: Carbidopa inhibits the growth hormone- and prolactin-suppressive effect of L-dopa in acromegalic patients. *J. Clin. Endocrinol. Metab.* 47:647, 1978.
10. Verde G., Oppizzi G., Colussi G., et al.: Effect of dopamine infusion on plasma levels of growth hormone in normal subjects and in acromegalic patients. *Clin. Endocrinol.* 5:419, 1976.
11. Peillon F., Cesselin F., Bression D., et al.: In vitro effect of dopamine and L-dopa on prolactin and growth hormone release from human pituitary adenomas. *J. Clin. Endocrinol. Metab.* 49:737, 1979.
12. Wass J.A.H., Thorner M.O., Morris D.V., et al.: Long-term treatment of acromegaly with bromocriptine. *Br. Med. J.* 1:875, 1977.
13. Patel Y.C.: Growth hormone stimulates hypothalamic somatostatin. *Life Sci.* 24:1589, 1979.
14. Tannenbaum G.S. Evidence for autoregulation of growth hormone secretion via the central nervous system. *Endocrinology* 107:2117, 1980.
15. Berelowitz M., Harris S.L., Frohman L.A.: Modification of somatostatin

(SRIF) homeostasis by growth hormone (GH): Effect of GH excess and deficiency on hypothalamic SRIF content and release and tissue SRIF distribution. 62nd Annual Meeting, Endocrine Society, Washington, D.C., June 18–20, 1980.

16. Berelowitz M., Szabo M., Firestone S., et al.: Somatomedin C (Sm-C) effects on hypothalamic somatostatin (SRIF) and pituitary growth hormone (GH) release in vitro: Evidence for a negative feedback role in the regulation of GH secretion. *Clin. Res.* 28:28, 760A, 1980.

17. Hagen T.C., Lawrence A.M., Kirsteins L.: Preliminary studies of plasma growth hormone releasing activity during medical therapy of acromegaly. *Horm. Metab. Res.* 10:310, 1978.

18. Besser G.M., Mortimer G.H., McNeilly A.S., et al.: Long-term infusion of growth hormone release inhibiting hormone in acromegaly: Effects on pituitary and pancreatic hormones. *Br. Med. J.* 4:622, 1974.

19. Giustina G., Peracchi M., Reschini E., et al.: Dose-response study of the inhibiting effect of somatostatin on growth hormone and insulin secretion in normal subjects and acromegalic patients. *Metabolism* 24:807, 1975.

20. Faglia G., Beck-Peccoz P., Ferrari C., et al.: Plasma growth hormone response to thyrotropin-releasing hormone in patients with active acromegaly. *J. Clin. Endocrinol. Metab.* 36:1259, 1973.

21. Faglia G., Beck-Peccoz P., Travaglini P., et al.: Elevations in plasma growth hormone concentration after luteinizing hormone-releasing hormone (LRH) in patients with active acromegaly. *J. Clin. Endocrinol. Metab.* 37:338, 1973.

22. Ishibashi M., Yamaji T.: Effect of thyrotropin-releasing hormone and bromoergocriptine on growth hormone and prolactin secretion in perfused pituitary adenoma tissues of acromegaly. *J. Clin. Endocrinol. Metab.* 47:1251, 1978.

23. Faglia G., Paracchi A., Ferrari C., et al.: Evaluation of the results of trans-sphenoidal surgery in acromegaly by assessment of the growth hormone response to thyrotropin-releasing hormone. *Clin. Endocrinol.* 8:373, 1978.

24. Dabek J.T.: Bronchial carcinoid tumour with acromegaly in two patients. *J. Clin. Endocrinol. Metab.* 28:329, 1974.

25. Uz Zafar M.S., Mellinger R.C., Fine G., et al.: Acromegaly associated with a bronchial carcinoid tumor: Evidence for ectopic production of growth hormone-releasing activity. *J. Clin. Endocrinol. Metab.* 48:66, 1979.

26. Shalet S.M., Beardwell C.G., MacFarlane I.A., et al.: Acromegaly due to production of a growth hormone releasing factor by a bronchial carcinoid tumour. *Clin. Endocrinol.* 10:61, 1979.

27. Leveston S.A., McKeel D.W. Jr., Buckley P.J., et al.: Acromegaly and Cushing's syndrome associated with a foregut carcinoid tumor. *J. Clin. Endocrinol. Metab.* 52:682, 1981.

28. Frohman L.A., Szabo M., Berelowitz M., et al.: Partial purification and characterization of a peptide with growth hormone-releasing activity from extrapituitary tumors in patients with acromegaly. *J. Clin. Invest.* 65:43, 1980.

29. Rinderknecht E., Humbel R.E.: The amino acid sequence of human in-

sulin-like growth factor I and its structural homology with proinsulin. *J. Biol. Chem.* 253:2769, 1978.

30. Svoboda M.E., Van Wyk J.J., Klapper D.G., et al.: Purification of somatomedin-C from human plasma: Chemical and biological properties, partial sequence analysis, and relationship to other somatomedins. *Biochemistry-USA* 19:790, 1980.

31. Furlanetto R.W., Underwood L., Van Wyk J.J., et al.: Estimation of somatomedin-C levels in normals and patients with pituitary disease by radioimmunoassay. *J. Clin. Invest.* 60:648, 1977.

32. Rinderknecht E., Humbel R.E.: Primary structure of human insulin-like growth factor II. *FEBS Lett.* 89:283, 1978.

33. Clemmons D.R., Van Wyk J.J., Ridgway E.C., et al.: Evaluation of acromegaly by radioimmunoassay of somatomedin-C. *N. Engl. J. Med.* 301:1138, 1979.

34. Daughaday W.H., Trivedi B., Kapadia M.: Measurement of IGF-II by a specific radioreceptor assay in serum of normal individuals, patients with abnormal GH secretion and patients with tumor associated hypoglycemia. *J. Clin. Endocrinol.* 53:289, 1981.

# Surgical Treatment of Acromegaly: Results in 140 Patients

EDWARD R. LAWS, JR., M.D., RAYMOND V. RANDALL, M.D. AND CHARLES F. ABBOUD, M.D.

*Departments of Neurologic Surgery, Endocrinology/ Metabolism, and Internal Medicine, Mayo Medical School, Mayo Clinic, Rochester, Minnesota*

ACTIVE ACROMEGALY is a relentlessly progressive illness with dire consequences for the patient. The original clinical description of acromegaly was published by Pierre Marie[1] in 1886 and subsequent clinicopathologic correlations by Benda[2] and others showed that the disease was caused by a tumor of the pituitary gland. By 1909, the stage was set for Harvey Cushing[3] to treat an acromegalic patient by "partial hypophysectomy." He used a transsphenoidal approach, and the patient had excellent resolution of symptoms and signs. Cushing treated some 70 acromegalics by transsphenoidal surgery until he abandoned this approach in 1927. For many years thereafter, surgical management in the United States consisted primarily of craniotomy. Acromegalics were at considerable risk because of the lack of steroid replacement therapy and antibiotics, and because of the need for the surgeon to traverse the large frontal sinuses so characteristic of the acromegalic skull. For these reasons, most patients with acromegaly were treated by radiation therapy unless the tumor was large enough to threaten vision by compression of the optic nerves and chiasm.

The transsphenoidal approach to the sella turcica was revived and popularized by Guiot[4] in France, and Hardy[5] contributed the concept of selective microsurgical removal of small pituitary adenomas with preservation of normal gland and its function. With these surgical

225

techniques and proper perioperative management,[6] transsphenoidal microsurgery has become the treatment of choice for the majority of patients with acromegaly.

## Material and Methods

The Mayo Clinic series consists of 140 patients with acromegaly treated by transsphenoidal surgery from November, 1972, through February, 1981. The tumors have been classified according to their size and biologic characteristics. Microadenomas appeared in 36 (26%) patients, diffuse adenoma in 68 (49%), invasive adenoma in 33 (24%), and hyperplasia in 2. Microadenomas are those intrasellar lesions 10 mm or less in diameter. Diffuse adenomas are those that essentially fill the sella but remain enclosed by the dura mater—they may have suprasellar extension. Invasive adenomas are those tumors that invade dura mater, bone, or both—a category defined at surgery. Two patients had pituitary hyperplasia. Eighty-one men and 59 women with an age range of 16 to 75 (mean age, 43.7) were followed up for a mean of 23 months.

All patients were operated on with a standard surgical technique,[7] the goal in most cases being the removal of all tumor and preservation of normal gland.

Clinical and follow-up data were available on all patients with a range of one month to eight years (average, 23 months). Currently, attempts are made to perform dynamic endocrine testing on each patient before and after surgery.[8] A surgical "cure" is defined as a postoperative human growth hormone (hGH) level that suppresses to $\leq 3$ ng/ml during a glucose tolerance test. The most consistent data available, however, continue to be basal fasting hGH levels, and these figures are used as well for an overall view of the series.

## Results

The preoperative mean basal levels of hGH (ng/ml) were as follows: microadenomas, 29.1; diffuse adenomas, 56.2; invasive adenomas, 65.2; and hyperplasia, 23.

Clinical improvement, the least sensitive criterion for surgical success, occurred in all but three of the patients with acromegaly. Little, if any, clinical improvement in acromegalic features occurred in the six patients with gigantism and acromegaly.

Postoperative hGH values were as follows: of 34 patients with microadenomas, 22 (65%) were "cured" (two of these required pituitary replacement); 22 (65%) had a level $\leq$ 5 ng/ml; and 31 (91%) had a level $\leq$ 10 ng/ml. Of 66 patients with diffuse adenomas, 36 (54.5%) were "cured" (two of these required pituitary replacement); 43 (65%) had a level $\leq$ 5 ng/ml; and 53 had a level $\leq$ 10 ng/ml. Of 33 patients with invasive adenomas, 17 (51.5%) were "cured" (one of these required pituitary replacement) and 23 (70%) had a level $\leq$ 10 ng/ml. Complications of surgery included cerebrospinal fluid rhinorrhea (1), intraoperative bleeding (2), carotid artery injury (1), anterior cerebral artery injury (1), postoperative bleeding (2), postoperative sinusitis (1), nasal septal perforation (1), and diabetes insipidus (4); there were no deaths.

## Discussion

The signs and symptoms and age and sex distribution are similar to those in other reports of acromegaly. It is interesting to note that signs and symptoms of mass effect are relatively uncommon (8% of our patients had them), which indicates that early diagnosis is the rule.

The classification of tumors as microadenomas, diffuse adenomas, and invasive adenomas correlates well with the basal preoperative GH levels, suggesting a biologic progression from small, relatively inactive tumors to large, active, and invasive lesions.

The results of surgery clearly suggest that transsphenoidal surgery is most effective when the treated patient has a small, noninvasive lesion producing GH levels $\leq$ 50 ng/ml. This was also stressed by Balagura[9] in his review of Guiot's patients.

Only one patient in this series who appeared initially to be "cured" has developed recurrent active acromegaly, and no patient with mass effect has developed recurrence of the tumor or the symptoms. Postoperative radiotherapy has generally been recommended for those patients with invasive tumors, those with major suprasellar extension, and those with significantly elevated postoperative GH levels.

Very few of the patients who were treated by transsphenoidal microsurgery alone developed postoperative pituitary insufficiency as a result of the surgical procedure.

The role of bromocriptine in the management of acromegaly has not yet been defined. Large doses offer some measure of control of elevated GH levels in about 75% of patients and probably will prevent further enlargement of the tumor, but normal GH levels and dynamics are achieved in only about 25% of patients. The drug can be useful, in some patients with persistent postoperative elevations of GH levels, as adjunctive therapy to subsequent radiation.

A review of published reports of other forms of therapy for acromegaly[10, 11] reveals that transsphenoidal surgery provides the most effective current means of control of the disease and carries minimal morbidity. Results should improve further as more patients with small tumors and early disease are detected and treated.

## REFERENCES

1. Marie P.: Sur deux cas d'acromégalie: Hypertrophie singulière non congénitale des extrémités supérieures, inférieures et céphalique. *Rev. Med. Liege* 6:297, 1886.
2. Benda C.: Beitrage zur normalen und pathologischen histologie der menschlichen hypophysis cerebri. *Berl. Klin. Wochenschr.* 37:1205, 1900.
3. Cushing H.: Partial hypophysectomy for acromegaly. *Ann. Surg.* 50:1002, 1909.
4. Guiot G., Thibaut B.: L'extirpation des adénomes hypophysaires par voie trans-sphénoïdale. *Neurochirurgia (Stuttg)* 1:133, 1959.
5. Hardy J., Wigser S.M.: Trans-sphenoidal surgery of pituitary fossa tumors with televised radiofluoroscopic control. *J. Neurosurg.* 23:612, 1965.
6. Laws E.R. Jr., Abboud C.F., Kern E.B.: Perioperative management of patients with pituitary microadenoma. *Neurosurgery* 7:566, 1980.
7. Laws E.R. Jr.: Transsphenoidal approach to lesions in and about the sella turcica—operative technique, in Schmidek H.H., et al. (eds): *Current Techniques in Operative Neurosurgery.* New York: Grune & Stratton, 1977, pp 161–172.
8. Abboud C.F., Laws E.R. Jr.: Clinical endocrinological approach to hypothalamic disease. *J. Neurosurg.* 51:271, 1979.
9. Balagura S., Derome P., Guiot G.: Acromegaly: Analysis of 132 cases treated surgically. *Neurosurgery.* 8:413, 1981.
10. Laws E.R. Jr., Piepgras D.G., Randall R.V., et al.: Neurosurgical management of acromegaly: Results in 82 patients treated between 1972 and 1977. *J. Neurosurg.* 50:454, 1979.
11. Laws E.R. Jr.: Transsphenoidal microsurgery in the management of acromegaly, in Smith (ed): *Neuro-Ophthalmology Focus, 1980.* New York: Masson Publ., 1980. pp 289–293.

# Acknowledgment

The authors are grateful to Mrs. Connie Hoeft for her expert assistance in preparing the manuscript.

# The Chemistry and Physiology of Prolactin

E.A. COWDEN, M.D., I. LANCRAJAN, M.D., AND
H.G. FRIESEN, M.D.

*Department of Physiology, Faculty of Medicine,
University of Manitoba, Winnipeg, Canada*

## Introduction

ALTHOUGH it had been established in the late 1920s that the anterior pituitary contained some agent that stimulated milk secretion in the developed mammary gland, Riddle et al.[1] first used the term prolactin (PRL) in 1933 to describe the distinct anterior pituitary hormone that stimulated crop "milk" production when injected into pigeons or ring doves. Ovine PRL was isolated and purified by 1937[2] and in species other than primates little difficulty was encountered in identifying distinct lactogenic hormones in pituitary extracts by the use of appropriate bioassays.[3, 4]

Because of its apparent antiquity, versatility of action, and physiologic evolution in vertebrate phylogeny, PRL received considerable attention from comparative endocrinologists, neuroendocrinologists, and zoologists. Until the early 1970s there was considerable doubt whether the human pituitary gland secreted a separate PRL molecule at all. In retrospect, several factors contributed to the difficulty in identifying human PRL (hPRL): (1) GH is present in 100-fold excess of PRL in the human pituitary, (2) GH and PRL have many physical and chemical properties in common, and (3) human GH (hGH) has considerable lactogenic activity. Nevertheless, there were both compelling clinical data[5, 6] to suggest the separate existence of hPRL and the very astute and courageous speculation of Forbes and her colleagues[7] that the amenorrhea-galactorrhea syndrome might be due to the presence of a PRL-secreting tumor of the pituitary gland.

0-8151-3530-0/82/006-229-236-$03.75

The controversy of course was resolved with the isolation and purification of hPRL,[8,9] based on the key immunologic differences between that molecule and hGH. A sensitive and specific radioimmunoassay for PRL was subsequently developed.[10] Thus, over the past ten years it has been possible for the clinician to study human PRL status in health and disease and gain some appreciation of its relevance in clinical practice.

## Source of hPRL

Human prolactin is secreted by the anterior pituitary, which contains between 100 and 500 μg hPRL per gland,[11] and the pituitary thus initially provided the sole source of hPRL for purification. However, the observation that in early pregnancy PRL concentrations in amniotic fluid were greatly in excess of those in either maternal or fetal serum[12,13] caused speculation on its origin. It now seems clear that human decidua[14] and even nonpregnant late-luteal-phase endometrium[15] can secrete hPRL that is chemically and immunologically indistinguishable from human pituitary PRL, and thus amniotic fluid now provides a useful source of the hormone as well.

## Physiologic Control of PRL Secretion

The physiologic control of PRL secretion is dealt with in detail in other parts of this volume and the subject has been extensively reviewed.[16-18] In summary, control of PRL secretion is effected predominantly under the inhibitory influence of dopamine (PIF), which reacts with specific dopamine receptors on pituitary lactotrophs.[19] There is also evidence for one or more prolactin-releasing factors (PRF), and PRL may exert negative feedback control over its own secretion. That there are, moreover, extensive central connections of neurons directly involved in the control of PRL secretion emphasizes the fact that the widely differing psychic, physical, chemical, and pharmacologic stimuli that have been observed in vivo to affect PRL status may do so by interaction at any of several sites.

## PRL Secretion in Health and Disease

Scientific interest in a particular field fluctuates greatly from time to time as new approaches or applications burst upon the scene. This phenomenon is aptly illustrated by a survey of literature on PRL. The identification of the hormone as a separate pituitary product in the human, subsequent ability to measure prolactin in serum under physiologic conditions, and the recognition of hyperprolactinemia as an important clinical entity have sparked enormous interest in PRL in the past decade.

Early in this explosion of knowledge came the recognition that not all patients who have elevated PRL levels have galactorrhea,[20] and conversely, that patients with profuse galactorrhea may have normal PRL concentrations.[21] It was quickly ascertained that elevated PRL levels could arise under numerous physiologic circumstances (Table 1), but it has taken rather longer to fully appreciate the variety of factors, such as sex, age, circadian rhythm, pulsatility of secretion, stress, and drug ingestion, that may affect PRL status, even in healthy individuals.[22, 23]

Only rarely has deficiency of PRL been reported,[24, 25] and in the adult it seems to be associated with little if any morbidity.

By contrast, pathologic hyperprolactinemia (see Table 1) is common. Indeed, it may be the most frequent hypothalamic-pituitary disorder seen in clinical practice, commonly presenting as it does with oligoamenorrhea and infertility in females and impotence in males.[26-28] The exact mechanism whereby elevated prolactin levels cause hypogonadism remains obscure, but certainly there is impairment of cyclic gonadotrophin release,[29] and at the level of the female gonad suppression of ovarian steroid secretion may be involved.[30, 31]

In the male, hyperprolactinemia may diminish peripheral conversion of testosterone to its more potent metabolite dihydrotestosterone and thus contribute to male hypogonadism.[32]

TABLE 1.—HYPERPROLACTINEMIA: A CLASSIFICATION

| PHYSIOLOGIC FACTORS | PATHOLOGIC FACTORS |
|---|---|
| Newborn | Hypothalamic disorders |
| Pregnancy | Pituitary disorders |
| Nursing mothers | Hypothalamic—pituitary stalk "irritation" |
| | Head injury |
| Stress | Primary hypothyroidism |
| Sleep-related nocturnal rhythm | Renal disease |
| Drugs | Idiopathic |
|   Dopamine receptor blockers | |
|     Phenothiazines | |
|     Metoclopramide | |
|   Dopamine depleting agents | |
|     α-methyl dopa | |
|     Reserpine | |
|   Others | |
|     Estrogens | |
|     TRH | |

## PRL: Physiologic Function and Mechanisms of Action

Despite the fact that men and women have remarkably similar basal PRL concentrations, the only physiologic function of PRL for which there is direct evidence is a lactogenic one.[33] It has been clearly demonstrated that the hormone increases casein production by primed mammary tissue by both increasing the rate of transcription of mRNA coding for casein and prolonging its half-life. The search for a nonlactogenic function for PRL in the human continues to evoke considerable interest, of course, particularly in view of the wide diversity of physiologic functions served by the hormone in the animal kingdom.[34]

It is now generally accepted that PRL initiates its action by binding to a cell surface receptor[35] that appears to be a very large glycoprotein molecule composed of several subunits. After PRL binds to its receptor, the complex is internalized, but it is not yet clear whether its biologic action is mediated by a second intracellular messenger. Prolactin binding may also be demonstrated in the Golgi apparatus,[36] but whether this represents receptor en route for degradation and disposal or receptor that is newly synthesized remains unclear, as does its physiologic significance.

In any event, traditionally it was thought that the magnitude of biologic response in a given tissue was governed only by the concentration of hormone, such as PRL. Since the discovery of hormone receptors and the demonstration that these are dynamically controlled by trophic factors, it is clear that receptors themselves may play a major role in determining the sensitivity of target tissues to hormones in the blood—a speculation particularly attractive to the clinician, who not infrequently encounters patients with circulating hormone levels that do not appear to correlate with anticipated biologic responses.

## Molecular Heterogeneity of Circulating PRL

Although heterogeneity in molecular size of immunologically detected hPRL in blood, amniotic fluid, pituitary extracts, and cerebrospinal fluid is well established, the nature, source and interrelationships between the various molecular species are poorly understood.[37-39] Three major immunoreactive peaks have been consistently identified with chromatographically determined molecular weights of 170,000 daltons, 48,000 daltons, and 23,000 daltons. The formal identity of these molecules has yet to be established, but recently it has been demonstrated that each of these forms is detectable in normal human sera and that each species is biologically active.[40]

This has been possible by the use of a new and exceedingly sensitive bioassay for lactogenic hormones that is of particular interest to the clinician. Since the assay has a sensitivity equal to or exceeding conventional radioimmunoassays for PRL, it allows, for the first time, a direct comparison of immunologic and biologic activity of PRL at physiologic concentrations.[41] The assay is based on the specific ability of lactogenic hormones to stimulate replication of a rat lymphoma cell line in suspension culture. The assay is more sensitive, less time-consuming, less manpower intensive, and has a greater sample capacity than conventional bioassays.

Recently, in the mouse[42] and the rat,[43] species of PRL have been identified in pituitary extracts and in circulation that have biologic activity in excess of immunologic activity. Indeed, it has also been reported that a newly identified PRL moiety—a 16k posttranscriptionally cleaved molecule[44]—may have distinct functions from the longer recognized 23k intact molecule.[45] In the human, structural and functional heterogeneity of PRL molecules has long been a matter of speculation, and in a preliminary study using the new lymphoma cell bioassay and conventional radioimmunoassay, some individuals have been identified in whom lactogenic activity exceeds immunologically measured PRL levels. There are also patients in whom the reverse is true: their elevated immunologically detected PRL levels are not associated with comparable biologic activity.

## Chemistry and Genetic Structure of hPRL

Pituitary PRL has now been purified from a number of amphibian, avian, and mammalian species. The human hormone is composed of 199 amino acids with three disulfide bonds. The complete amino acid sequence of hPRL was first reported in 1977.[46] More recently, the nucleotide sequence of the complementary DNA (cDNA) for hPRL has been described.[47] Earlier reports that PRL might be "the" ancestral pituitary hormone, a hormone derived from a primordial peptide by gene duplication and evolving into placental lactogen and GH,[48] appear to have been substantiated, and it seems that the PRL molecule probably diverged from GH and placental lactogen (PL) some 300 million years ago, while GH and PL diverged a mere 56 million years ago! It is also interesting that while the genes for GH and PL are now localized on chromosome 17, the prolactin gene is found on chromosome 6.

The possibility that previously unsuspected forms of PRL may exist and have considerable physiologic and pathologic significance is, as previously discussed, a topical one and is supported by the fact that the PRL gene is enormous—about 11 kilobases (kb) in size compared to 2.6 and 2.8 for GH and PL genes, while all three peptide molecules are of comparable size.[49]

## Conclusion

Measurement of serum prolactin concentration is now an essential part of the routine investigation of patients with suspected hypothalamic-pituitary dysfunction and in the past decade a knowledge of prolactin status in health and disease has become necessary for a wide spectrum of clinicians, from neurosurgeons to nephrologists.

We have certainly advanced considerably in the last few years, but clearly, much remains to be elucidated, and our continued study of both the chemistry and physiology of this latest but not least pituitary hormone should be productive for some time to come.

REFERENCES

1. Riddle O., Bates, R.W., Dykshorn S.W.: The preparation, identification and assay of prolactin—a hormone of the anterior pituitary. *Am. J. Physiol.* 105:191, 1933.
2. White A., Catchpole H.R., Long C.N.H.: A crystalline protein with high lactogenic activity. *Science* 86:82, 1937.
3. Nicoll C.S.: Bioassay of prolactin: Analysis of the pigeon crop-sac response to local prolactin injection by an objective and quantitative method. *Endocrinology* 80:641, 1967.
4. Frantz A.G., Kleinberg D.L.: Prolactin: Evidence that it is separate from growth hormone in human blood. *Science* 170:745, 1970.
5. Rimoin D.L., Holzman G.B., Merimee T.J., et al.: Lactation in the absence of human growth hormone. *J. Clin. Endocrinol. Metab.* 28:1183, 1968.
6. Peake G.T., McKeel D.W., Jarett L., et al.: Ultrastructural, histologic and hormonal characterization of a prolactin-rich human pituitary tumor. *J. Clin. Endocrinol. Metab.* 29:1383, 1969.
7. Forbes A.P., Henneman P.H., Griswold G.C., et al.: Syndrome characterized by galactorrhea, amenorrhea and low urinary FSH: Comparison with acromegaly and normal lactation. *J. Clin. Endocrinol. Metab.* 14:265, 1954.
8. Friesen H., Guyda H., Hardy J.: Biosynthesis of human growth hormone and prolactin. *J. Clin. Endocrinol. Metab.* 31:611, 1970.
9. Hwang P., Friesen H.G., Hardy J., et al.: Biosynthesis of human growth hormone and prolactin by normal pituitary glands and pituitary adenomas. *J. Clin. Endocrinol. Metab.* 33:1, 1971a.
10. Hwang P., Guyda H., Friesen H.: A radioimmunoassay for human prolactin. *Proc. Natl. Acad. Sci. U.S.A.* 68:1902, 1971b.

11. Friesen H.G., McNeilly A.S.: Nature of prolactin and its measurement, in Martini L., et al. (eds): *Clinical Neuroendocrinology.* New York: Academic Press, 1977.
12. Tyson J.E., Hwang P., Guyda H., et al.: Studies of prolactin secretion in human pregnancy. *Am. J. Obstet. Gynecol.* 113:14, 1972.
13. Clements J.A., Reyes F.I., Winter J.S.D., et al.: Studies on human sexual development: IV. Fetal pituitary and serum and amniotic fluid concentrations of prolactin. *J. Clin. Endocrinol. Metab.* 44:408, 1977.
14. Riddick D.H., Kusmik W.F.: Decidua: A possible source of amniotic fluid prolactin. *Am. J. Obstet. Gynecol.* 127:187, 1977.
15. Maslar I.A., Kaplan B.M., Luciano A.A., et al.: Prolactin production by the endometrium of early human pregnancy. *J. Clin. Endocrinol. Metab.* 51:78, 1980.
16. Tindal J.S.: Hypothalamic control of secretion and release of prolactin. *J. Reprod. Fertil.* 39:437, 1974.
17. Tindal J.S.: Control of prolactin secretion, in Jeffcoate S.L., et al. (eds): *The Endocrine Hypothalamus.* New York: Academic Press, 1978.
18. Neill J.D.: Neuroendocrine regulation of prolactin secretion, in Martini L., et al. (eds): *Frontiers in Neuroendocrinology.* New York: Raven Press, 1980, vol 6, pp 129–155.
19. Cronin M.J., Cheung C.Y., Wilson C.B., et al.: $^3$H Spiperone binding to human anterior pituitaries and pituitary adenomas secreting prolactin, growth hormone and adrenocorticotropic hormone. *J. Clin. Endocrinol. Metab.* 50:387, 1980.
20. Friesen H., Hwang P., Guyda H., et al.: A radioimmunoassay for human prolactin, in Boyns A.R., et al. (eds): *Prolactin and Carvinogenesis: Fourth Tenovus Workshop.* Cardiff: Alpha Omega Alpha, 1972.
21. Frantz A.G., Kleinberg D.L., Noel G.: Studies on prolactin in man. *Recent Prog. Horm. Res.* 28:527, 1972.
22. Jeffcoate S.L.: Diagnosis of hyperprolactinaemia. *Lancet* 2:1245, 1978.
23. Cowden E.A., Ratcliffe W.A., Beastall G.H., et al.: Laboratory assessment of prolactin status. *Ann. Clin. Biochem.* 16:113, 1979.
24. Turkington R.W.: The clinical endocrinology of prolactin. *Adv. Intern. Med.* 18:363, 1972.
25. Carlson H.E., Brickman A.S., Bottazzo G.F.: Prolactin deficiency in pseudohypoparathyroidism. *N. Engl. J. Med.* 296:140, 1977.
26. Jacobs H.S., Franks S., Murray M.A.F., et al.: Clinical and endocrine features of hyperprolactinaemic amenorrhoea. *Clin. Endocrinol. (Oxf.)* 5:439, 1976.
27. Franks S., Nabarro J.D.N., Jacobs H.S.: Prevalence and presentation of hyperprolactinaemia in patients with "functionless" pituitary tumours. *Lancet* 1:778, 1977.
28. Carter J.N., Tyson J.E., Tolis G., et al.: Prolactin-secreting tumors and hypogonadism in 22 men. *N. Engl. J. Med.* 299:847, 1978.
29. Tyson J.E., Khojandi M., Huth J., et al.: Inhibition of cyclic gonadotropic secretion by endogenous human prolactin. *Gynecology* 121:375, 1974.
30. McNatty K.P., Savers R.S., McNeilly A.S.: A possible role for prolactin in control of steroid secretion by the human graafian follicle. *Nature* 250:653, 1974.
31. McNeilly A.S.: Paradoxical prolactin. *Nature* 284:212, 1980.

32. Magrini G., Ebiner J.R., Burckhardt P., et al.: Study on the relationship between plasma prolactin levels and androgen metabolism in man. *J. Clin. Endocrinol. Metab.* 43:944, 1976.
33. Guyette W.A., Matusik R.J., Rosen J.M.: Prolactin-mediated transcriptional and posttranscriptional control of casein gene expression. *Cell* 17:1013, 1979.
34. Nicoll C.S.: Physiological actions of prolactin, in Greep R.O., et al. (eds): *Handbook of Physiology: Section 7. Endocrinology*. Washington, D.C.: American Physiological Society, 1974, vol 4, part 2.
35. Shiu R.P.C., Friesen H.G.: Regulation of prolactin receptors in target cells, in Lefkowitz R.J. (ed): *Receptor Regulation*. London: Chapman and Hall, 1980.
36. Posner B.I., Josefsberg Z., Bergerson J.M.: Intracellular polypeptide hormone receptors. *J. Biol. Chem.* 254:11294, 1979.
37. Suh H.K., Frantz A.G.: Size heterogeneity of human prolactin in plasma and pituitary extracts. *J. Clin. Endocrinol. Metab.* 39:928, 1974.
38. Fang V.S., Refetoff S.: Heterogeneous human prolactin from a giant pituitary tumor in a patient with panhypopituitarism. *J. Clin. Endocrinol. Metab.* 47:780, 1978.
39. Garnier P.E., Aubert M.L., Kaplan S.L., et al.: Heterogeneity of pituitary and plasma prolactin in man: Decreased affinity of "big" prolactin in a radioreceptor assay and evidence for its secretion. *J. Clin. Endocrinol. Metab.* 47:1273, 1978.
40. Cowden E.A., Friesen H.G., Gout P.W., et al.: Biologically active circulating prolactin in uremia. *Clin. Res.* 28:695A, 1980.
41. Tanaka T., Shiu R.P.C., Gout P.W., et al.: A new sensitive and specific bioassay for lactogenic hormones: Measurement of prolactin and growth hormone in human serum. *J. Clin. Endocrinol. Metab.* 51:1058, 1980.
42. Sinha Y.N.: Molecular size variants of prolactin and growth hormone in mouse serum: Strain differences and alterations of concentrations of physiological and pharmacological stimuli. *Endocrinology* 107:1959, 1980.
43. Asawaroengchai H., Russell S.M., Nicoll C.S.: Electrophoretically separable forms of rat prolactin with different bioassay and radioimmunoassay activities. *Endocrinology* 102:407, 1978.
44. Mittra I.: A novel "cleaved prolactin" in the rat pituitary: Part 1. Biosynthesis, characterization and regulatory control. *Biochem. Biophys. Res. Commun.* 95:1750, 1980.
45. Mittra I.: A novel "cleaved prolactin" in the rat pituitary: Part 11. In vivo mammary mitogenic activity of its N-terminal 16K moiety. *Biochem. Biophys. Res. Commun.* 95:1760, 1980.
46. Shome B., Parlow A.F.: Human pituitary prolactin (hPRL): The entire linear amino acid sequence. *J. Clin. Endocrinol. Metab.* 45:1112, 1977.
47. Cooke N.E., Coitt D., Shine J., et al.: The nucleotide sequence of human prolactin cDNA. *J. Biol. Chem.* In press.
48. Schwartz T.B.: What you always wanted to know about prolactin but were afraid to ask, in Schwartz T.B. (ed): Year Book of Endocrinology. Chicago: Year book Medical Publishers, Inc., 1973.
49. Chien Y., Thompson E.B.: Genomic organization of rat prolactin and growth hormone genes. *Proc. Natl. Acad. Sci. U.S.A.* 77:4583, 1980.

# The Amenorrhea-Galactorrhea Syndrome: Clinical Features

ANNE P. FORBES, M.D.

*Clinical Professor of Medicine Emerita, Harvard University Medical School, Honorary Consultant, Massachusetts General Hospital*

In 1954 we described 15 patients with amenorrhea and persistent lactation whom we had seen with Dr. Fuller Albright in his clinic.[1] Our report was by no means the first, since we were able to refer to five prior articles on the syndrome. Argonz and del Castillo's[2] paper appeared the year before ours, and they, as well as we, referred to Frommel[3] who had written about the syndrome 72 years before they did, citing Chiari[4] who had described the same disorder 27 years before that. The 1954 article nevertheless provides a good starting point for a discussion of the clinical features of the syndrome, as we can now reexamine each of the seven major points that it made and see how all but one of them have had to be modified with time.

Our first premise, that the disease was distinct from acromegaly, was based on the appearance of the patients and the fact that they had normal levels of serum phosphorus. Acromegaly may be associated with amenorrhea and galactorrhea but by the time that gonadal function has been compromised in acromegaly, there is an elevated serum phosphorus.[5] In 1954 there were no good specific assays for GH or prolactin. The two hormones have so much in common physiologically, structurally, and immunologically that it was another 16 years before their separate identities could be proved. The distinction from acromegaly was confirmed by Frantz and Kleinberg[6] in 1970, when they developed a sensitive bioassay for prolactin and, by using a highly specific antibody to GH, which is lactogenic in its own right, were able to separate the two hormones. It turned out that 30% to

0-851-3530-0/82/006-237-254-$03.75

40% of acromegalics produce excessive prolactin,[7, 8] but that GH is not elevated in patients with the galactorrhea-amenorrhea syndrome.[8] None of our original 15 patients subsequently developed acromegaly.

The cardinal feature of the syndrome pointed out by us and our predecessors was galactorrhea. The lactation followed pregnancy in only one of the 15 patients, nine of whom had never been pregnant. The chronicity of the galactorrhea was impressive. Six of our patients had lactated for more than 12 years. Patient I.R. has now been lactating for more than 40 years, patient J.R. stopped spontaneously after 14 years, and patient M.F. after 25 years. Yet, although all our patients had galactorrhea, because that was how we identified the syndrome, we might have suspected that this feature was not invariably present since one of our patients had had amenorrhea for two years before galactorrhea was observed and another patient, who continued to have amenorrhea, had ceased to lactate five years before we saw her.

We now know that somewhat less than a third of patients with the amenorrhea-galactorrhea syndrome have galactorrhea. Jacobs et al.[9] noted galactorrhea in only 37% of patients with amenorrhea and hyperprolactinemia. Franks and Nabarro[10] found galactorrhea in only 28% of a series of patients with pituitary tumor and hypersecretion of prolactin. Molitch and Reichlin[11] summarized the literature on the incidence of hyperprolactinemia in women with amenorrhea. They collected 654 patients with amenorrhea without galactorrhea from seven reported series. Of these, 12.8% had hyperprolactinemia. Galactorrhea may or may not accompany the amenorrhea caused by oral contraceptives, phenothiazines, and other drugs. Kleinberg et al.[8] studied 235 patients who presented with galactorrhea and noted that in a number of them amenorrhea had preceded the galactorrhea for months to years. Thus although galactorrhea is easily missed by both patients and doctors, and although it is not rare but common when systematically looked for, it is nevertheless more often absent than present in the amenorrhea-galactorrhea syndrome.

Galactorrhea is the exception in the hyperprolactinemic syndrome in males.[12] Since prolactin cannot initiate lactation except in mammary tissue adequately primed by estrogen and progesterone, it is not surprising that most males with hyperprolactinemia do not lactate. Only 13 of the 235 patients with galactorrhea studied by Kleinberg et al. were male and most of them had a history of estrogen treatment, Klinefelter's syndrome, or other cause for gynecomastia. The infrequency of galactorrhea in male patients explains why none of the early reports of the syndrome mention the existence of the hyper-prolactinemia syndrome in males. Even when it became possible to measure prolactin the syndrome was not looked for in men except when there was galactorrhea or an obvious, usually a large, pituitary tumor. Most of the male patients reported therefore have had ma-croadenomas, not microadenomas. Carter et al.,[12] in presenting a se-ries of male patients with the hyperprolactinemia syndrome, makes the point that the tumors were more advanced and loss of pituitary functions was more frequent in them than in female patients. Male patients without detectable tumors were not at first recognized. When it was found that hyperprolactinemia in men causes impaired testosterone production, impotence, and decreased spermatogenesis and that bromocriptine treatment can often reverse these effects,[13] it became mandatory to look for hyperprolactinemia in males with unexplained impotence or infertility, hence less advanced cases of the syndrome began to emerge. Saidi et al.[14] treated 11 males with de-creased or absent spermatogenesis and marginally elevated prolac-tins and obtained striking increases in plasma testosterone and in sperm count with bromocriptine.

The third feature by which we characterized our syndrome was amenorrhea, yet one of the 15 patients had irregular menses, not amenorrhea, while two more had had galactorrhea for six and two years respectively before their periods ceased. Seventy-six of the 235 patients with galactorrhea studied by Kleinberg and Frantz had "id-iopathic galactorrhea" without amenorrhea and eight patients with galactorrhea associated with pituitary tumor had menses, albeit ir-regular in most of them. In some of the patients with both galactor-rhea and amenorrhea the galactorrhea had preceded the amenor-rhea. We now know that many patients with the hyperprolactinemia syndrome have oligoamenorrhea rather than amenorrhea and some have an even more subtle disorder, regular ovulatory periods with a defective luteal phase.[15] The fact that amenorrhea is not necessary for the clinical definition of the amenorrhea-galactorrhea syndrome has important implications for the investigation of infertility. It may be of interest that our patient J.R., who had irregular periods, had four pregnancies during the 13 years of our observation of her but at least two pregnancies ended in spontaneous abortion. The galactor-rhea continued throughout these pregnancies. Carter et al.[16] mention a high abortion rate in patients with prolactinomas who conceive on bromocriptine therapy and then stop treatment as soon as pregnancy occurs.

Despite the many exceptions that have been pointed out, hypoestrinism remains the rule in hyperprolactinemia. It was considered a cardinal feature of the syndrome by Argonz and del Castillo, although one of their patients also had oligomenorrhea, not amenorrhea, and another had one normal pregnancy during the 15 years in which she had galactorrhea and infrequent periods. The hypoestrinism was demonstrated in our cases by failure of all but one patient to have withdrawal bleeding following a course of progesterone. It has since been well documented by measurements of plasma estradiol.[9, 11, 17, 18]

Two mechanisms are currently offered as explanation for decreased ovarian function in hyperprolactinemia. One is a direct action of prolactin on ovarian follicles to inhibit steroidogenesis. The ovary has receptors for prolactin; in fact, it takes up more isotopically labelled prolactin than does mammary tissue.[19] McNatty et al.[20] found the mean concentration of prolactin in ovarian follicular fluid slightly higher than that in blood. As follicles enlarged the concentration fell while the total content of the follicle remained the same. Small amounts of prolactin were necessary for steroidogenesis by isolated granulosa cells while concentrations above 20 ng/ml inhibited the synthesis of progesterone.

The second mechanism offered is a direct action of prolactin on the hypothalamic LRF releasing mechanism. In hyperprolactinemia the hypothalamus becomes less sensitive to the negative feedback effect of estrogen,[21] as well as to its positive, LH-releasing, action.[22] Thus LH levels may be low and mid-cycle LH surges absent in hyperprolactinemia, while the integrity of the pituitary gonadotropin-producing cells can be demonstrated by a normal response to exogenous LRF.[23]

We compared the amenorrhea of our 15 patients to that of a series of normal nursing mothers whom we studied. The normal mothers who were amenorrheic also failed to flow following progesterone injections. Nevertheless, nursing mothers, like patients with the amenorrhea-galactorrhea syndrome, may or may not have amenorrhea. Often they have amenorrhea for three or four months, then resume menstruation despite continuing to nurse their babies. From the studies of Rolland et al.[24] we know that the resumption of estrogen production in the nursing mothers coincides with a decrease in prolactin, which falls steadily after the early postpartum period despite continued lactation. It remains slightly above the normal for nonlactating women until weaning is complete. Delvoye[25] studied mothers in central Africa who nurse their babies for one to two years. Serum prolactins were still slightly elevated 15 months postpartum and 80% to

85% of the mothers were still amenorrheic. The birth spacing among these women was 36 to 39 months.

FSH levels rise to normal follicular phase levels within one to two weeks after delivery. The fact that estradiol levels remain low for months after FSH has returned to normal accords with the theory that prolactin interferes directly with ovarian steroidogenesis. The fact that the FSH does not rise to high levels in the face of deficient production of estrogen accords with the theory that prolactin interferes with the negative feedback control of the hypothalamus by estrogen.

In 1954 we supposed that when a patient had amenorrhea associated with a pituitary tumor, the amenorrhea must be the result either of destruction of the gonadotropin-producing cells or of blockage of their access to stimuli coming from the hypothalamus. Neither mechanism would be necessarily reversed by the removal of tumor tissue. The realization that amenorrhea or infertility in most patients with pituitary tumor is caused not by an anatomical defect but by the reversible metabolic action of prolactin has completely altered the outlook for fertility and the approach to management of patients with the amenorrhea-galactorrhea syndrome. The further realization that these same metabolic actions of prolactin are responsible for the physiologic infertility accompanying normal lactation cannot help but raise hopes of finding a harmless way to produce a similar infertility at will.

The absence of ovarian steroidogenesis in physiologic lactation, since it usually lasts for a few months only, is not likely to be associated with important side effects of estrogen deficiency. The more rapid involution of the uterus in nursing than in nonnursing mothers is considered beneficial and is entirely reversible. Even in the amenorrhea-galactorrhea syndrome, where uterine atrophy, as pointed out by Frommel, is very marked and may last for years, it does not seem to be a bar to resumption of fertility when ovulation is restored by treatment. Dyspareunia is mentioned in a number of reports of the amenorrhea-galactorrhea syndrome and is presumably based on atrophic changes in the vagina. Those changes are likewise readily reversible. The effects of chronic estrogen deficiency on bone are less benign. Klibanski et al.[26] have recently pointed out a measurable degree of osteopenia in patients with the amenorrhea-galactorrhea syndrome. They noted also that the degree of osteoporosis correlated with the degree of estrogen deficiency among the patients.

Our series provides no information on this point. Although several of the patients have been followed for as long as twenty years, they have received adequate estrogen replacement therapy for most of that time. Our index patient, I.R., was treated cyclically with estrogen, sometimes in high dosage, for 30 years. Estrogen diminished the galactorrhea, which resumed in force four or five days after each course was stopped, so that the patient had estrogen withdrawal lactation as well as estrogen withdrawal uterine bleeding once a month. We now know that this treatment might have been stimulating prolactin production by the pituitary at the same time that it was inhibiting the effect of prolactin on the breast. In 1960 the patient developed hypertension and reserpine was added to her therapy. It did not make the galactorrhea any better or worse. In 1973, because of an episode of congestive failure, the estrogen was stopped. After that the galactorrhea became more troublesome. On one or two occasions swelling and pain in one or other breast was relieved only by breast pumping. The patient resorted to regular visits to the obstetric service of her local hospital for breast pumping. We now know that this maneuver alone can perpetuate the syndrome.[18]

Microadenomas have been identified in some patients whose galactorrhea followed pregnancy or prolonged use of oral contraceptives, leading to the suggestion that estrogen therapy could cause or accelerate the development of a prolactinoma.[11] Since estrogen stimulates pituitary lactotropes in vitro and since it can cause prolactinomas in rats,[28] it has been assumed that the enlargement of the normal pituitary and of some prolactinomas that occurs in pregnancy is caused by the increase in circulating estrogen. It is therefore of interest that patient I.R., whose routine skull x-rays made in the 1950s showed no evidence of tumor, had polytomes in 1974 that showed the sella still normal in size and configuration. By then she had had galactorrhea and amenorrhea for 43 years and had received estrogen for 19 years. In 1975 a prolactin assay was obtained and showed 5.4 ng/ml, which constitutes further evidence against an unrecognized prolactinoma.

The fourth feature of the syndrome that we emphasized in 1954 was a low urinary FSH. The assay used was the mouse uterine weight assay, a test not highly specific for FSH but to some extent a measure of total urinary gonadotropins. In normal men and women the test was always positive for at least 6.5 MU/24 hours and usually for 13. It might or might not be positive for 26 MU/24 hours and was negative for 52. Of our 15 patients nine had no demonstrable gonadotropin in the urine and three had more than 6.5 but less than 13 MU/24 hours, which is at the lower limit of the normal range. The values were in contrast to those of the normal nursing mothers who excreted more than 13 MU/24 hours in every case and up to 52 in some. The values were as high in nursing mothers as in a comparable group of mothers who did not breast-feed; moreover, they were as high in the first few weeks of lactation, when, as we now know, prolactin levels are very high, as they were some months later. Rolland et al.[24] had radioimmunoassays specific for FSH and LH available to them. They found that FSH is suppressed during pregnancy, presumably by the high levels of circulating estrogen, but returns to normal about a month after delivery whether or not the mother is nursing. LH, on the other hand, remains at low levels and the duration of LH suppression appears to be related to nursing and to the duration of elevated prolactin. At this stage, according to Crystle et al.[28] the administration of exogenous estrogen will effect the hypothalamic release of LHRF, indicating that the low LH is the result of underproduction of estrogen by the inhibited ovary rather than of inability of the hypothalamus to respond to the LH-releasing stimulus of an estrogen peak. In the amenorrhea-galactorrhea syndrome it is not surprising that the patients who do not have amenorrhea do not have an abnormally low FSH. Some of the patients who do have amenorrhea, particularly those with pituitary tumors, do have a diminished FSH, but others, like the normal lactating woman, have normal levels of FSH with low LH or LH that remains at preovulatory levels without ovulatory surge and luteal phase elevation.

Another feature that characterized many of our patients, although we did not consider it an invariable feature of the syndrome, was evidence of mild hyperfunction of the adrenal glands. Weight gain, seborrhea or acne, and some degree of hirsutism had appeared at the same time as the galactorrhea in several patients. The level of urinary 17 ketosteroids in those patients was above average for their age although not outside the normal range. In Jacobs'[9] series of 30 women with "functionless" pituitary tumors and secondary amenorrhea, hirsutism was the presenting complaint of four patients. Five of 20 patients in Seppälä and Hirvonen's[29] series of patients with secondary amenorrhea and prolactin levels greater than 30 ng/ml, were hirsute. Lavric[30] reported two patients with irregular periods and galactorrhea who complained of obesity and hirsutism and had large, sclerocystic ovaries. Lamotte[31] reported a patient with galactorrhea, irregular menses, and infertility who had "orange-sized" ovaries. Mulla[32] reported a similar patient who resumed periods and became pregnant following wedge resection of the ovaries. Thorner[33] stated that a "subset" of patients with hyperprolactinemia have a disorder of androgen production simulating the polycystic ovary syndrome.

It so happens that the ovaries were examined in three of our 15 patients who had obesity and hirsutism as well as galactorrhea and amenorrhea. The ovaries in all three were found to be small and atrophic.

As McNatty et al.[20] showed, a concentration of prolactin greater than 20 ng/ml is inhibitory to steroid production by human ovarian granulosa cells. There is also good evidence that an excess of prolactin inhibits testosterone production by the testis,[12] although a small amount may be permissive.[34] It seems likely that excessive androgen production in patients with hyperprolactinemia originates in the adrenal gland rather than in the ovary. Plasma dehydroepiandrosterone sulfate is elevated in patients with the galactorrhea-amenorrhea syndrome.[35-37] Moreover, ovarian androgen production in the polycystic ovary (PCO) syndrome is associated with an increased output of LH, whereas LH is usually diminished in the hyperprolactinemia syndromes. Recently Quigley et al.[38] measured prolactin levels in women with the PCO syndrome. Although the patients did not have hyperprolactinemia, infusions of dopamine caused more LH suppression in the patients than in normal people. The authors hypothesized that the elevated LH in women with polycystic ovaries resulted from tonic positive feedback to the hypothalamus caused by chronically elevated estrogen, and that dopaminergic cells are subject to modulation by estrogen. The authors described acute experiments and do not report a clinical trial of bromocriptine therapy in the PCO syndrome. We must await the results of such trials before speculating further on the relation of the PCO syndrome to the amenorrhea-galactorrhea syndrome.

The last condition laid down for the definition of the amenorrhea-galactorrhea syndrome was, in 1954, a presumptive one, namely hypersecretion of prolactin. At that time the chromophobe cell was thought not to be a secretory cell and in the two of our six patients with enlarged sellas who underwent operation the tumor tissue was found to be chromophobic. We assumed that the chromophobe cells were "preeosinophilic" secretory cells making prolactin and we further assumed that the patients who did not have tumors, because they had the same disease, were also making too much prolactin. The presumption has been considered a shrewd guess. Was it in fact correct? It has proved to be true in the main for patients with tumors. Most patients with galactorrhea and pituitary tumors have prolactin levels greater than 200 ng/ml; levels above 300 ng/ml make the diagnosis of tumor almost certain. There are, however, enough patients with the syndrome who have verified tumors but do not have very high prolactin levels so that tumor cannot be excluded by the absence of a high prolactin. Although tumor patients rarely have prolactin levels below the upper limit of normal, many have levels between 20 and 150 ng/ml, which are also seen in patients who have the syndrome without any evidence for tumor. A number of tests of suppression and stimulation have been explored in the hope of finding one to which tumor patients respond differently from patients without tumor.[8, 9, 18, 39] Most of them do not reliably distinguish between tumors and other causes of the syndrome. Among these are chlorpromazine stimulation, stimulation by insulin-induced hypoglycemia, suppression by L-dopa, the gonadotropin response to luteinizing hormone releasing factor and the prolactin response to TRF. Müller et al.[40] reported that Nomifensine causes a drop in prolactin in nursing mothers and in patients with galactorrhea without tumor but not in patients with prolactinomas. The fact that prolactinomas can be suppressed by dopamine agonists like normal pituitary cells, although it makes diagnosis more difficult, is, of course, extremely fortunate for the patients. The medical treatment of prolactinoma is discussed elsewhere in this symposium.

Tumors can cause overproduction of prolactin in two ways: first, by providing an excess of prolactin producing cells, and second, by interfering with the supply of PIF to the tumor itself and to surrounding normal pituitary tissue. A microadenoma that does not impinge on the stalk and is too small to seriously distort anatomical relationships illustrates the first mechanism only. A craniopharyngioma, which does not contain secretory cells but can destroy hypothalamic nuclei or cut them off from the pituitary portal circulation or both, serves as an example of the second mechanism. Kapcala et al.[41] found from 20 to 60 ng/ml of prolactin in three patients with craniopharyngioma. Since the same patients had preservation of thyroid and adrenal function, they postulated that the tumors had not interrupted the portal circulation but were causing hypothalamic damage.

So far our guess was a good one, but since the radioimmunoassay of prolactin has become generally available, more and more exceptions have emerged to prove the rule. More than half of patients with galactorrhea without amenorrhea have prolactins in the normal range and so do most patients with the empty sella syndrome and a significant portion of those whose galactorrhea follows a pregnancy (the Chiari-Frommel syndrome) or is caused by tranquilizers or by oral contraceptives or hypothyroidism. Thus hyperprolactinemia, the most central feature of the syndrome, like all the other features by which the syndrome was defined, is absent about half the time. Nevertheless, the concept that the amenorrhea-galactorrhea syndrome is caused by prolactin should not be immediately abandoned merely because some patients' prolactins fall within the normal range. In the first place it may be that the accepted normal range is too wide. The normal range is arrived at by averaging spot determinations, usually single determinations, on healthy people. Because any kind of stress can cause prolactin release, most surveys of normal people are likely to contain some high values. Friesen's[42] comparison of assays made on hospital patients compared with assays on healthy blood donors illustrates this point. It is also possible that round-the-clock determination of prolactin would pick up differences that are missed by single determinations. Kleinberg et al.[8] carried out such round-the-clock studies in six patients. They found higher than normal rises during sleep in two patients whose waking values fell within the normal range. It is therefore possible that some "euprolactinemic" patients with the amenorrhea-galactorrhea syndrome produce too much prolactin but that our tests are not thorough enough to show it. When prolactin is measured in normal mothers it is found to be well above the normal nonpregnant level for the first two or three postpartum weeks. Peaks of prolactin secretion follow each breast feeding in about 30 minutes. After about three weeks prolactin levels decline toward normal but there continue to be peaks following feedings. Finally prolactin returns to nearly prepregnant levels and there are no more peaks after suckling.[24, 25] Meanwhile milk production is undiminished or even augmented. We might consider the possibility that those patients with the amenorrhea-galactorrhea syndrome who do not have elevated prolactins had them at one time, when their disease began.

Aono et al.[43] found that large postsuckling peaks in prolactin are characteristic of mothers who have abundant milk and nurse successfully. The poorer milk producers who have smaller peaks are generally primipara with small or inverted nipples, which offer a less good hold for the baby and are therefore less effectively stimulated. The role of afferent stimuli from the chest wall in causing prolactin secretion is illustrated by the many patients with galactorrhea that has been provoked by disease or surgery of the chest wall.[44, 45] Kolodny et al.[46] found that stimulation of the nipples caused brief peaks of prolactin secretion in normal nonpuerperal women and sometimes even in men. Only the occasional patient with galactorrhea regularly pumps or manually expresses milk, since for some reason most galactorrhea patients do not experience the breast pain and engorgement that invariably occur in the nursing mother if the milk is not regularly removed. Except for this difference, the euprolactinemic galactorrhea patient might be compared to the normal mother late in lactation, when the serum prolactin is near normal while milk production and amenorrhea continue. The explanation often offered for these manifestations of hyperprolactinemia in the face of normal prolactin levels is that the mammary tissue has become more sensitive to prolactin. This might be another way of saying that it had developed more prolactin receptors. Perhaps there is a change in distribution among the various target organs of the prolactin that circulates. Hayden et al.[47] found, for instance, that oophorectomy influences the amount of prolactin which is bound to mammary tissue. One could hypothesize that under certain conditions more prolactin than usual is taken up by the mammary gland or ovary and less by the uterus and liver. One might also hypothesize a change in the proportion of "big" and "little" prolactins that would not be revealed by radioimmunoassay.[48]

The reason for wishing to believe that prolactin is responsible for all varieties of the galactorrhea-amenorrhea syndrome is that such remarkable benefits can be had by treatment with a dopamine agonist. Most therapeutic trials of bromocriptine have been made in patients selected for hyperprolactinemia. A few investigators, however, have treated patients with amenorrhea or galactorrhea and normal serum prolactin levels. Tolis and Naftolin[49] treated three patients, one with anorexia nervosa, one with a reactive depression, and one with the postpill syndrome, who had amenorrhea and low serum prolactin levels. All three resumed normal ovulatory periods. Sepälä et al.[50] reported success in treating four similar patients with plasma prolactins less than 15 ng/ml. Van der Steeg and Bennink[51] treated 19 normoprolactinemic women with postpill amenorrhea and 14 of them ovulated. The mean prolactin level of the responders was even lower than in the nonresponders.

We know that about 12% of all patients with secondary amenorrhea without galactorrhea have elevated prolactins and that 90% of such patients resume ovulation and fertility on bromocriptine treatment. We do not know how many of the 86% of patients with secondary amenorrhea who do not have hyperprolactinemia would respond similarly. Patients with galactorrhea or amenorrhea who are known to have pituitary adenomas but do not have hyperprolactinemia respond to treatment. It is reasonable to suppose that they have the same disease as patients with pituitary adenoma who do have hyperprolactinemia. It might therefore be reasonable to abandon all of the original criteria for the definition of the amenorrhea-galactorrhea syndrome and redefine it as any form of amenorrhea, galactorrhea, or infertility, in either a female or a male, that can be reversed by a dopamine agonist or by any other means of suppressing or counteracting prolactin secretion.

With this new definition it no longer serves any purpose to classify patients as having the Chiari-Frommel or the Argonz-del Castillo or the Forbes-Albright syndrome. Be it said for Argonz and del Castillo and for Forbes, Henneman, and Albright that they never supposed that they were describing different syndromes in the first place.

To conclude this historical review, it might be worthwhile to mention the outcome in the 15 patients who were followed for many years in a time when no medical treatment for the syndrome was available. No patient who did not have evidence for a tumor in 1954 subsequently developed tumor. Of those who did have tumor, three ceased to lactate following pituitary surgery but continued to be amenorrheic. One patient ceased to lactate and had return of menses following pituitary irradiation, but although she desired a pregnancy was never able to conceive. She had had a miscarriage followed by sterility for four years before she developed amenorrhea and galactorrhea. Of the two patients whose galactorrhea had been associated with thyrotoxicosis, one became myxedematous after treatment and took thyroid replacement treatment irregularly. Galactorrhea continued for eight years, during which time she had two miscarriages and four full-term pregnancies. Fifteen years after that, although she was still undertreated with thyroid, her menses were regular and there had been no recurrence of galactorrhea. Polytomes of the sella showed a rather large volume (1,260 cu mm) with focal erosion of the cortex. The TSH was found to be greater than 50 $\mu$U/ml. The serum prolactin was measured six years after that and was 6.0 ng/ml. No cause has emerged for the galactorrhea and amenorrhea in three patients. One of the three had been lactating for 43 years when last seen. The two others had stopped lactating spontaneously after respectively, six and 25 years of lactation.

In all, 15 patients were observed through 195 years of lactation and 248 years of amenorrhea. Two of them developed fibrocystic disease of the breast. The association of galactorrhea with fibrocystic disease has been reported.[52] Although they have now reached a mean age of 47 years, none of the patients has developed carcinoma of the breast. The absence of breast carcinoma in so small a group of women can very easily occur by coincidence. It is nevertheless mentioned because it raises the question, Is hyperprolactinemia protective against breast cancer?

There are many experiments that show that prolactin causes or favors the development of mammary tumors in rats and mice. The search for a like relationship in humans, however, has not met with much success. Although it has been reported that thyroid disorders are more common in patients with breast carcinoma than in the general population,[53] and although it stands to reason that patients with thyroid insufficiency who have elevated TSHs would be likely to have elevated prolactins, it turns out that the association with thyroid disease has been questioned[54] and that women with carcinoma of the breast do not, in fact, have high serum prolactins.[52, 55, 56] It was tempting to assume that the remissions in breast carcinoma that followed hypophysectomy might be ascribed, not only to the removal of GH and of adrenal and ovarian hormones but also to the removal of prolactin. Ehni and Eckles'[57] reports of an almost equal percentage of remissions following pituitary stalk section, a maneuver that causes hyperprolactinemia while eliminating adrenal and ovarian function,[58] casts doubt upon this reasoning. Epidemiologic studies show that cancer of the breast has a much lower incidence in some countries where prolonged breast-feeding is the rule. Even in this country, early pregnancy and breast-feeding are associated with a somewhat lower incidence.[59] With the recent surge of interest in prolactinomas, and the recognition of the ubiquity of these benign tumors, many hundreds of cases have been reported. It may be that the absence of reports of an association between prolactinoma and breast cancer is significant.

To summarize, I have been asked for a definition of the clinical features of the amenorrhea-galactorrhea syndrome and have not found one. The syndrome appears to have the shape of an ameba. One pseudopod has engulfed many cases of female infertility that were not understandable or treatable before. By the same token, a pseudopod is reaching out in the direction of the control of female fertility. That pseudopod may be considered as a double-headed, perhaps one should say a double-footed, one, since there are two classes of mechanisms that can cause the amenorrhea-galactorrhea syndrome. It may arise from interference with prolactin inhibiting factor or from stimulation, or simulation of prolactin releasing factor. We already have drugs which act in each of these ways.[60, 61] Another pseudopod reaches toward the hitherto frustrating problem of oligospermia in men. There are hints that one of the pseudopods may throw some much needed light on the polycystic ovary syndrome. Treatment of hyperprolactinemic syndromes with bromocryptine constitutes a pseudopod that may prove to be successful medical treatment for many pituitary tumors. If ever we acquire the means not only to turn the amenorrhea-galactorrhea syndrome off but to turn it on to the desired degree, we might have a safe and physiologic means of contraception and perhaps some degree of protection from mammary cancer. I submit, in conclusion, that this shapeless syndrome, with its shifting boundaries, has so far taught us only a small part of all it has to teach.

## Appendix

A hard and fast definition of the clinical features of the amenorrhea-galactorrhea syndrome is no longer possible. The 15 patients who were observed in Fuller Albright's clinic and reported in 1954:

1. Did not have acromegaly, as judged by their appearance and normal levels of serum phosphorus. The distinction from acromegaly was confirmed in 1970 by Kleinberg and Frantz, who used a sensitive bioassay for prolactin with removal of GH by immunoprecipitation (1). Since Friesen developed a specific radioimmunoassay for prolactin we know that prolactin is elevated in 30% of acromegalics but GH is not elevated in the galactorrhea-amenorrhea syndrome (3).

2. Had galactorrhea, in 13 cases nonpuerperal. Galactorrhea is no longer essential for the diagnosis of the syndrome. Franks (4) found galactorrhea in only 28% of patients with pituitary tumors and hypersecretion of prolactin. Galactorrhea is frequently absent in the amenorrhea and hyperprolactinemia syndrome caused by oral contraceptives, phenothiazines, hypothyroidism, and other causes of the syndrome.

3. Amenorrhea. Now also not a necessary feature. There may be irregular periods, oligomenorrhea or regular periods with a short or defective luteal phase. In Frantz's series of 235 patients with galactorrhea there were 76 without amenorrhea, eight patients with pituitary tumor and galactorrhea still menstruated, and in a number of patients with both amenorrhea and galactorrhea the galactorrhea had preceded the amenorrhea by months to years.

4. Had low or absent FSH by mouse uterine weight bioassay. FSH is not decreased in patients who continue to menstruate and not in all patients without menses. Hyperprolactinemia may be associated with a normal preovulatory level of LH with failure of midcycle LH surge.

5. Had evidence of mild hyperactivity of the adrenal cortex, consisting of obesity, seborrhea, slight hirsutism, and 17 ketosteroid ex-

cretion above average although not outside the normal range. Although there has since been some clinical[29, 35, 36] and experimental evidence for increased androgen production in hyperprolactinemia, the majority of patients reported since 1954 have not had the above features.

6. Pituitary tumor in seven of 15 patients. Although radiologic methods in 1954 might have failed to reveal microadenomata that could be demonstrated today, it is most unlikely that all of the 15 original patients had tumors. Two of the 15 are still followed after 27 years and have developed no evidence of tumor. Obviously, when the syndrome is caused by hypothyroidism or drug ingestion, and reversed by removing the cause, tumor need not be implicated.

7. Were presumed to have hypersecretion of prolactin. Since radioimmunoassay for prolactin has become available we know that even hyperprolactinemia may be absent in the amenorrhea-galactorrhea syndrome. Serum prolactin may be normal in postcontraceptive amenorrhea-galactorrhea, drug-induced galactorrhea, the Chiari-Frommel syndrome, and the empty sella syndrome.

8. Were compared with healthy nursing mothers who had amenorrhea. FSH levels were normal in the mothers, although estrogen production was presumably decreased, since the administration of progesterone did not result in withdrawal flow. We now know that prolactin levels are increased early in lactation but decrease as lactation continues and may be in the normal prepregnancy range after a few months despite continued suckling.

## REFERENCES

1. Forbes A.P., Henneman P.H., Griswold G.C., et al.: Syndrome characterized by galactorrhea, amenorrhea and low urinary FSH: Comparison with acromegaly and normal lactation. *J. Clin. Endocrinol. Metab.* 14:265, 1954.

2. Argonz J., del Castillo E.B.: A syndrome characterized by estrogenic insufficiency, galactorrhea and decreased urinary gonadotropin. *J. Clin. Endocrinol. Metab.* 13:79, 1953.

3. Frommel R.: Uber puerpale Atrophie des Uterus. *Ztschr. Geburtsh. Gynakol.* 7:305, 1882.

4. Chiari J.: Bericht uber die in den Jahren 1848 bis inclusive 1851 an der gynakologischen Abteilung in Wien beobachteten Frauenkrankheiten im engern Sinne des Wortes, in Chiari J., Braun C., Spath J.: *Klinik der Geburtshilfe und Gynakologie.* Erlanger Verlag von Ferdinand Enke, 1855, p 362.

5. Reifenstein E.C. Jr., Kinsell L.W., Albright F.: Observations on the use of the serum phosphorus level as an index of pituitary growth hormone activity: The effect of estrogen therapy in acromegaly, abstracted. *Endocrinology* 39:71, 1946.

6. Frantz A.G., Kleinberg D.L.: Prolactin: Evidence that it is separate from growth hormone in human blood. *Science* 170:745, 1970.
7. Franks S., Jacobs H.S., Nabarro J.D.N.: Prolactin concentrations in patients with acromegaly: Clinical significance and response to surgery. *J. Clin. Endocrinol.* 5:63, 1976.
8. Kleinberg D.L., Noel G.L., Frantz A.G.: Galactorrhea: A study of 235 cases, including 48 with pituitary tumors. *N. Engl. J. Med.* 296:589, 1977.
9. Jacobs H.S., Franks S., Murray M.A.F., et al.: Clinical and endocrine features of hyperprolactinemic amenorrhea. *Clin. Endocrinol. (Oxf.)* 5:439, 1976.
10. Franks S., Nabarro J.D.N.: Prolactin secretion in patients with chromophobe adenoma of the pituitary: Incidence and presentation of hyperprolactinemia: Results of surgical treatment. *Ann. Clin. Res.* 10:157, 1978.
11. Molitch M.E., Reichlin S.: The amenorrhea, galactorrhea and hyperprolactinemia syndromes, in Stollerman G.H. (ed): *Advances in Internal Medicine*. Chicago: Year Book Medical Publishers, Inc., 1980.
12. Carter J.N., Tyson J.E., Tolis G., et al.: Prolactin-secreting tumors and hypogonadism in 22 men. *N. Engl. J. Med.* 299:847, 1978.
13. Thorner M.O., Besser G.M.: Bromocriptine treatment of hyperprolactinemic hypogonadism. *Acta Endocrinol. [Suppl.](Copenh.)* 216:131, 1978.
14. Saidi K., Wenn R.V., Sharif F.: Bromocriptine for male infertility. *Lancet* 1:250, 1977.
15. Seppälä M., Hirvonen E., Ranta T.: Hyperprolactinemia and luteal insufficiency. *Lancet* 1:229, 1976.
16. Carter J.N., Gomez F., Friesen H.G.: Human prolactin and the galactorrhea-amenorrhea syndrome, in Givens J.R. (ed): *Endocrine Causes of Menstrual Disorders*. Chicago: Year Book Medical Publishers, Inc., 1977.
17. Bohnet H.G., Dahlén H.G., Wuttke W., et al.: Hyperprolactinemic anovulatory syndrome. *J. Clin. Endocrinol. Metab.* 42:132, 1976.
18. Biller B.J., Boyd A. III, Molitch M.E., et al.: Galactorrhea Syndromes, in Post K.D., Jackson I.M.D., Reichlin S. (eds): *The Pituitary Adenoma*. New York: Plenum Publ., 1980.
19. Posner B.I., Kelly P.A., Shiu R.P.C., et al.: Studies of insulin growth hormone and prolactin binding: Tissue distribution, species variation and characterization. *Endocrinology* 95:521, 1974.
20. McNatty K.P., Sawers R.S., McNeilly A.S.: A possible role for prolactin in control of steroid secretion by the human Graafian follicle. *Nature* 250:653, 1974.
21. Glass M.R., Shaw R.W., Butt W.R., et al.: An abnormality of oestrogen feedback in amenorrhea-galactorrhea. *Br. Med. J.* 3:274, 1975.
22. Aono T., Miyake A., Shioji T., et al.: Impaired LH release following exogenous estrogen administration in patients with amenorrhea-galactorrhea syndrome. *J. Clin. Endocrinol. Metab.* 42:696, 1976.
23. Besser G.M., Thorner M.O.: Prolactin and gonadal function. *Pathol. Biol. (Paris)* 23:779, 1975.
24. Rolland R., Lequin R.M., Schellekens L.A., et al.: The role of prolactin in the restoration of ovarian function during physiological lactation. *Clin. Endocrinol.* 4:15, 1975.
25. Delvoye P., Delogne-Desnoek J., Robyn C.: Serum prolactin in long-lasting lactation amenorrhea. *Lancet* 2:288, 1976.

26. Klibanski A., Neer R.M., Beitins I.Z., et al.: Decreased bone density in hyperprolactinemic women. *N. Engl. J. Med.* 303:1511, 1980.
27. Kwa H.G., Gugten A.A., Verhofstad F.: Radioimmunoassay of rat prolactin, prolactin levels in plasma of rats with spontaneous pituitary tumors, primary estrone-induced tumors or pituitary tumor transplants. *Eur. J. Cancer* 5:571, 1969.
28. Crystle C.D., Sawaya G.A., Stevens V.C.: Effects of ethinyl estradiol on the secretion of gonadotropins and estrogens in postpartum women. *Am. J. Obstet. Gynecol.* 116:616, 1973.
29. Seppälä M., Hirvonen E.: Raised serum prolactin levels associated with hirsutism and amenorrhea. *Br. Med. J.* 4:144, 1975.
30. Lavric M.V.: Galactorrhea and amenorrhea with polycystic ovaries. *Am. J. Obstet. Gynecol.* 104:814, 1969.
31. Lamotte M.: Le syndrome amenorrhée-galactorrhée. *Nouv. Presse Med.* 74:1025, 1966.
32. Mulla N.P.: Chiari-Frommel syndrome: Report of a case. *Ohio State Med. J.* 61:358, 1965.
33. Thorner M.O.: Hyperprolactinemia: Current concepts of management including medical treatment with bromocriptine. *Adv. Biochem. Psychopharmacol.* 23:165, 1980.
34. Hafiez A.A., Lloyd C.W., Bartke P.: The role of prolactin in the regulation of testis function: The effects of prolactin and luteinizing hormone on the plasma levels of testosterone and adrostenedione in hypophysectomized rats. *J. Endocrinol.* 52:327, 1972.
35. Bassi F., Giusti G., Borsi L., et al.: Plasma androgens in women with hyperprolactinemic amenorrhea. *Clin. Endocrinol.* 6:5, 1977.
36. Carter J.N., Tyson J.E., Warne J.L., et al.: Adrenocortical function in hyperprolactinemic women. *J. Clin. Endocrinol. Metab.* 45:973, 1977.
37. Vermculen A., Suy E., Rubens R.: Effect of prolactin on plasma DHEA(s) levels. *J. Clin. Endocrinol. Metab.* 44:1222, 1977.
38. Quigley M.E., Rakoff J.A., Yen S.S.C.: Increased luteinizing hormone sensitivity to dopamine inhibition in polycystic ovary syndrome. *J. Clin. Endocrinol. Metab.* 52:231, 1981.
39. Boyd A.E. III., Reichlin S., Turksoy R.N.: Galactorrhea-amenorrhea syndrome: Diagnosis and therapy. *Ann. Intern. Med.* 87:165, 1977.
40. Müller E.E., Genazanni A.R., Murru S.: Nomifensine: Diagnostic test in hyperprolactinemic states. *J. Clin. Endocrinol. Metab.* 47:1352, 1978.
41. Kapcala L.P., Molitch M.E., Post K.D., et al.: Galactorrhea, oligoamenorrhea and hyperprolactinemia in patients with craniopharyngiomas. *J. Clin. Endocrinol. Metab.* 51:798, 1980.
42. Friesen H.G.: Bromocriptine treatment of hyperprolactinemic disorders. *Adv. Biochem. Psychopharmacol.* 23:147, 1980.
43. Aono T., Shioji T., Shoda T., et al.: The initiation of human lactation and the prolactin response to suckling. *J. Clin. Endocrinol. Metab.* 44:1101, 1977.
44. Moreley J.E., Dawson M., Hodgkinson H., et al.: Galactorrhea and hyperprolactinemia associated with chest wall injury. *J. Clin. Endocrinol. Metab.* 45:931, 1977.
45. Herman V., Kalk W.J., deMoor N.G., et al.: Serum prolactin after chest wall surgery: elevated levels after mastectomy. *J. Clin. Endocrinol. Metab.* 52:148, 1981.

46. Kolodny R.C., Jacobs L.S., Daughaday W.H.: Mammary stimulation causes prolactin secretion in non-lactating women. *Nature* 238:284, 1972.
47. Hayden T.J., Bonney R.C., Forsyth I.A.: Ontogeny and control of prolactin receptors in the mammary gland and liver of virgin, pregnant and laboratory rats. *J. Endocrinol.* 80:259, 1979.
48. Garnier P.E., Aubert M.L., Kaplan S.L., et al.: Heterogeneity of pituitary and plasma prolactin in man: Decreased affinity of "big" prolactin in a radioreceptor assay and evidence for its secretion. *J. Clin. Endocrinol. Metab.* 47:1273, 1978.
49. Tolis G., Naftolin F.: Induction of menstruation with bromocriptine in patients with euprolactinemic amenorrhea. *Am. J. Obstet. Gyneçol.* 126:426, 1976.
50. Sepälä M., Unnerus H.A., Hirvonen E., et al.: *J. Clin. Endocrinol. Metab.* 43:474, 1976.
51. Van der Steeg H.J., Bennink H.J.T.C.: Bromocriptine for induction of ovulation in normoprolactinemic post-pill anovulation. *Lancet* 1:502, 1977.
52. Latteri M., Bajardi G., Cashglione C., et al.: Prolactin in pathology of the breast. *Minerva Med.* 71:1915, 1980.
53. Bogardus G.M., Finley J.W.: Breast cancer and thyroid disease. *Surgery* 49:461, 1961.
54. Hedley A.J., Spiegelhalter D.J., Jones S.J., et al.: Breast cancer in thyroid disease: Fact or fallacy? *Lancet* 1:131, 1981.
55. Mittra I., Hayward J.L.: Hypothalamic pituitary prolactin axis in patients with breast carcinoma. *Lancet* 1:889, 1974.
56. Franks S., Ralph D.N.L., Seagroatt V., et al.: Prolactin concentration in patients with breast carcinoma. *Br. Med. J.* 4:320, 1974.
57. Ehni G., Eckles N.E.: Interruption of the pituitary stalk in the patient with mammary cancer. *J. Neurosurg.* 16:628, 1959.
58. Turkington R.W., Underwood L.E., Van Wyk J.J.: Elevated serum prolactin levels after pituitary stalk section in man. *N. Engl. J. Med.* 285:707, 1971.
59. Wynder E.L., Bross I.J., Hirayama J.: A study of the epidemiology of cancer of the breast. *Cancer* 13:559, 1960.
60. Boyd A.E. III, Reichlin S.: Neural control of prolactin secretion in man. *Psychoneuroendocrinology* 3:113, 1978.
61. Aono T., Shioji T., Kinugasa T., et al.: Clinical and endocrinological analyses of patients with galactorrhea and menstrual disorders due to sulpiride and metoclopramide. *J. Clin. Endocrinol. Metab.* 47:1352, 1978.

# Medical Management of Prolactinomas

## G.M. BESSER, M.D.

Department of Endocrinology, St. Bartholomew's
Hospital, London, England

SINCE THE FIRST REPORTS in 1970 and 1971 of the occurrence in the human of prolactin as a physiologically important pituitary hormone, and the realization of its potential role in gonadal dysfunction,[1-3] it has become apparent that hyperprolactinemia, far from being rare, is an extraordinarily common pathogenetic accompaniment of hypogonadism in both males and females.[3, 4] Among the many causes of pathologic hyperprolactinemia (Table 1), it is now increasingly realized that tumors of pituitary prolactin-secreting cells (lactotrophs) are common.[4-6] Thus, pituitary tumors may consist merely of localized collections of hyperplastic lactotrophs in the lateral wing of the pituitary, often without a true capsule, which collections constitute so-called microadenomas if they are less than 1 cm in diameter,[7] or macroadenomas. It is the massive macroadenomas that may occasionally develop large extrasellar extension that may grow upwards to compress the visual pathways and the hypothalamus, or extend laterally across the cavernous sinus, displacing the carotid siphon and pressing on the oculomotor nerve.

Patients with prolactinomas often manifest features of hypogonadism, such as menstrual disorders or amenorrhea in women, and impotence in men. In the past it was assumed that patients with pituitary tumors and hypogonadism suffered from gonadotrophin deficiency. It is now realized that this is rather uncommon. The majority of these tumors are prolactinomas; since the gonadotrophin reserve is often normal despite the hypogonadism, it would appear that the hyperprolactinemia is the cause of the deficient gonadal function.

255

0-8151-3530-0/82/006-255-273-$03.75

TABLE 1.—Causes of Pathologic Elevation of Circulating Prolactin

| |
|---|
| Pituitary and hypothalamic diseases |
|   Pituitary tumors |
|     Pure prolactin-secreting prolactinomas—microadenomas or macroadenomas |
|     Mixed hormone producers—prolactin with GH or ACTH |
|   Hypothalamic diseases |
|     Granulomatous diseases, craniopharyngioma, meningioma, glioma, pinealoma, ischemia |
|   Pituitary stalk lesions |
|     Section, head injury, meningitis |
|   Drugs |
|     Dopamine depleting agents, e.g., methyldopa, reserpine |
|     Dopamine receptor blocking agents, e.g., phenothiazines, such as chlorpromazine, perphenazine, trifluoperazine; benzamides, e.g., metoclopramide, sulpiride; pimozide; haloperidol |
|     Estrogens |
|     Opiates, e.g., metenkephalin, β-endorphin, opium alkaloids |
|   Hypothyroidism |
|   Chronic renal failure, including long-term hemodialysis |
|   Idiopathic—may have pituitary microadenomas too small to alter the pituitary fossa contour on x-ray |

This is borne out by clinical results following reduction of raised prolactin levels using dopamine agonists; then gonadal function returns very quickly to normal.[8, 9] Clear evidence has accrued recently that as raised prolactin levels associated with prolactinomas are lowered with dopamine agonist therapy, the pituitary tumor shrinks, often very dramatically. As it shrinks, any deficient pituitary function may improve and indeed normalize as the previously compressed normal pituitary regains functional contact with the hypothalamus.

## Clinical Features of Hyperprolactinemia

The cardinal clinical feature in women with hyperprolactinemia is menstrual dysfunction usually with infertility, whether or not there is evidence of the presence of a pituitary tumor. Secondary amenorrhea is the classical menstrual disturbance and an incidence of hyperprolactinemia of between 13% and 30% is reported in unselected patients with secondary amenorrhea.[4, 10] However, the amenorrhea may be primary and the hyperprolactinemia, particularly when due to a prolactinoma, may be a cause of delayed puberty. Alternatively, in an important group, menstruation may be completely regular. The latter patients present with infertility and on investigation show an absence of the midcycle surge in serum luteinizing hormone necessary for ovulation; alternatively, they ovulate and have an inadequate luteal phase of the cycle with a progesterone rise that is too small or is poorly sustained.[4, 10, 11] The reported incidence of inappropriate lactation depends on the enthusiasm with which it is sought. Overall, the incidence of galactorrhea is reported as varying between 30% and 80%.[4, 10] Clearly, many patients have clinically significant hyperprolactinemia without milk in the breasts; sometimes venous engorgement or hypertrophy of Montgomery's tubercles is present. A few patients show signs of mild virilism, such as acne, hirsutism, greasy skin, and clitoromegaly and may have clinical or biochemical features of polycystic ovarian disease.[9, 11] Patients with microadenomas are indistinguishable clinically from patients with other causes of hyperprolactinemia on clinical grounds. Amenorrhea occurs in a higher proportion of patients with obvious pituitary tumors, however, than in patients without evidence of a tumor.[9-11]

Male patients with prolactinomas usually present with relative or absolute impotence. While they may show signs of testosterone deficiency such as a decrease in the frequency of shaving, or decreased secondary sexual hair with testicular shrinkage, these features are unusual. The most common presentation of male patients with hyperprolactinemia is relative or absolute impotence in an otherwise normal male. Galactorrhea is even less common in men than women. Gynecomastia, if present, is minimal, although there often is a collection of fat rather than glandular tissue around the breast. It is of interest that a higher proportion of males with hyperprolactinemia present with macroadenomas and extrasellar extensions to their pituitary tumors than is encountered in women. It would seem that symptoms are present longer in men with hyperprolactinemia than in women before they seek medical advice and that any pituitary tumor is likely, therefore, to be more advanced.[10]

## Investigation

Serum prolactin measurements must be made in any patient presenting with menstrual dysfunction or regular menstruation with infertility when there is no obvious local cause in the internal genitalia. Similar measurements must be made in men presenting with impotence. Since prolactin is normally secreted in a pulsatile fashion, and this is even more marked in many patients with hyperprolactinemia due to prolactinomas, more than one sample must be obtained in order to establish the overall average level. It is our normal practice to obtain at least three venipuncture samples in the morning, apart from the time of clinical examination to obtain an average level. Although it was originally believed that frequent sampling through an indwelling venous cannula might get over the problem of a venipuncture-stress-induced rise in prolactin levels, this does not appear to be the case. Clinically relevant information is more often provided by repeated outpatient venipuncture samples.[12] Clearly, routine straight lateral and anteroposterior radiography of the skull must be carried out to provide an assessment of the pituitary fossa. It is essential for this to be augmented with tomography of the pituitary fossa when the outline is not absolutely clear. The clinical significance of minor radiologic changes has caused some controversy.[13–15] It is now generally accepted that the presence of blisters larger than 3 mm or major asymmetry between the two sides of the fossa is likely to indicate the presence of a prolactinoma within it. Several classifications of the radiologic abnormalities seen on x-ray of the pituitary fossa are available. One that our group introduced[16] and that is generally being adopted is of particular relevance to the significance of changes in patients likely to be treated medically and who wish to be fertile. This classification is shown in Table 2.

In our clinical practice we suspect a pituitary tumor (SPT) to be present in a patient with hyperprolactinemia and fossa abnormalities of B3 to B5. Prolactinoma patients tend to have higher circulating prolactin levels than patients with other causes of hyperprolactinemia but this is not always so. The presence of prolactinomas is unusual in patients with prolactin levels less than 100 ng/ml (2,000 mU/L), but we have seen much lower values (Fig 1). Each laboratory must establish not only its own normal range (ours is less than 18

TABLE 2.—PITUITARY FOSSA CLASSIFICATION FROM SKULL RADIOGRAPHS*

| GRADE† | LATERAL VIEW | POSTEROANTERIOR VIEW | INTERPRETATION |
|---|---|---|---|
| BO | Single contour | Flat floor: no blistering | Normal |
| B1 | Less than 1-mm difference between contours | Minimal slope: less than 1-mm dip | Probably normal |
| B2 | 1–3-mm difference between contours; less than 3 mm blister | 1–3-mm dip | Possibly abnormal |
| B3 | Over 3-mm blister | Asymmetry over 3 mm | Abnormal |
| B4 | Double contour throughout | Asymmetry over 3 mm | Abnormal |
| B5 | Both sides of fossa expanded in all directions (ballooned fossa) | | Abnormal |

If the cortex is eroded then the fossa is classified as above but "E" is added—for example, B4E.

*Adapted from Thorner M.O., et al.: *Br. Med. J.* 2:771, 1979.

†B: St. Bartholomew's Hospital. Grades B3 to B5 are regarded as "suspected pituitary tumors" for the purpose of this chapter.

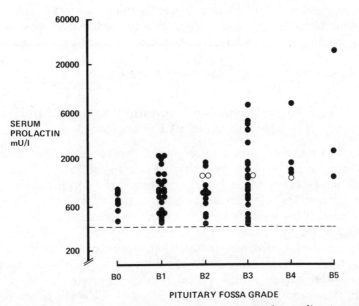

**Fig 1.**—Serum prolactin concentration in patients grouped according to grade of radiologic abnormality of pituitary fossa. *Dotted line,* upper limit of normal range (360 mU/l or 18 ng/ml). *Open circles,* minimum values obtained from undiluted sera. (From Thorner M.O., et al.: *Br. Med. J.* 2:771, 1979. Used by permission.)

ng/ml or 360 mU/L, depending on the standard) but also the relevant range of the different diagnostic groups, as methodology and antisera differ widely.

In addition, patients with pituitary tumors require complete endocrine assessment to exclude partial or complete deficiencies of other hormones, such as impaired ACTH, TSH, or gonadotrophin secretion, by standard tests such as insulin-induced hypoglycemia and the intravenous (IV) gonadotrophin-releasing or thyrotrophin-releasing hormone tests.[10] ACTH and TSH deficiencies are rare in patients with prolactinomas who have never received surgical treatment. Gonadotrophin deficiency is unusual in prolactinoma patients. Indeed, normal or excessive gonadotrophin responses to the releasing hormone, despite the apparent hypogonadism, are characteristic. LH deficiency is particularly unusual in microadenomas and in less than one third of the patients with macroadenomas (grade B4 and B5 fossae). The presence of a normal or excessive LH response to gonadotrophin-releasing hormone test is of good prognostic value and in such patients return to normal gonadal function is expected when prolactin levels are reduced to normal by means of dopamine agonist therapy.[10] Impaired gonadotrophin responses suggest the patient may fail to regularly menstruate or ovulate when prolactin is lowered. This is not an absolute finding, however, since patients with even massive pituitary tumors may show such shrinkage of the tumor that normal pituitary function ensues on long-term medical treatment.

## Physiologic Basis for Dopamine Agonist Medical Management of Prolactinomas

Normal control of prolactin secretion involves tonic inhibition of its synthesis and secretion by a hypothalamic inhibitory factor.[3] Evidence suggests that the most important prolactin-inhibiting factor coming from the hypothalamus is dopamine[3, 17] and that all physiologic stimuli responsible for alterations in prolactin secretion can be accounted for by alterations in the degree of tonic inhibition by this catecholamine neurotransmitter. Dopamine can be found in the region of the median eminence in nerve terminals in close apposition to the capillary loops of the portal capillary system of the pituitary stalk; it is present in the capillary blood of the stalk in appropriate concentrations and there are specific dopaminergic receptor mechanisms in the anterior pituitary, lactotroph cells.[17] While most of this physiologic data had been obtained from animals, particularly rats,

**Fig 2.**—Dispersed cells from a human prolactin-secreting microadenoma suspended in Bio-Gel beads and perfused in a column. Prolactin secretion is inhibited when dopamine or bromocriptine is added to the medium. Details of the technique are given by Yeo et al.[17]

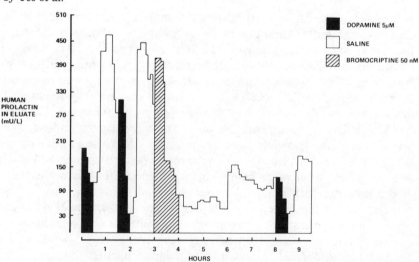

similar receptor systems sensitive to dopaminergic inhibition of prolactin secretion can be demonstrated using human prolactinoma cells (Fig 2). Good data exist that γ-aminobutyric acid (GABA)-sensitive prolactin-inhibiting mechanisms and specific receptors exist on the anterior pituitary cells as well, although a higher order of magnitude of GABA-ergic inhibition is required to produce prolactin suppression.[18] It is not clear whether GABA-ergic mechanisms are of physiologic relevance, although it seems likely that they are.[18] Prolactin-raising factors coming from the hypothalamus are also a possibility, particularly since thyrotrophin-releasing hormone will increase prolactin secretion. Their physiologic relevance is unclear. In summary, it may therefore be assumed that the dominant and specific mechanism for the control of prolactin, from both normal and tumorous cells, resides in a dopaminergic system, both dopamine and dopaminergic agonists being capable of powerful inhibition of prolactin secretion.

## Dopamine Agonist Medical Therapy

Dopamine itself and its precursor, L-dopa, are too short-acting to be effective agents for the medical management of hyperprolactinemia. However, a number of long-acting dopamine agonists have been used in hyperprolactinemia and these are usually related to the ergot alkaloids. Drugs used clinically have included bromocriptine, lergotrile, lisuride, and pergolide, and a number of others show promise.[19-23] To date, however, only bromocriptine has had extensive clinical use. In 1972 the first description of bromocriptine in clinical practice, with its property to lower prolactin in the human being, heralded a major change in the management of hypogonadal patients with hyperprolactinemia, with or without pituitary tumors.[8] The drug is now in widespread use throughout the world, and experience with it has been uniform. Bromocriptine (2-Br-α-ergocryptine) is a long-acting dopamine agonist that shows persistent suppression of prolactin secretion long after the drug has left the cell, presumably due to persistent receptor occupancy[8, 16, 17, 24] (see Fig 2; Figs 3 and 4). Oral administration of bromocriptine rapidly lowers prolactin levels in prolactinoma patients as well as in other causes of hyperprolactinemia. In the majority of patients, 2.5 mg given three times a day suffices to lower the prolactin levels to normal range, although higher doses (10, 15, or even up to 40 mg per day) rarely are required. The levels should be lowered into the normal range but not rendered undetectable, since very low prolactin levels as well as very high ones

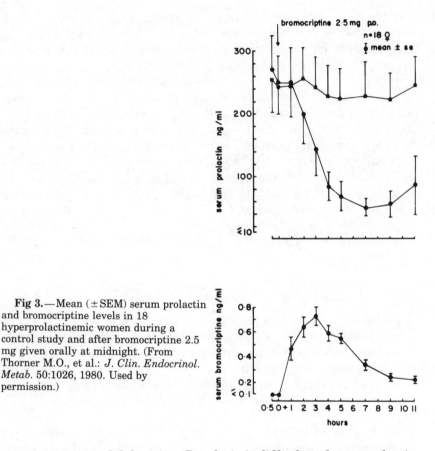

**Fig 3.**—Mean (±SEM) serum prolactin and bromocriptine levels in 18 hyperprolactinemic women during a control study and after bromocriptine 2.5 mg given orally at midnight. (From Thorner M.O., et al.: *J. Clin. Endocrinol. Metab.* 50:1026, 1980. Used by permission.)

may impair gonadal function. Rarely is it difficult to lower prolactin levels to normal.

Unless gonadotrophin reserve is grossly impaired, regular ovulatory menstrual cycles return rapidly, irrespective of the cause of the hyperprolactinemia[16, 24] (Fig 5). The first one or two cycles may not be ovulatory, but soon ovulatory menstruation supervenes, as documented by adequately maintained progesterone levels in the luteal phase. In idiopathic hyperprolactinemia, over 80% of patients show return of regular menstruation within two months, but the response of pituitary tumor patients may be somewhat slower: 60% of the latter resume regular menstruation within three months, followed by a slow increase in the proportion of responders thereafter. A small proportion (about 10%) of patients with macroadenomas fail to resume normal menstruation, particularly if they have been subject to sur-

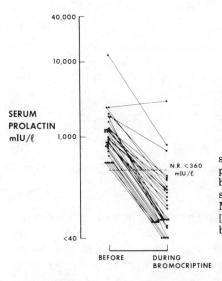

SERUM
PROLACTIN
mIU/ℓ

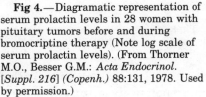

**Fig 4.**—Diagramatic representation of serum prolactin levels in 28 women with pituitary tumors before and during bromocriptine therapy (Note log scale of serum prolactin levels). (From Thorner M.O., Besser G.M.: *Acta Endocrinol.* [*Suppl. 216*] *(Copenh.)* 88:131, 1978. Used by permission.)

gical manipulation before treatment; this failure appears to be due to associated persisting gonadotrophin deficiency.

Once regular menstruation has supervened, 50% of patients wishing to conceive do so within two months after beginning attempts to do so (Fig 6). It is now our practice with prolactinoma patients who wish to conceive and fail to do so within three months to add clomiphene (100 to 300 mg per day for five days each month, starting on

**Fig 5.**—Cumulative percentage of 40 amenorrhoeic women, 26 of whom had suspected pituitary tumors *(S.P.T.)* and 14 of whom had idiopathic hyperprolactinemia *(I.H.)*, showing return to regular menstrual cycles related to months of bromocriptine therapy. (From Thorner M.O., Besser G.M.: *Acta Endocrinol.* [*Suppl. 216*] *(Copenh.)* 88:131, 1978. Used by permission.)

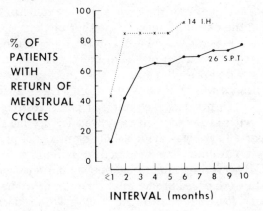

% OF PATIENTS WITH RETURN OF MENSTRUAL CYCLES

INTERVAL (months)

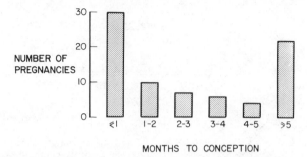

MONTHS TO CONCEPTION

**Fig 6.**—Interval to conception (months) in 80 pregnancies in 68 patients treated for hyperprolactinemia with bromocriptine.

the second day of the cycle, with 5,000 units of human chorionic gonadotrophin given intramuscularly on day 12). Hyperprolactinemia patients usually respond readily to clomiphene once prolactin levels are lowered. Conceptions following bromocriptine therapy are not associated with any increase in the incidence of either abortion or fetal abnormality, and multiple ovulation does not appear to occur any more frequently than would be expected in a normal population. In other words, pituitary-ovarian relationships return rapidly to normal.

In male patients with hyperprolactinemia, hypogonadism rapidly resolves. Normal potency returns quickly. In both male and female patients any galactorrhea disappears usually within a few days of the commencement of treatment.

## Alterations in the Mass of Pituitary Tumors

Recent evidence suggests that not only do prolactin levels return to normal with the use of bromocriptine therapy, but the mass of any pituitary tumor present may be dramatically reduced. Apart from isolated reports of resolution of visual defects in patients with large prolactinomas and suprasellar extensions, the first review of a large number of patients was that of Wass et al.[26] These authors reported on 69 patients with prolactin-secreting or GH-secreting pituitary tumors treated with bromocriptine, followed for six months up to six and a half years. There was evidence of shrinkage of pituitary tumor in 23% of these patients. This occurred in patients with pure prolactin or pure GH-secreting tumors as well as patients with mixed lesions. The data were based predominantly on improvement in the size of the pituitary fossa on routine radiology. This report is likely to underestimate the incidence of shrinkage of the soft tissues of the tumor, since it is recognized that in the majority of patients whose pituitary tumors shrink, a "partially empty" fossa is found without alteration in the overall radiologic size of the fossa. It can only be in the minority of patients that the fossa itself shrinks on skull x-ray. Wass and colleagues also reported that, not only did the pituitary fossa size shrink, but sometimes pituitary function improved with the resolution of hypopituitarism.

We have now followed up this observation by closely monitoring a group of patients with massive pituitary tumors and large extrasellar extensions associated with headache, visual field defects, or oculomotor nerve palsies, and often hypopituitarism. Prior to this study, such patients in our practice would have been submitted to emergency neurosurgical decompression of the tumor mass.

The patients all have computerized tomographic (CT) scanning and contrast radiography (either pneumoencephalography or metrizamide cisternography) with full dynamic pituitary function tests before and at three months after the commencement of bromocriptine therapy. To date we have followed 16 such patients, and by three months all but two have shown a clear and often dramatic reduction in the pituitary tumor mass, and resolution, often complete, of the extrasellar extension. When this response has been seen at three months medical treatment has been continued and progressive shrinkage of the tumor back into the fossa has been found. Such complete resolution of extrasellar extensions has allowed external conventional radiotherapy to be performed; thus surgery was avoided. In addition to the reduction in the mass of pituitary tumors, five patients who had had hypopituitarism before treatment showed return to normal of pituitary function. Presumably, as the tumor shrinks, the hypothalamus is able once more to regain functional communication and control of the normal pituitary gland.

An example of the changes in the radiology is shown in Fig 7, A-C. The patient was a man with hyperprolactinemia who also had acromegaly, field defects in the upper outer quadrant, diabetes insipidus, pituitary hypothyroidism, low gonadotrophin and circulating testosterone levels, and a low plasma cortisol both at rest and during insulin-induced hypoglycemia. A CT scan before treatment showed the presence of a large suprasellar extension (see Fig 7,A). On bromocriptine therapy his visual field defects disappeared within two months, and serial CT scanning over 11 months showed virtually complete disappearance of the large suprasellar extension (see Fig 7,B). His replacement therapy was stopped, he was shown no longer to have any evidence of diabetes insipidus, and his thyroid and gonadal func-

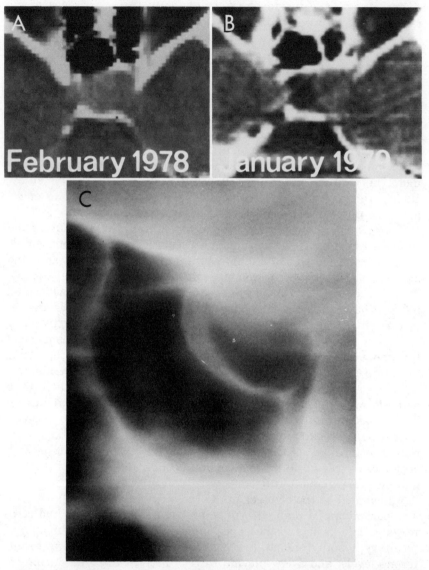

**Fig 7.**—**A,** sellar region on CT scanning before bromocriptine therapy, and **B,** after 11 months of treatment in an acromegalic, hyperprolactinemic patient showing shrinkage of suprasellar extension to the tumor. **C,** after a further 22 months metrizamide cisternography showed a partially empty fossa; a midline tomographic cut is illustrated. (**A** and **B** from Wass J.A.H., et al.: *Lancet* 2:66, 1979. Used by permission.)

tion was now normal. His circulating plasma cortisol under basal conditions had become normal and the cortisol rose normally during insulin-induced hypoglycemia. The patient received no treatment other than bromocriptine. It is evident that, not only did his tumor shrink, but that his pituitary function had become entirely normal. One year later a metrizamide cisternogram showed that the fossa was two thirds empty and only a small residual pituitary shadow was present (see Fig 7,C).

With this sort of evidence, it is now realistically possible to suggest that patients with prolactin-secreting tumors should receive a trial of medical treatment with bromocriptine before neurosurgery even if such tumors are massive and have large extrasellar extensions. With such a trial the majority of patients will show rapid shrinkage of their pituitary tumor, resolution of pressure symptoms on neighboring structures, and improvement in pituitary function. Unlike neurosurgery, where there is risk of inducing hypopituitarism, dopamine agonist therapy of pituitary tumors restores normal gonadal function without the risk of hypopituitarism; in fact, pituitary function improves with this measure.

## Side Effects

In the treatment of hyperprolactinemia, side effects are very rare once patients are established on bromocriptine. However, they are common at the start of treatment unless care is taken in the introduction of therapy. These initiating side effects consist of posturally related dizziness, anorexia, and vomiting, but may be completely avoided. Puerperal patients given bromocriptine to suppress lactation do not get these symptoms and may be started on full dosage immediately. All other patients must build the dose up slowly and all the doses must be taken *during,* not after, meals to avoid side effects. We start with half a tablet (1.25 mg) taken after retiring to bed at night and during a snack (a sandwich and glass of milk). After two days, the patient takes one whole tablet (2.5 mg) in the same way, and two or three days later, if all is well, takes it instead during the evening meal. At intervals of two to three days, one extra tablet is added during breakfast and then during lunch until the normal dose of 2.5 mg three times daily is taken *during* food. Some particularly sensitive patients may still get symptoms at any particular dose level, in which case the dose is lowered by one step and increments are taken even more slowly (one or two weekly). Serum prolactin levels may be followed after the patient is on 5 and 7.5 mg per day (a

48-hour delay from the start of a particular dose suffices) in order to use the lowest dose possible of this expensive drug to maintain normal levels. If 7.5 mg per day (three tablets) is insufficient to achieve normal levels, then the drug is slowly increased further. This is rarely required.

## Ablative Therapy Directed at the Pituitary

Attempts may be made to ablate the prolactinoma instead of, or in addition to, using bromocriptine. If the tumor is small, its transsphenoidal selective removal may be attempted. When successful, this results in the fall of prolactin levels to normal and the resumption of normal gonadal function without the loss of other pituitary secretions. Results vary markedly from center to center.[11] Unfortunately, it is difficult to ascertain from published series the incidence of persistent hyperprolactinemia or postsurgical hypopituitarism, because patients have often not been followed for long and are not repeatedly subjected to basal or dynamic pituitary function tests or documentation of the thyroid, adrenal, and gonadotrophin reserve: in particular, the incidence of ovulation postoperatively is poorly documented, properly established by regular progesterone measurements in the second half of the cycle. It is inadequate to simply provide reports of just the occurrence of menstruation that may well be anovular, or of changes in basal body temperature, which is insufficient evidence of an adequate luteal phase. Because gonadotrophin deficiency, especially of LH, is particularly at risk in any ablative cause of partial hypopituitarism, it is a worrisome feature of this form of therapy in these patients, who often are young.

## Pregnancy, Bromocriptine Therapy, and Pituitary Tumors

Patients with hyperprolactinemia treated with bromocriptine become highly fertile and conceive readily and those with pituitary tumors are no different from others in this respect, provided they are not gonadotrophin-deficient. Among the first 70 women we treated, 36 wished to conceive and 31 did so, six twice, one thrice, often despite prolonged periods of antecedent infertility. The interval-to-conception range was two weeks to five months in pituitary tumor patients, eight weeks being the most common interval. We have supervised 125 pregnancies in patients treated with bromocriptine and approximately one third of them have been in patients considered to have pituitary tumors. There is no evidence that bromocriptine is associated with an increase in multiple births, fetal abnormalities, or increased abortion rates, either in our own data or the series collected to date.[16, 28] Nevertheless, the longest follow-up of the newborn has been some eight years. We therefore still tell our patients to discontinue bromocriptine as soon as pregnancy is confirmed.

One major unresolved management problem relates to the undoubted danger of rapid enlargement of pituitary tumors during pregnancy. Complications following bromocriptine therapy, such as severe headaches, visual field loss, blindness, or simply changes of the fossa, were first reported after successful pregnancy induction with gonadotrophins but are now being reported with increasing frequency.[16, 29] The risk of worsening of a pituitary tumor during pregnancy in a patient who has had a microadenoma (a grade B3 or lower fossa) is, however, small and appears to be of the order of 0.5%; in patients with larger tumors (those that correspond to our grades of B4 or B5) the risk appears to be much greater and of the order of 25%.[29] For this reason we believe that prophylactic radiotherapeutic treatment directed at the pituitary fossa should be given to patients with significant hyperprolactinemia (above 100 ng/ml or 2,000 mU/L), who have fossa grades of B4 or B5 but no evidence of a partially empty fossa, before they are allowed to conceive on bromocriptine therapy for hyperprolactinemia. If a suprasellar extension exists it should be treated first. Although we initially suggested that this should involve surgical removal of the suprasellar extension, we now treat the patient with bromocriptine to shrink this part of the tumor before administering the radiotherapy. We have never encountered any evidence of tumor growth in prolactinoma patients during pregnancy when this has been preceded by radiotherapy. Such growth has been described often in patients not treated so at other centers. We have ourselves seen six patients who have become pregnant with pituitary tumors but in whom pregnancy was not planned and preceded by radiotherapy. Of these, two developed field defects.[16]

External pituitary radiotherapy appears to be entirely safe and is apparently not associated with hypopituitarism, at least within the time scale required for completion of a family. We have had no problem with it during the ten years we have regularly used bromocriptine. We have used a 4-meV linear accelerator with a three-field technique, individual planning, and full isodosimetry. Treatment was localized to the pituitary, and irradiation of surrounding structures was kept to a minimum. For each patient an individually constructed skin-tight plastic head and shoulder cast was constructed to allow fixation of the patient and accurate localization of the irradiation fields. Treatment was given over five weeks in 26 fractions up to a total tumor dosage of 4,500 rad. It is essential to avoid administration of more than 200 rad per fraction, since then radiation-induced neural damage appears to be unrecorded. Over 200 pituitary tumor patients have been treated over a span of 20 years with this technique, and no radiotherapy-induced complications have been encountered in our center.[16]

Should we be presented with a patient treated elsewhere for a prolactinoma with bromocriptine and who has not had radiotherapy, but who has developed an enlarging tumor with significant neighborhood signs or symptoms, it would be our policy to use bromocriptine as urgent treatment, since it is now well established that this will shrink the tumor during pregnancy. Alternatively, radioactive seeds of yttrium could be implanted in the pituitary, transfrontal hypophysectomy carried out, or termination of pregnancy effected.[30] If the patient can be taken through to term then the tumor will shrink again once the baby is delivered and the level of circulating estrogens falls.

## Conclusions

Hyperprolactinemia is a common cause of hypogonadism and infertility in women. It also occurs in men when it causes impotence. Prolactinomas occur in about one third of these patients and the tumors are usually small (microadenomas). Less commonly they are larger and may occasionally cause neighborhood problems with pressure on the surrounding vital structures. This occurs more commonly in men. Residual pituitary function is usually intact, although hypopituitarism, particularly of gonadotrophins, may occur. The use of dopamine agonists, such as bromocriptine, as medical therapy lowers circulating prolactin levels by a direct action on the pituitary cells. In association with the resolution of the hyperprolactinemia, the mass of the pituitary tumor usually shrinks. As shrinkage of the tumor mass occurs, residual pituitary function, if initially impaired, usually returns to normal. Occasionally, hypopituitarism may persist but this is most likely to occur if surgical treatment has also been attempted. For this reason surgical treatment should be avoided whenever possible. Bromocriptine therapy alone does not result in permanent cure because hyperprolactinemia will resume when this medical treatment is stopped. While the patient is on treatment, however, the prime objects of treatment of pituitary tumors are fulfilled: reduction of tumor mass, resolution of hyperprolactinemia, maintenance or improvement in residual pituitary function, and absence of recurrence.

Normal gonadal function is rapidly restored and regular ovulatory menstruation resumes; in men, potency is restored, unless gonadotrophin deficiency persists. Even if hormonal replacement appears necessary initially, then such replacement should be stopped after six months because by this time normal pituitary function has often returned. Women become highly fertile and conception occurs readily in prolactinoma patients. Except in microadenoma patients, when the risk is small, prolactinoma patients are exposed to the risk of rapid enlargement of their pituitary tumors when they become pregnant (pituitary fossa grades 4 and 5). This risk (one in four) appears to be safely resolved with external pituitary irradiation. This is carefully given from a linear accelerator (4,500 rad delivered in 26 doses). Side effects of bromocriptine are rare providing the drug is introduced slowly and the tablets are swallowed with food.

## Other Uses of Dopamine Agonist Therapy

Dopamine agonists raise GH levels in normal people but lower them in the majority (about 80%) of patients with acromegaly. This has provided a very useful form of medical management to augment ablative therapy directed to the pituitary in acromegalic patients. We have now treated over 100 acromegalic patients with external pituitary radiotherapy associated with bromocriptine to lower GH levels during the interval required for the radiotherapy to lower GH levels into the normal range.[31, 32] The chemical and biochemical responses are dramatic, with shrinkage of skin and restitution of normal facial features, shrinkage of hands and feet, cessation of sweating and headache, improvement in potency, menstrual function, and abolition of diabetes mellitus in the majority of patients; as with prolactinoma patients, the tumor also shrinks. The introduction of dopamine agonist therapy for acromegaly represents a major advance in the management of this otherwise often intractable condition.

## Acknowledgments

The work reported in this chapter has been carried out in association with many colleagues, particularly Professors Lesley H. Rees, A.E. Jones, and C.R.W. Edwards, and Drs. J.E. Dacie, M. Charlesworth, M.O. Thorner, J.A.H. Wass, and P.J.A. Moult. It has been supported by the Medical Research Council, the Joint Research Board of St. Bartholomew's Hospital, and the Peel Medical Research Trust. The author is grateful to the editors and authors associated with the acknowledged, previously published illustrations and tables for permission to reproduce them here.

## REFERENCES

1. Frantz A.G., Kleinberg D.L.: Prolactin: Evidence that it is separate from growth hormone in human blood. *Science* 170:745, 1970.
2. Forsyth I.A., Besser G.M., Edwards C.R.W., et al.: Plasma prolactin activity in inappropriate lactation. *Br. Med. J.* 3:225, 1971.
3. Thorner M.O.: Prolactin: Clinical physiology and the significance and management of hyperprolactinaemia, in Martini L., et al. (eds): *Clinical Neuroendocrinology*. New York: Academic Press, 1977, pp 319–361.
4. Thorner M.O.: Prolactin, in Besser G.M. (ed): *Clinics in Endocrinology and Metabolism*. Philadelphia: W.B. Saunders Co., 1977, vol 6, pp 201–222.
5. Costello R.T.: Subclinical adenoma of the pituitary gland. *Am. J. Pathol.* 12:205, 1936.
6. Hardy J.: Ten years after the recognition of pituitary microadenomas, in Faglia G., et al. (eds): *Pituitary Microadenomas*. New York: 1980, vol 29, pp 7–14.
7. Peillon F., et al.: Microadenomas, structure and function, in Faglia G., et al. (eds): *Pituitary Microadenomas*. New York: 1980, vol 29, pp. 91–106.
8. Besser G.M., Parke L., Edwards C.R.W., et al.: Galactorrhoea: Successful treatment with reduction of plasma prolactin levels by bromergocryptine, *Br. Med. J.* 3:669, 1972.
9. Thorner M.O., Besser G.M.: Bromocriptine treatment of hyperprolactinaemic hypogonadism. *Acta Endocrinol. [Suppl. 216] (Copenh.)* 88:131, 1978.
10. Thorner M.O., et al.: Hyperprolactinaemia and gonadal function: results of bromocriptine treatment, in Crosignani P.G., et al. (eds): *Prolactin and Human Reproduction*, Serono Symposia. London: Academic Press, 1977, vol 11, pp. 285–301.
11. Thorner M.O., et al.: Hyperprolactinaemia, current concepts of management including medical therapy with bromocriptine, in Goldstein M., et al. (eds): *Ergot Compounds and Brain Function: Neuroendocrine and Neuropsychiatric Aspects*. New York: Raven Press, 1980, pp. 165–189.
12. Moult P.A., Dacie J.E., Rees L.H., et al.: Prolactin pulsatility in patients with gonadal dysfunction. *Clin. Endocrinol.* 14:387, 1981.
13. Swanson H.A., du Boulet G.: Borderline variants of the normal pituitary fossa, *Br. J. Radiol.* 48:366, 1975.
14. Besser G.M.: The pituitary fossa—normal or abnormal? *Br. J. Radiol.* 49:652, 1976.
15. Burrow G.N., Wortzman G., Rewcastle N.E., et al.: Microadenomas of the pituitary and abnormal sellar tomograms in an unselected autopsy series. *N. Engl. J. Med.* 304:156, 1981.
16. Thorner M.O., Edwards C.R.W., Charlesworth M., et al.: Pregnancy in patients presenting with hyperprolactinaemia, *Br. Med. J.* 2:771, 1979.
17. Yeo T., Thorner M.O., Jones A., et al.: The effects of dopamine, bromocriptine, lergotrile and metoclopramide on prolactin release from continuously perfused columns of isolated rat pituitary cells. *Clin. Endocrinol. (Oxf.)* 10:123, 1979.

18. Grossman A., Delitala G., Yeo T., et al.: Gaba and muscimol inhibit the release of prolactin from dispersed rat anterior pituitary cells. *Neuroendocrinology* 32:145, 1981.
19. Besser G.M., et al.: Clinical neuroendocrine relationships in normal and disordered prolactin secretion, in Fuxe K., et al. (eds): *Central Regulation of the Endocrine System,* Nobel Symposium 42. New York: Plenum Publishing, 1979, pp. 457–472.
20. Delitala G., Yeo T., Grossman A., et al.: A comparison of the effects of four ergot derivatives on prolactin secretion by dispersed rat pituitary cells. *J. Endocrinol.* 87:95, 103.
21. Grossman A., Yeo T., Delitala G., et al.: Two new dopamine agonists that are long acting in vivo but short acting in vitro. *Clin. Endocrinol. (Oxf.)* 13:595, 1978.
22. Thorner M.O., Ryan S.N., Wass J.A.H., et al.: Effect of the dopamine agonist lergotrile mesylate on circulating anterior pituitary hormones in man. *J. Clin. Endocrinol. Metab.* 47:372, 1978.
23. Delitala G., Wass J.A.H., Stubbs W.A., et al.: Effect of lisuride hydrogen maleate, an ergot derivative on anterior pituitary hormone secretion in man. *Clin. Endocrinol. (Oxf.)* 11:1, 1979.
24. Thorner M.O., Besser G.M.: Bromocriptine treatment of hyperprolactinaemic hypogonadism. *Acta Endocrinol. [Suppl. 216] (Copenh.)* 88:131, 1978.
25. Thorner M.O., Schran H.F., Evans W.S., et al.: A broad spectrum of prolactin suppression by bromocriptine in hyperprolactinaemic women: A study of serum prolactin and bromocriptine levels after acute and chronic administration of bromocriptine. *J. Clin. Endocrinol. Metab.* 50:1026, 1980.
26. Wass J.A.H., Moult P.J.A., Thorner M.O., et al.: Reduction of pituitary tumor size in patients with prolactinomas and acromegaly treated with bromocriptine with or without radiotherapy. *Lancet* 2:66, 1979.
27. Thorner M.O., et al.: Hyperprolactinemia, current concepts of management including medical therapy with bromocriptine, in Goldstein M., et al. (eds): *Ergot Compounds and Brain Function: Neuroendocrine and Neuropsychiatric Aspects.* New York: Raven Press, 1980, pp. 165–189.
28. Griffith R.W., Turkalj I., Braun P.: Outcome of pregnancy in mothers given bromocriptine. *Br. J. Clin. Pharmacol.* 5:227, 1978.
29. Gemzell C., Wang C.F.: Outcome of pregnancy in women with pituitary adenomas. *Fertil. Steril.* 31:363, 1979.
30. Franks S., Nabarro J.D.N., Jacobs L.: Prevalence and presentation of hyperprolactinaemia in patients with "functionless" pituitary tumors. *Lancet* 1:778, 1977.
31. Wass J.A.H., Thorner M.O., Morris D.V., et al.: Long-term treatment of acromegaly with bromocriptine. *Br. Med. J.* 1:875, 1977.
32. Besser G.M., Wass J.A.H., Thorner M.O.: Acromegaly—Results of long term treatment with bromocriptine. *Acta Endocrinol. [Suppl. 216] (Copenh.)* 88:187, 1978.

# Transsphenoidal Microsurgery for Prolactinomas

MIGUEL A. FARIA, JR., M.D. AND GEORGE T. TINDALL, M.D.

*Division of Neurosurgery, Department of Surgery, Emory University School of Medicine, Atlanta Georgia*

## Introduction

THREE YEARS AFTER PUBLICATION of reports from our institution on the results of transsphenoidal microsurgery in 37 patients with prolactin-secreting pituitary adenoma (prolactinoma), new developments are beginning to have an impact on the management of these tumors. Prominent among these developments have been the increasing roles of computerized tomography (CT), especially the updated models of scanners in diagnosis,[14] and bromocriptine in treatment.[25, 39, 45, 51, 54] The capability of the updated scanner to diagnose tumors as small as 5 mm has led to reassessment of the diagnostic workup of these patients, particularly reassessment of the continued use of sellar polytomography.[14, 63] While bromocriptine relieves symptoms in most and shrinks the tumor in many patients, the drug does not appear to eradicate the tumor completely and its ultimate role in treatment remains to be defined.

This chapter deals with 100 women with the amenorrhea-galactorrhea (A-G) syndrome associated with a prolactinoma who were treated by transsphenoidal microsurgery. The results of surgery in terms of its effect on serum prolactin (PRL) levels and symptomatology and the various issues and controversies involving the manage-

Research for this study was supported by a grant from the Lyndhurst Foundation, Chattanooga, Tennessee.

ment of this tumor, particularly in view of recent developments, are discussed in this chapter.

## Historical Background

Horsley[13, 50] was probably the first surgeon to operate successfully on a pituitary tumor. He used a transcranial approach. But because of frequent complications—hemorrhage, brain injury, and inadequate exposure of the tumor—craniotomy for pituitary tumor in the early 1900s was usually unsuccessful; operative mortality was as high as 70% to 80%.[13]

The first successful transsphenoidal operation for a pituitary tumor was performed by Schloffer[13, 59] in 1907. His approach was modified by Hirsch and later, Cushing, who reported an operative mortality rate of 5.5% in a total of 231 transsphenoidal operations.[13, 32, 50] However, technical drawbacks of the transsphenoidal operation, e.g., inadequate visualization with poor exposure of these tumors, lack of magnification, etc., resulted in a relatively high rate of recurrence and thus discouraged many surgeons. High recurrence rates together with improvement and modification of craniotomy techniques resulted in a significant decline in usage of the transsphenoidal approach in the 1920s.[28, 45] Craniotomy became the procedure of choice, and as late as 1971, Ray and Patterson[58] reported a 1.2% operative mortality in 146 patients with chromophobe adenomas treated by this approach. Thus the intracranial approach became and remained the operative procedure of choice until the mid 1960s, when Guiot[26] and Hardy[28, 31] rekindled interest in the transsphenoidal operative technique by the adoption of two major innovations—the operating microscope and televised fluoroscopy. Hardy[28] in particular showed that it was possible to remove small tumors and preserve pituitary glandular function in the majority of patients. Currently, the transsphenoidal microsurgical operation with its low morbidity and mortality is the method of choice for the definitive treatment of most pituitary tumors, including prolactinomas. Using this approach, many neurosurgeons have confirmed Hardy's observations that hyperfunctional pituitary tumors can usually be totally removed with sparing of the pituitary gland in most patients and restoration of normal hormonal function in some patients after removal of the tumor.[4, 28, 29, 30, 52, 53, 70, 76]

Recently several reports have advocated medical treatment of pituitary adenomas associated with hyperprolactinemia with bromocriptine and have demonstrated not only reduction of PRL levels to normal but also regression (but not eradication) of tumor along with symptomatic improvement.[39, 45, 48, 54, 55, 64, 68, 73]

## Operative Technique

Operative technique, which has been described previously,[70] is similar to that performed by Hardy.[27, 28, 31] The authors have modified the initial part of the operation such that the approach is made unilaterally alongside the nasal septum and the septum is spared rather than removed.[69]

Because many tumors associated with abnormalities in PRL secretion are small (i.e., <10 mm in diameter), it is important that the pituitary gland not be damaged during the dural opening. Lacerations in the gland with attendant subcapsular bleeding make it extremely difficult, if not impossible, to detect the subtle differences that exist between normal gland and small tumors and that must be determined if the surgeon is to successfully remove the tumor and spare the gland. Also, the less the gland is manipulated the greater the chance for preservation of pituitary function postoperatively. The dura mater can be opened safely by making a slow, deliberate incision with a No. 11 blade on an appropriate bayonet knife holder under relatively high magnification. Once an adequate opening is made, it can be enlarged appropriately with fine angled microscissors.

After removal of the tumor, absolute alcohol was applied to the tumor bed for five minutes. Alcohol was used only when the diaphragm sellae-tumor capsule was intact, thus providing a barrier between the subarachnoid space and the tumor site. Adipose tissue taken from the abdominal wall was inserted loosely into the tumor bed to prevent prolapse of the optic chiasm into the sella turcica. After withdrawal of the speculum, the incision in the gingival mucosa was closed with a single catgut suture. Soft airway tubes were inserted into each nostril in order to reapproximate the nasal mucosa, and the patient was then allowed to recover from anesthesia. The nasal tubes were removed after 24 hours.

## Case Material and Methods

Over a seven-year period (August, 1973 through March, 1981) a total of 631 patients have undergone transsphenoidal microsurgery operations (Table 1) at Emory University Affiliated Hospitals. Surgery was performed for pituitary tumors in 351 patients. Included in the latter group were 139 women who had a prolactinoma and who

TABLE 1.—TRANSSPHENOIDAL
PITUITARY MICROSURGERY AT EMORY
UNIVERSITY AFFILIATED HOSPITALS,
1973–1981

| INDICATION FOR SURGERY | | NO. OF PATIENTS |
|---|---|---|
| Hypophysectomy | | |
| Breast | | 132 |
| Prostate | | 80 |
| Other | | 28 |
| Tumors | | |
| Adenomas | | |
| Nonfunctional | | 147 |
| Functional | | 204 |
| HGH (acromegaly) | 50 | |
| ACTH (Cushing's) | 12 | |
| (Nelson's) | 3 | |
| Prolactin | 139 | |
| Other | | 40 |
| Total | | 631 |

presented with impairment of the menstrual cycle and, usually, galactorrhea. In this chapter we present the results obtained in 100 patients from this latter group in whom there was a follow-up period of at least six months. The age of these women ranged from 16 to 47 years (average, 27).

All patients underwent testing for pituitary function (Table 2) before and ten days after surgery. These studies were believed to be the minimum studies that would provide accurate assessment of general pituitary and pituitary-target organ function.[11, 37, 70] PRL reserve was determined both by chlorpromazine[11, 71] and thyrotropin-releasing hormone (TRH) (Thypinone).[1, 11, 37] The normal basal value of PRL ranges from 5 to 25 ng/ml. A less than twofold increase at the peak response after chlorpromazine or TRH is considered to show loss of pituitary reserve if the baseline PRL value is low and loss of hypothalamic control if the baseline is high.[37]

## Neurodiagnostic Studies

Over the period of this study, neurodiagnostic evaluation has undergone periodic evolution. All patients underwent sellar polytomography.[40, 72] As will be discussed later, the results of surgery correlated with the preoperative levels of PRL, and for this reason, we divided the patients into two groups: Group 1 had preoperative PRL levels less than 200 ng/ml and Group 2 had levels greater than 200 ng/ml.

TABLE 2.—MINIMAL DATA ENDOCRINOLOGIC TESTING FOR
PITUITARY TUMORS

| TESTS | NORMAL VALUES (FEMALE) |
|---|---|
| Anterior pituitary function | |
| Pituitary-gonad axis | |
| Follicle-stimulating hormone (FSH) | 5–20 IMU/ml |
| Luteinizing hormone (LH) | 2–30 IMU/ml |
| Estradiol (females) | 2–7 ng/100 ml |
| Testosterone | 20–80 ng/100 ml |
| Pituitary-thyroid axis | |
| Thyroid-stimulating hormone (TSH) | 4.5–11.5 µg/100 ml |
| Total thyroxine | 1.0–2.3 ng/100 ml |
| Free thyroxine | <6 µU/ml |
| Pituitary-adrenal axis | |
| Serum A.M. cortisol | 6–18 µg/100 ml |
| 24-hour urinary 17- | 1.1–8.6 mg/24 hr |
| hydroxycorticosteroid and 17- | 1–18 mg/24 hr |
| ketosteroid excretion | |
| Metyrapone test if values are low | |
| Prolactin reserve | |
| Chlorpromazine provocative | |
| TRH provocative | |
| Posterior pituitary function | |
| Simultaneous serum and urine | |
| osmolalities after 8–12-hr period of | |
| water deprivation | |

A close correlation between tumor size and preoperative levels of PRL was observed (Table 3). Of 72 women in Group 1, only 14 (19%) had tumors greater than 1 cm, while 24 (86%) of 28 women in Group 2 had tumors greater than 1 cm. The results of polytomography were interesting. As shown in Table 4, only 40% of the 72 patients in Group 1 had abnormal polytomography. The decision to operate on patients with negative polytomes was made on the basis of clinical and endocrine findings, and more recently with visualization of the tumor (coronal view) on an updated CT scanner (made by General Electric Co., Medical Systems Division, Milwaukee, Wisconsin). Once considered a vital part of the evaluation of patients with pituitary adenoma, polytomography[36, 72] may diminish in importance in future diagnostic protocols.

Conventional CT scanning techniques (i.e., slices made at an angle 15 to 25 degrees from the canthomeatal line) utilizing 5- to 8-mm cuts both with and without intravenous (IV) contrast media enhancement in our series, as shown in Table 4, gave the following results: 75 patients had negative studies; nine patients had a definite intrasellar abnormality; and 11 patients had evidence of parasellar and/or supra-

TABLE 3.—RELATIONSHIP OF SERUM PROLACTIN
AND TUMOR SIZE (CM)

| | NO. OF PATIENTS | <1.0 | >1.0 |
|---|---|---|---|
| Group 1 | | | |
| Prolactin <200 | 72 | 58 (81%) | 14 (19%) |
| Group 2 | | | |
| Prolactin >200 | 28 | 4 (14%) | 24 (86%) |

TABLE 4.—RELATIONSHIP OF SERUM PROLACTIN
AND RESULTS OF POLYTOMOGRAPHY

| | NO. OF PATIENTS | NORMAL | ABNORMAL |
|---|---|---|---|
| Group 1 | | | |
| Prolactin <200 | 72 | 32 (44%) | 40 (56%) |
| Group 2 | | | |
| Prolactin >200 | 28 | 3 (11%) | 25 (89%) |

sellar extension. As expected, the majority of patients in whom conventional CT scanning was abnormal were in Group 2 and all had tumors that were 1 cm or greater in diameter (Table 5).

Prior to February, 1980, CT scans were obtained using either the EMI or the GE scanner (Model CT 8800 Body Scanner, made by General Electric Co., Medical Systems Division, Milwaukee, Wisconsin). The GE scanner has since been updated to provide better imaging of intrasellar lesions. The current technique involves serial 1.5-mm coronal cuts through the sella turcica with contrast enhancement. The diagnosis was made by identifying subtle changes, e.g., upward bowing of the pituitary gland, sloping of the sella floor, deviation of the stalk, focal alterations in the gland, etc. To date, 22 patients in the present series with prolactinomas have been studied using the updated scanner. Of this total, 14 (Table 6) showed an intrasellar ab-

TABLE 5.—RESULTS OF CONVENTIONAL CT
SCANNING OF 95 PATIENTS

| FINDING | TOTAL NO. OF PATIENTS | GROUP 1 | GROUP 2 |
|---|---|---|---|
| Negative | 75 | 61 | 14 |
| Intrasellar abnormality | 9 | 1 | 8 |
| Suprasellar, parasellar extension | 11 | 7 | 4 |

TABLE 6.—CORRELATION OF UPDATED GE SCANNER
DIAGNOSIS WITH PATHOLOGIC FINDINGS

| GE SCANNER DIAGNOSIS (NO. OF PATIENTS) | PATHOLOGIC DIAGNOSIS (NO. OF PATIENTS) |
|---|---|
| Pituitary adenoma (14) | Pituitary adenoma (9); hyperplasia (4); no tumor (1) |
| No tumor (6) | Pituitary adenoma (6) |
| Empty sella turcica (2) | Empty sella turcica (1); hyperplasia (1) |
| Total 22 | Total 22 |

normality and at surgery and on subsequent histologic examination a pituitary adenoma was found in nine of these 14. Examples of the CT findings in these patients are shown in Figures 1 and 2. Pituitary hyperplasia was found in four of the 22 patients and no tumor could be identified in one. Six of the twenty-two patients had CT scans that were interpreted as normal, but because strong clinical and endocrinologic findings were consistent with a prolactinoma, surgery was performed. In all of these six patients a pituitary adenoma was found

**Fig 1.**—Contrast-enhanced CT scan in coronal projection shows an area of radiolucency in right side of sella approximately 6 mm in diameter *(arrows),* which at surgery was found to be a microadenoma.

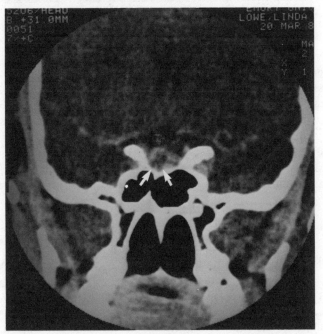

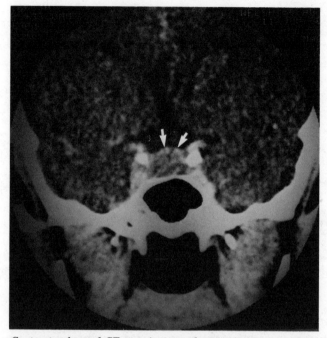

**Fig 2.**—Contrast-enhanced CT scan in coronal projection in a patient with a PRL level of 540 ng/ml. A tumor that measures 1.5 cm in greatest diameter is visualized as a radiodense intrasellar mass with bulging of diaphragmatic sella *(arrows).*

at surgery and histologically. In addition, in two of the 22 patients an empty sella was diagnosed by CT scan, but because of the possibility of a concomitant microadenoma and an empty sella, surgery was performed. One patient had no tumor (empty sella) and the other had a partially empty sella in association with pituitary hyperplasia. Thus we believe that the fourth-generation (high-resolution) CT scanners will become a useful modality for studying patients with the A-G syndrome and suspected microadenoma, even though further experience is still needed with this technique.

## Pathology

Histologically, the adenomas in our series were classified as chromophobe in 36 patients, eosinophilic in 17, mixed types in 4; and 43 patients were simply classified as having pituitary adenomas. Calcospherites, which are spherical calcified concretions (either concentric laminations or irregular aggregates of smaller concretions), were seen in 16 patients in our series. These structures are seen more often in prolactinoma than any other type of pituitary adenoma.[66]

Ultrastructurally, PRL cells have been described as pleomorphic cells with branching and processes. Their granules have been described as being sparse and measuring 50–100 nm in diameter. Prolactinomas may also demonstrate their hormone-secreting character by immunofluorescence.[60, 61, 66] Robert[60] used electron microscopy to study 132 patients with prolactin-secreting adenomas and showed that the cells contain scarce dense secretory granules that may reach up to 500–600 nm. In four of her patients in whom immunoperoxidase technique for prolactin was performed at the ultrastructural level, the secretory granules stained with antiadenomatous prolactin serum.

## Clinical Findings

Amenorrhea was present in 97 patients and some disturbance in the menstrual cycle was found in the remaining three. Sixty-two patients in Group 1 and twenty-two patients in Group 2 also had galactorrhea. Headaches occurred in 27 patients and impairment in visual acuity and/or fields was present in 21.

A total of 39 (45%) of 86 patients in whom a history of birth control prophylaxis was recorded had been taking oral contraceptives (OCs) and had developed the A-G syndrome immediately after discontinuation of these medications; some of these women actually became symptomatic while still taking the drugs. Twenty-nine patients had never taken OC, and eighteen had taken the drugs some time in their past. Because the incidence of OC usage in this population is estimated at 37.6%,[22] our results do not show a significant relationship between OC usage and the A-G syndrome (45% vs 37.6%). Therefore we are in agreement with Keye et al.[36] and in disagreement with Teperman et al.[67] in regard to the significance of OC usage and the development of microadenomas.

The follow-up period ranged from six months to seven years. Of the 21 patients with impairment in visual acuity and/or visual fields, there was significant improvement in 19 and no change in two. Vision did not worsen in any patient.

## Effects of Surgery on Amenorrhea, Galactorrhea, and PRL Levels

The results of surgery correlated with the preoperative level of PRL. Preoperatively, these values ranged from 25 to 192 ng/ml in Group 1 and from 210 to 6,600 in Group 2. As shown in Tables 7 and

TABLE 7.—EFFECT OF SURGERY ON AMENORRHEA AND
GALACTORRHEA

| FINDING | NO. OF PATIENTS | RESUMED PERIODS | STOPPED GALACTORRHEA |
|---|---|---|---|
| Group 1 | | | |
| Prolactin <200 | 72 | 56 (78%) | 45 (75%) |
| Group 2 | | | |
| Prolactin >200 | 28 | 11 (39%) | 12 (55%) |

TABLE 8.—EFFECTS OF SURGERY ON PRL
LEVELS

| FINDING | NO. OF PATIENTS | NO. NORMAL ON 10TH POSTOPERATIVE DAY |
|---|---|---|
| Group 1 | | |
| Prolactin <200 | 72 | 55 (76%) |
| Group 2 | | |
| Prolactin >200 | 28 | 13 (46%) |

8, the postsurgical results in Group 1 were significantly better.
Among both groups, galactorrhea persisted in a few patients even
through postoperative PRL values returned to normal. There was also
a good correlation between tumor size and preoperative PRL levels.
Of 72 women in Group 1, only 14 (19%) had a tumor that measured
1 cm or larger. On the other hand, of 28 women in Group 2, 24 (86%)
had tumors of that size or larger.

Interestingly, some women had return of menses despite slight elevation of postoperative serum PRL, and conversely, some had persistent amenorrhea with normal postoperative levels. These data are
shown in Table 9. Postoperatively, 60 women (51 patients in Group 1

TABLE 9.—RELATIONSHIP OF POSTOPERATIVE
PRL LEVEL TO CESSATION OF AMENORRHEA
FOLLOWING SURGERY

| FINDING | GROUP 1 (72 PATIENTS) | GROUP 2 (28 PATIENTS) |
|---|---|---|
| Resumed periods, normal PRL | 51 (71%) | 9 (32%) |
| Resumed periods, elevated PRL | 5 ( 7%) | 2 ( 7%) |
| Amenorrhea normal PRL | 5 ( 7%) | 4 (14%) |
| Amenorrhea elevated PRL | 11 (15%) | 13 (47%) |

and nine in Group 2) resumed menses and had normal PRL levels, whereas seven women (five in Group 1 and two in Group 2) resumed menses despite persistently elevated prolactin levels. Nine women (five in Group 1 and four in Group 2) remained amenorrheic despite normal PRL levels, whereas twenty-four (11 in Group 1 and 13 in Group 2) remained amenorrheic with persistently elevated PRL levels.

Thirteen patients have become pregnant and have delivered eleven normal babies, two normal twins and one abnormal baby (multiple congenital anomalies—probably unrelated to the mother's pituitary disorder).

Postoperatively, the PRL response to chlorpromazine returned to normal in 19 (26%) of the 72 patients in Group 1 and in only one (4%) of the 28 patients in Group 2 (Table 10). The TRH provocative test was performed on 28 patients preoperatively and 27 patients postoperatively. All but two patients had an abnormal PRL response to TRH in Group 1. Postoperatively, the prolactin response to TRH returned to normal in ten (41%) of the 17 patients in Group 1 and in two (20%) of the ten patients in Group 2 (see Table 10). Thus, while both tests appear to be reliable indicators of PRL reserve preoperatively, the TRH provocative test seems to be a more sensitive indicator of recovery of PRL reserve postoperatively.

## RECURRENT TUMORS

Five patients needed further therapy for persistent or recurrent tumors. Two women were reoperated on via the transsphenoidal approach. One patient who had a persistently elevated and gradually rising PRL level (in the range of 2,000 ng/ml) over a two-year period had a surprisingly negative exploration. The other patient underwent reoperation for mass effect (e.g., bitemporal hemianopia and panhy-

TABLE 10.—PREOPERATIVE AND POSTOPERATIVE RESULTS OF THE CHLORPROMAZINE AND TRH TEST

| FINDING | CHLORPROMAZINE PROVOCATIVE | | TRH PROVOCATIVE | |
| --- | --- | --- | --- | --- |
| | Abnormal Preoperative | Normal Postoperative | Abnormal Preoperative | Normal Postoperative |
| Group 1 Prolactin <200 | 70/72 (97%) | 19/72 (26%) | 18/20 (90%) | 10/17 (41%) |
| Group 2 Prolactin >200 | 28/28 (100%) | 1/28 (4%) | 8/8 (100%) | 2/10 (20%) |

popituitarism), and a large mass was subtotally removed via the transsphenoidal approach. A third patient had craniotomy and postoperative radiation; a fourth patient was given radiotherapy alone. The fifth patient currently is being followed closely for persistent postoperative hyperprolactinemia (i.e., 70 ng/ml) due possibly to remaining tumor.

Serial PRL determinations were obtained in 30 patients in Group 1 and in 11 in Group 2 at intervals ranging from six months to seven years following surgery. We arbitrarily decided that a 15% change in either direction from the ten-day postoperative PRL value is significant. Patients in whom values remained below 25 ng/ml were considered to be normal. Of the 30 Group 1 patients, follow-up serum PRL determinations showed no change in 20, a further decrease in six, and a significant increase in four. In the 11 Group 2 patients, five showed no change, two a significant decrease, and four a significant increase.

### Preservation of Endocrine Function

The surgeon believed that gross total tumor removal was accomplished in 97 and subtotal removal in three of the 100 patients. The pituitary gland was identified and spared in the majority of patients. However, preoperative and postoperative endocrinologic evaluation provided a more accurate assessment than gross observations of the status of pituitary function following transsphenoidal microsurgery.

Complete preoperative and postoperative data were available for 97 of the 100 patients and thus permitted an evaluation of the effect of surgery on the pituitary-target organ axes (i.e., pituitary-gonadal, pituitary-adrenal, pituitary-thyroidal); these data are summarized in Table 11. In 50 (77%) of 65 women with normal preoperative pituitary-target organ axes, normal function was preserved in all axes.

TABLE 11.—Preoperative and Postoperative Endocrine Values

| FINDING | TOTAL NO. OF PATIENTS | GROUP 1 PRL <200 (72 PATIENTS) | GROUP 2 PRL >200 (28 PATIENTS) |
|---|---|---|---|
| Normal preoperatively | 65 | 54 | 11 |
| Normal postoperatively | 50 | 41 | 9 |
| Deficient 1 or more axes | 15 | 13 | 2 |
| Abnormal preoperatively | | | |
| (i.e., deficit 1 or more axes) | 32 | 17 | 15 |
| Improvement postoperatively | 11 | 8 | 3 |
| No change postoperatively | 19 | 12 | 7 |
| Worsened postoperatively | 2 | 2 | 0 |

Of the remaining 15 women (23%) with a deficit in one or more axes postoperatively, the resultant deficits were distributed as follows: two patients had deficits in two axes (thyroidal and gonadal axes in both); the other 13 all had deficits in one axis (the thyroidal axis in one and the gonadal axis in 12). Fortunately, the deficits were temporary in the majority, as shown by the fact that of these 15 patients, only two required replacement therapy for longer than six months. Thus, even in those patients with postoperative pituitary-target organ axes deficits, the deficiencies were short-lived. Furthermore, of 32 women with deficits in one or more axes preoperatively, 11 (34%) improved in one or more of these axes postoperatively: one patient had a normal thyroid axis, whereas ten women had normal gonadal axes postoperatively.

These results indicate that transsphenoidal microsurgical removal of a pituitary tumor can be accomplished in the majority of cases without damaging a functionally intact gland, and in some cases of prolactinomas associated with the A-G syndrome, pituitary-target organ function can be improved or restored to normal.

## Complications

Postoperative complications were relatively few in this series. One patient developed maxillary sinusitis, which was successfully treated with a course of antibiotics. Another patient developed cerebrospinal fluid (CSF) rhinorrhea that was treated with reoperation and packing of the sphenoid sinus with an abdominal fat graft. Three patients experienced superficial abdominal wound infections, which were successfully treated with a course of antibiotics and local wound care. Sixty patients had transient diabetes insipidus, which was self-limited in most patients or required only one or two doses of pitressin tannate in oil (5 units delivered intramuscularly) in the immediate postoperative period. Only three patients had permanent but partial diabetes insipidus, which has required treatment with desmopressin acetate or pitressin injections.

There were no deaths, but one patient developed several life-threatening complications. She was a 27-year-old woman with the A-G syndrome who also had panhypopituitarism and a bitemporal hemianopia. She had received irradiation as primary treatment at another institution. At our hospital, she underwent two transsphenoidal operations separated by an interval of eight months. Following the second operation she developed CSF rhinorrhea, which ultimately required a lumbar subarachnoid-peritoneal shunt. She subsequently developed a sellar and parasellar cryptococcal abscess that required a third transsphenoidal procedure for drainage.

## Bromocriptine

Bromocriptine has been used extensively in clinical trials in Europe and Canada in women with amenorrhea and/or galactorrhea associated with hyperprolactinemia. An extensive literature relative to its use in experimental as well as clinical trials already exists.*

It has proved to be effective in the majority of patients in reducing elevated PRL levels to normal and reversing the symptoms (amenorrhea, galactorrhea, and infertility) associated with the hyperprolactinemia due to the tumor. Tumor regression as measured by CT scan, reconstitution of the sella on plain x-rays, or pneumoencephalography has been reported in some patients.[39, 45, 64] In fact, pregnancies have occurred in some of these patients.[5] However, it is important to recognize that although bromocriptine can cause a dramatic reduction in size of prolactinomas and symptomatic improvement, the drug does not eradicate the tumor, a fact emphasized by a study conducted by Weiss.[74] He treated 20 patients with prolactinomas with bromocriptine for two years; 19 patients had resolution of amenorrhea with a marked reduction of hyperprolactinemia. When the drug was withdrawn, however, amenorrhea returned in all patients and PRL levels returned to their pretreatment levels.

The enthusiasm among some clinicians over these initial results with bromocriptine in prolactinomas has led to the suggestion that the drug can be used as primary treatment for these lesions, and that surgery can be reserved for those patients in whom actual tumor regression fails to occur.[55] In our opinion, this approach is inappropriate, as there are inadequate data currently available to support this recommendation. For instance, one of the major gaps in existing knowledge in this field is the fact that there are no systematic pathologic studies of prolactinomas removed from patients who have received either short- or long-term bromocriptine.[79] In virtually all reported cases of tumor regression caused by bromocriptine, assessment of the regressive changes was based on either clinical data (symptomatic improvement, return of menses, return of elevated PRL level to normal, and/or cessation of galactorrhea) or radiologic evidence (reconstitution of the bone of the floor of the sella turcica, a CT scan that fails to reveal a tumor shown to be present prior to the admin-

---

*References 2, 6, 8, 9, 12, 17–21, 24, 25, 34, 35, 38, 41–44, 47, 48, 51, 52, 54–56, 65, 68, 73, 77, 78.

istration of bromocriptine, and/or a decrease on serial pneumoencephalography). No study has yet assessed structural or biologic changes in prolactinomas after the administration of bromocriptine and compared these changes in tumor from "control" patients who have received no bromocriptine.

At the present time, despite the sporadic case reports of successful medical treatment of patients treated with bromocriptine for prolactinomas,[39, 45, 54, 64, 68, 73] we are reluctant to recommend the use of this drug as primary therapy for this tumor. The many advantages of transsphenoidal microsurgery with its low morbidity and mortality does not warrant the use of a drug that as yet has not been proved to eradicate the tumor. On the other hand, bromocriptine may prove useful in effecting *preoperative* shrinkage in patients with large tumors in terms of facilitating their total removal. Additionally, the drug probably will find a use in patients who have had transsphenoidal surgery for prolactinomas and in whom hyperprolactinemia persists because of persistent tumor and/or stalk damage.

## Discussion

Pituitary tumors that autonomously secrete PRL as their sole endocrine abnormality have been termed prolactinomas and have been estimated to account for approximately 70% of chromophobe adenomas.[23, 25] Currently, prolactinomas are the most frequently diagnosed functional pituitary tumors, and represent approximately 25% of all pituitary tumors.[52, 53] As indicated by Hardy,[29] these tumors are usually located in the lateral aspect of the pituitary gland, which was true for most of our patients.

A number of workers have reported results of transsphenoidal microsurgery for prolactinomas (Table 12). Hardy et al.[30] showed that transsphenoidal surgery for these tumors was followed by a return of PRL level to normal in 59 (74%) of 80 patients. In 50 (63%) of them, menses returned, and 29 (36%) became pregnant. Similar beneficial results were obtained by Chang et al.,[7] who reported return of menses in 16 of 17 women with PRL microadenomas and in two of seven with adenomas larger than 1 cm in diameter (macroadenomas). The wide range of surgical results obtained in various surgical series of patients with prolactinomas who were treated by transsphenoidal surgery[3, 7, 15, 16, 25, 30, 57, 70, 75] reflects, among other variables, differences in patient selection. In several series,[3, 7, 15, 30] the results were better among patients harboring microadenomas than among those with larger tumors. Tindall et al.[70] reported normalization of PRL levels

TABLE 12.—Summary of Published Surgical Series
of Treatment of Hyperprolactinemia

| SERIES | EVALUABLE PATIENTS* | PRL NORMALIZED POSTOPERATIVELY (% OF PATIENTS) |
|---|---|---|
| Chang et al.[7] | 23 | 11 (48) |
| Hardy et al.[30] | 80 | 59 (74) |
| Tindall et al.[70] | 36 | 24 (67) |
| Derome et al.[15] | 71 | 17 (24) |
| Post et al.[57] | 30 | 21 (70) |
| Aubourg et al.[3] | 90 | 39 (43) |
| Domingue et al.[16] | 91 | 62 (68)† |
| Present series | 100 | 69 (69) |

*Evaluable patients refer to those in whom preoperative and
postoperative data was complete, and in whom the follow-up period was, in the opinion of the authors, adequate for analysis of
the results of surgery.
†In this series, resolution of amenorrhea after a follow-up period of 18 months following transsphenoidal surgery was considered a "therapeutic success." Preoperative and postoperative
PRL levels were not reported.

following transsphenoidal surgery in 19 of 26 patients whose preoperative PRL level was <200 ng/ml and in only 3 of 11 patients in
whom the preoperative PRL level was >200 ng/ml. In the series of
Hardy et al.,[30] normalization of serum PRL following transsphenoidal
surgery occurred in 90% of localized microadenomas, 53% of enclosed
adenomas, and 43% of invasive adenomas. Domingue et al.[16] defined
"therapeutic failure" as failure of resolution of amenorrhea to occur
until follow-up had extended for at least 18 months. Therapeutic failure was encountered in 32% (29 of 91) of their patients with prolactinomas. They found that therapeutic failure occurred in patients who
had higher preoperative serum PRL levels (i.e., PRL levels >200 ng/
ml) and in those in whom total removal was not achieved. Normal
menstruation was restored in 31 of 32 patients with preoperative PRL
values <200 ng/ml, but in only three of nine patients with preoperative levels >200 ng/ml in the group of women studied by Keye and
associates.[36] Aubourg et al.[3] reported the results of transsphenoidal
surgery in 90 patients with prolactinomas and found that those patients who were cured had a distinctly lower mean PRL level (<200
ng/ml) than those who were not cured. Of those patients whose adenomas were larger than 10 mm in diameter, only 39% were cured.
In their series, PRL levels increased with the size of the adenoma,
and those patients harboring microadenomas associated with preoperative PRL determinations <200 ng/ml had the best prognosis, with
postoperative return of normal menses in 80%.

Interestingly, the normal menstrual cycle and fertility can be restored following transsphenoidal microsurgical removal of prolactinomas even when postoperative PRL values, although reduced, remain slightly or moderately elevated. In the present series, seven women resumed normal menses despite persistently elevated PRL levels, and nine women remained amenorrheic even though normal PRL levels were restored following tumor removal. Hardy et al.[29, 30] reported similar findings among 80 patients with prolactinomas undergoing transsphenoidal surgery. The fact that some women with PRL levels higher than normal will menstruate probably means that the endocrine mechanisms involved in this complicated process are capable at times of overcoming the inhibitory influence of a persistently mild elevated PRL level.

Persistent postoperative hyperprolactinemia with or without amenorrhea does not necessarily imply that viable tumor tissue remains.[1, 37] In most cases it seems more likely that the elevations are due to pituitary stalk impairment by the tumor and/or surgery, with resultant interference with the normal delivery of PRL inhibitory factor (PIF) to the adenohypophysis, which in turn allows an unrestrained release of PRL from the normal gland.[37] In such patients, PRL levels should continue to fall gradually or remain unchanged; the former would imply that the stalk is gradually regaining its capacity to deliver PIF and the latter, that it is permanently damaged. On the other hand, if PRL levels begin to rise, it is likely that the tumor has recurred and that a residual tumor fragment was probably responsible for the failure of PRL to return to normal in the immediate postoperative period. It is likely that serial CT scanning with one of the newer models will be useful in the follow-up evaluation of patients suspected of having recurrent tumors.[49]

Our experience supports the results of others[3, 30] in that there is a close correlation between the size of prolactinomas and serum PRL levels. In our series of 72 patients in Group 1 (whose PRL levels were <200 ng/ml), 58 patients (81%) had tumors <1 cm in diameter. On the other hand, of 28 patients in Group 2 (whose PRL levels were >200 ng/ml), only four patients (14%) had tumors <1 cm in size.

Both the TRH and the chlorpromazine stimulation tests have proved valuable in facilitating the diagnosis of prolactinomas.[11, 37] However, these tests may be abnormal in hypothalamic-pituitary disorders other than tumors. Before operation, 97% and 90% of Group 1 patients and 100% of Group 2 patients in our series had abnormal chlorpromazine and TRH provocative tests, respectively. Following surgery, 74% and 41% of Group 1 and 96% and 80% of Group 2 continue to have abnormal chlorpromazine and TRH tests.

In our experience, polytomography often proved unreliable in the detection of microadenomas. For instance, 44% of patients in Group 1 and 11% of those in Group 2 had normal polytomes despite the presence of prolactinomas that were subsequently confirmed at surgery and histologically. Since 81% of patients in Group 1 and 14% of patients in Group 2 had tumors that were <1 cm (microadenomas), the reliability of polytomography appears to correlate with the size of the tumor. The increasing use of the newer scanners will probably change the diagnostic protocol for the investigation of pituitary adenomas and microadenomas and it is likely that the use of polytomography of the sella turcica will diminish in future evaluation of these patients. Currently, we do not believe that cerebral angiography and pneumoencephalography are indicated in the management of these patients. With the development of metrizamide cisternography,[33] and in the future with coronal views on high-resolution scanners, the empty sella syndrome may be readily diagnosed without the use of pneumoencephalography.

The minimal criteria necessary in the workup of these patients who present with an A-G syndrome associated with hyperprolactinemia should include history and physical examination, at least two random PRL levels, either a TRH or chlorpromazine provocative test, high-resolution CT scanning if available, and/or sellar polytomography, although the latter recommendation is subject to change. Suprasellar extension can be determined with either conventional or high-resolution (coronal) CT scanning. Visual field examination and visual acuity testing are important to rule out subtle visual field impairment. Baseline anterior and posterior pituitary function tests (see Table 2) should also be obtained.

The present series emphasizes many of the advantages of the modern transsphenoidal microsurgical approach to pituitary tumors over other operative approaches such as craniotomy.* The low incidence of complications and a negligible mortality rate represent major advantages of the procedure. In our series of 100 patients, there were no deaths and the complications were relatively benign and not disabling, except for the one patient previously described who developed a CSF rhinorrhea and a cryptococcal sellar and parasellar abscess. The temporary diabetes insipidus is probably caused by transient edema of the pituitary stalk due to operative manipulation.[70] The rare occurrence of CSF rhinorrhea is related to the fact that pituitary tumors are separated from the subarachnoid space by the tumor pseudocapsule and diaphragm sella.

---

*References 4, 7, 26–32, 36, 46, 50, 53, 57, 59, 70, 75, 76.

Another significant advantage of transsphenoidal surgery over other operative approaches is that gross total removal of the majority of tumors, even those lesions that extend significantly above the upper limits of the sella turcica, can be accomplished with preservation of the pituitary gland in the majority of patients.[46, 70] Not only can pituitary function be maintained, but, as shown in the present study, certain hormonal functions may be restored following successful removal of the tumor by the transsphenoidal approach. In the authors' opinion, the ability to remove tumors and spare normal pituitary tissue with an operation that carries a low incidence of complications and rare mortality constitutes a major advance in pituitary tumor surgery.

In our opinion, *routine* postoperative irradiation following transsphenoidal microsurgical "gross total" removal of a pituitary tumor in every patient is not warranted. We would agree with those authors who recommend that irradiation should probably be reserved for patients with tumors associated with mass effect in whom recurrence becomes evident or for those who have an invasive tumor at the first operation.[10, 58, 62] On the other hand, because clinical data on the irradiation of prolactinomas in patients in whom the A-G syndrome is the main symptomatology is very limited,[62] and because hyperprolactinemia per se is not a health hazard,[10, 11] we do not advise routine irradiation of these tumors. Persistent postoperative hyperprolactinemia in patients who continue to have amenorrhea and galactorrhea on the basis of disruption of PIF pathways are good candidates for medical treatment with bromocriptine. Reliable patients with persistent hyperprolactinemia from suspected persistent or recurrent tumors not associated with mass effect can also be considered for bromocriptine therapy, provided close medical supervision is available.

## BIBLIOGRAPHY

1. Antunes J.L., Housepian E.M., Frantz A.G., et al.: Prolactin-secreting pituitary tumors. *Ann. Neurol.* 2(2):148, 1977.
2. Aronoff S.L., Daughaday W.H., Laws E.R., Jr.: Bromocriptine treatment of prolactinomas (letter). *N. Engl. J. Med.* 300:1391, 1979.
3. Aubourg P.R., Derome P.J., Peillon F., et al.: Endocrine outcome after transsphenoidal adenomectomy for prolactinoma: Prolactin levels and tumor size as predicting factors. *Surg. Neurol.* 14:141, 1980.
4. Becker D.P., Atkinson R., Sakalas R., et al.: Transsphenoidal microsurgery for acromegaly: Successful treatment with preservation of pituitary function. *Confin. Neurol.* 36:101, 1974.
5. Bergh T., Nillius S.F., Wide L.: Clinical course and outcome of pregnancies in amenorrheic women with hyperprolactinemia and pituitary tumors. *Br. Med. J.* 2:875, 1978.

6. Besser G.M., Mouk P.J.A.: Prolactinomas and their management, in Jacobs H.S. (ed): *Advances in Gynecological Endocrinology*, ed. 6. London: London Royal College of Obstetricians and Gynecologists, 1978, pp 234–247.

7. Chang R.J., et al.: Detection, evaluation, and treatment of pituitary microadenomas in patients with galactorrhea and amenorrhea. *Am. J. Obstet. Gynecol.* 128:356, 1977.

8. Billeter E., Fluckiger E.: Evidence for a luteolytic function of prolactin in the intact cyclic rat using a 2-Br-ergokryptine (CB 154). *Experientia* 27:464, 1971.

9. Carter J.N., Tyson J.E., Tolis G., et al.: Prolactin-secreting tumors and hypogonadism in 22 men. *N. Engl. J. Med.* 299:847, 1978.

10. Collins W.F.: Pituitary tumor management: An overview, in Tindall G.T., et al. (eds): *Clinical Management of Pituitary Disorders*. New York: Raven Press, 1979, pp 179–186.

11. Christy J.H.: Clinical and endocrinologic evaluation of patients with suspected pituitary tumors, in Tindall G.T., et al.(eds): *Clinical Management of Pituitary Disorders*. New York: Raven Press, 1979, pp 161–170.

12. Corenblum B., Webster B.R., Mortimer C.B., et al.: Possible antitumor effects of 2-bromo-ergocryptine (CB-154 Sandoz) in 2 patients with large prolactin-secreting pituitary adenomas. *Clin. Res.* 23:614A, 1975.

13. Cushing H.: Surgical experiences with pituitary disorders. *J.A.M.A.* 63:1515, 1914.

14. Cusick J.F., Houghton V.M., Hagen T.C.: Radiological assessment of intrasellar prolactin-secreting tumors. *Neurosurgery* 6:376, 1980.

15. Derome P.J., et al.: Adénomes à prolactine: Résultats du traitment chirugical. *Nouv. Presse Med.* 8:577, 1979.

16. Domingue J.N., Richmond I.L., Wilson C.B.: Results of surgery in 114 patients with prolactin-secreting pituitary adenomas. *Am. J. Obstet. Gynecol.* 137:102, 1980.

17. Ezrin C., Kovacs K., Horvath E.: Hyperprolactinemia. Morphologic and clinical considerations. *Med. Clin. N. Am.* 62:393, 1978.

18. Fluckiger E.: Effects of bromocriptine on the hypothalamo-pituitary axis. *Acta Endocrinol [Suppl.] (Copenh.)* 216:111, 1978a.

19. Fluckiger E.: Pharmacology of prolactin secretion, in Falbusch R., et al. (eds): *Treatment of Pituitary Adenomas*. Massachusetts, 1978a, pp 351–360.

20. Fluckiger E., Lutterbeck P.M., Wagner H.R., et al.: Antagonism of 2-Br-Ergokryptine-Methanesulfonate (CB154) to certain endocrine actions of centrally active drugs. *Experientia* 28:924, 1972.

21. Fluckiger E., Wagner H.R.: 2-Br- Ergokryptine: Beeinflussung von Fertilität und Laktation bei der Ratte. *Experientia* 24:1130–1131, 1968.

22. Ford K.: Contraceptive utilization among currently married women 15–44 years of age: United States 1973. *Monthly Vital Stat.* 7 (Suppl.): October 4, 1976.

23. Franks S., Jacobs H.S., Nabarro J.D.N.: Prolactin concentrations in patients with acromegaly: Clinical significance and response to surgery. *Clin. Endocrinol. (Oxf.)* 5:63, 1976.

24. Franks S., Jacobs H.S., Nabarro J.D.N.: Studies of prolactin secretion in pituitary disease. *J. Endocrinol.* 67:55, 1975.

25. Grisoli F., Vincentelli F., Jaquet P., et al.: Prolactin-secreting adenomas in 22 men. *Surg. Neurol.* 13:241, 1980.
26. Guiot G.: Transsphenoidal approach in surgical treatment of pituitary adenomas, in *Diagnosis of Pituitary Tumors.* New York: Elsevier North-Holland, 1973, pp 159–178.
27. Hardy J.: Transsphenoidal hypophysectomy. *J. Neurosurg.* 34:582, 1971.
28. Hardy J.: Transsphenoidal microsurgery of the normal and pathological pituitary. *Clin. Neurosurg.* 16:185, 1968.
29. Hardy J.: Transsphenoidal surgery of hypersecreting pituitary tumors, in Kohler P.O., et al. (eds): *Diagnosis and Treatment of Pituitary Tumors.* Amsterdam: Excerpta Medica, International Congress Series 303, 1973, pp 179–194.
30. Hardy J., Beauregard H., Robert F.: Prolactin-secreting adenomas: Transsphenoidal microsurgical treatment, in Robyn C., et al. (eds): *Progress in Prolactin Physiology and Pathology.* New York: Elsevier North-Holland, 1978, pp 361–370.
31. Hardy J., Wigser S.M.: Transsphenoidal surgery of pituitary tumors with televised radiofluoroscopic control. *J. Neurosurg.* 23:612, 1965.
32. Henderson W.R.: The pituitary adenomata. *Br. J. Surg.* 26:809, 1939.
33. Hoffman J.C., Tindall G.T.: Diagnosis of empty sella syndrome using Amipaque cisternography combined with computerized tomography. *J. Neurosurg.* 52:99, 1980.
34. Horrobin D.F.: Prolactin: Role in health and disease. *Drugs* 17:409, 1979.
35. Jacobs H.S.: Prolactin and amenorrhea. *N. Engl. J. Med.* 295:954, 1976.
36. Keye W.R., Chang R.J., Wilson C.B., et al.: Prolactin-secreting pituitary adenomas. *J.A.M.A.* 244:1329, 1980.
37. Kleinberg D.L., Noel G.L., Frantz A.G.: Galactorrhea: A study of 235 cases, including 48 with pituitary tumors. *N. Engl. J. Med.* 296:589, 1977.
38. Lamberti S.W.J., Seldenrath H.J., Kwa H.G., et al.: Transient bitemporal hemianopsia during pregnancy after treatment of galactorrhea-amenorrhea syndrome with bromocriptine. *Br. J. Clin. Pharmacol.* 5:227, 1978.
39. Landolt A.M., Wutrich R., Fellmann H.: Regression of pituitary prolactinoma after treatment with bromocriptine. *Lancet* 1:1082, 1979.
40. Littleton J.T.: *Tomography: Physical Principles and Clinical Application.* Baltimore: William & Wilkins Co., 1976, pp 810–815.
41. Lloyd H.M., Meares J.D., Jacobi J.: Effects of estrogen and bromocriptine on *in vivo* secretion and mitosis in prolactin cells. *Nature* 255:497, 1975.
42. MacLeod R.M., Lehmeyer J.E.: Studies on the mechanism of the dopamine-mediated inhibition of prolactin secretion. *Endocrinology* 94:1077, 1974.
43. MacLeod R.M.: Regulation of prolactin secretion, in Martini L., et al. (eds): *Frontiers in Neuroendocrinology.* New York: Raven Press, 1976, vol 4, pp 169–194.
44. Mashiter K., Adams E., Beard M., et al.: Bromocriptine inhibits prolactin and growth-hormone release by human pituitary tumours in culture. *Lancet* 2:197, 1977.
45. McGregor A.M., Scanlon M.F., Hall K., et al.: Reduction in size of a pituitary tumor by bromocriptine therapy. *N. Engl. J. Med.* 300:291, 1979.
46. McLanahan C.S., Christy J.H., Tindall G.T.: Anterior pituitary function

before and after transsphenoidal microsurgical resection of pituitary tumor. *Neurosurgery* 3:142, 1978.
47. Mehta A.E., Tolis G.: Pharmacology of bromocriptine in health and disease. *Drugs* 17:313, 1979.
48. Mroueh A.M., Siler-Khodr T.M.: Bromocriptine therapy in cases of amenorrhea-galactorrhea. *Am. J. Obstet. Gynecol.* 127:291, 1977.
49. Muhr C., Bergstrom K., Enoksson P., et al.: Follow-up study with computerized tomography and clinical evaluation 5 to 10 years after surgery for pituitary adenoma. *J. Neurosurg.* 53:144, 1980.
50. Nager F.R.: The paranasal approach to intrasellar tumors. *Laryngoscope* 55:361, 1940.
51. Nagulesparen M., Ang V., Jenkins J.S.: Bromocriptine treatment of males with pituitary tumors, hyperprolactinaemia, and hypogonadism. *Clin. Endocrinol. (Oxf.)* 9:73, 1978.
52. Nasr H., Mozaffarian G., Pensky J., et al.: Prolactin-secreting pituitary tumors in women. *J. Clin. Endocrinol. Metab.* 35:505, 1972.
53. Nielson K.D., Clark K.: Transsphenoidal microsurgery for selective removal of functional pituitary microadenomas. *Tex. Med.* 72(11):61, 1976.
54. Nillius S.J., Bergh T., Lundberg P.O., et al.: Regression of a prolactin-secreting pituitary tumor during long-term treatment with bromocriptine. *Fertil. Steril.* 30:710, 1978.
55. Parkes D.: Drug therapy: Bromocryptine. *N. Engl. J. Med.* 301:873, 878, 1979.
56. Pasteels J.L., Danguy A., Frerotte M., et al.: Inhibition de la sécrétion de prophylactine par l'ergocornine et la 2-Br-ergocryptine action directe sur l'hypophyse en culture. *Ann. Endocrinol. (Paris)* 32:188, 1971.
57. Post K.D., et al.: Results of selective transsphenoidal adenomectomy in women with galactorrhea-amenorrhea. *J.A.M.A.* 242:158, 1979.
58. Ray B.S., Patterson R.H. Jr.: Surgical experience with chromophobe adenomas of the pituitary gland. *J. Neurosurg.* 34:726, 1971.
59. Richards S.H., Thomas J.P., Kilby D.: Transethmoidal hypophysectomy for pituitary tumors. *Proc. R. Soc. Med.* 67:889, 1974.
60. Robert F.: Electron microscopy of human pituitary tumors, in Tindall G.T., et al. (eds): *Clinical Management of Pituitary Disorders.* New York: Raven Press, 1979, pp 113–131.
61. Robert F., Hardy J.: Prolactin-secreting adenomas: A light and electron microscopical study. *Arch. Pathol.* 99:625, 1974.
62. Sheline G.E.: Conventional radiation therapy in the treatment of pituitary tumors, in Tindall G.T., et al. (eds): *Clinical Management of Pituitary Disorders.* New York: Raven Press, 1979, pp 179–186.
63. Sherman B.M., Schlechte J., Halni N.S., et al.: Pathogenesis of prolactin-secreting pituitary adenomas. *Lancet* 2:1019, 1978.
64. Sokrinho I.G., Nunes M.C.P., Santos M.A., et al.: Radiological evidence for regression of prolactinoma after treatment with bromocriptine. *Lancet* 2:257, 1978.
65. Stahelin H., Bruckhardt-Vischer B., Fluckiger E.: Rat mammary cancer inhibition by a prolactin suppressor, 2-BR-Ergokryptine (CB 154). *Experientia* 27:915, 1971.
66. Takei Y.: Pathology of pituitary tumors and value of frozen section diagnosis, in Tindall G.T., et al. (eds): *Clinical Management of Pituitary Disorders.* New York: Raven Press, 1979, pp 93–112.

67. Teperman L., Vutterweit W., Zappulla R., et al.: Oral contraceptive history as a risk indicator in patients with pituitary tumors with hyperprolactinemia: A case comparison study of twenty patients. *Neurosurgery* 7:571, 1981.
68. Thorner M.O., Evans W.S., MacLeod R.M., et al.: Hyperprolactinemia: Current concepts of management including medical therapy with bromocriptine. *Adv. Biochem. Psychopharmacol.* 23:165, 1980.
69. Tindall G.T., Collins W.F., Kirchner J.A.: Unilateral septal technique for transsphenoidal microsurgical approach to the sella turcica. *J. Neurosurg.* 49:138, 1978.
70. Tindall G.T., McLanahan S., Christy J.H.: Transsphenoidal microsurgery for pituitary tumors associated with hyperprolactinemia. *J. Neurosurg.* 48:849, 1978.
71. Tolis G., Goldstein M., Friesen H.G.: Functional evaluation of prolactin secretion in patients with hypothalamic-pituitary disorders. *J. Clin. Invest.* 52:783, 1973.
72. Vezina J.L., Sutton T.J.: Prolactin-secreting pituitary microadenomas: roentgenologic diagnosis. *Am. J. Roentgenol. Radium Ther. Nucl. Med.* 120:46, 1974.
73. Wass J.A.H., Moult P.J.A., Thorner M.O., et al.: Reduction of pituitary-tumour size in patients with prolactinomas and acromegaly treated with bromocriptine with or without radiotherapy. *Lancet* 2:66, 1979.
74. Weiss M.: Personal communication, 1980.
75. Wilson Ch.B., Dempsey S.C.: Transsphenoidal microsurgical removal of 250 pituitary adenomas. *J. Neurosurg.* 48:13, 1978.
76. Wilson C.B., Rand R.W., Grollmus J.M., et al.: Surgical experience with a microscopic transsphenoidal approach to pituitary tumors and non-neoplastic parasellar conditions. *Calif. Med.* 117:1, 1972.
77. Yeo T., Thorner M.O., Jones A., et al.: The effects of dopamine, bromocriptine, lergotrile and metoclopramide on prolactin release from continuously perfused columns of isolated rat pituitary cells. *Clin. Endocrinol.* 10:123, 1979.
78. Yuen B.H.: Bromocriptine, pituitary tumours and pregnancy. *Lancet* 2:1314, 1978.
79. Zimmerman E.A., Defendini R., Frantz A.G.: Prolactin and growth hormone in patients with pituitary adenomas: A correlative study of hormone in tumor and plasma by immunoperoxidase technique and radioimmunoassay. *J. Clin. Endocrinol. Metab.* 38:577, 1974.

# The Great Debate: Medical vs. Surgical Treatment of Prolactinomas

G.M. BESSER, M.D.*

*Department of Endocrinology, St. Bartholomews
Hospital, London, England*

GEORGE T. TINDALL, M.D.†

*Chief, Division of Neurosurgery, Emory University,
Atlanta, Georgia*

## Argument of G. M. Besser, M.D.

I SHOULD LIKE TO DISCUSS ATTITUDES toward dopamine agonist therapy and what we regard as objectives for treatment of pituitary tumors. I would agree that it would be nice to reduce or remove the tumor mass, remembering that these are benign tumors. The very big ones may infiltrate the bone locally, but they do not distantly metastasize. Carcinomas are very rare. We would like to preserve anterior pituitary function and hopefully reverse pretreatment hypopituitarism. We would obviously like to correct hormone excess and the clinical syndrome that goes with it, and we wish to prevent recurrence. This is the context in which we have to consider the opportunity to treat the patient medically, surgically or, I suppose, to do nothing. Because the possibility of establishing the presence of prolactin-secreting pituitary tumors has only become real over the past ten years, this is the length of our experience with the medical

---

*Speaking in favor of medical treatment.
†Speaking in favor of surgical treatment.

0-8151-3530-0/82/0006-0299-0312-$03.75

treatment of this condition. I would remind you once again that prolactin was finally established to exist in the human, simultaneously
in the laboratories of Dr. Frantz and our own in 1970, as I shall show
you. It is a recent story, but it is a story of ten years of experience
that has relied heavily on routine radiography supplemented by polytomography when necessary to outline the fossa. It is only recently
that we have had advantage of the use of the computerized tomographic (CT) scanner and, very recently for us, of the new, high-resolution scanners using the very thin slices.

Let me define our grading of the routine radiology and when we
regard a suspected pituitary tumor to be present.* The grading is
from zero to five. We regard as a normal appearance on the straight
lateral view of a single contour to the fossa and a flat floor with no
blistering. B-1 is one with an asymmetrical blister of less than 1 mm,
which is probably normal. The B-2 is where the asymmetrical blisters between 1 and 3 mm or a dip of 1 to 3 mm is possibly abnormal.
A B-3 is a blister of over 3 mm, which we regard as abnormal. B-4 is
where the asymmetry occupies the whole of one side of the fossa. And
a B-5, of course, is a balloon fossa. B-3 to B-5 we regard as almost
certainly indicative of the presence of what we have conventionally
called tumors, but some of them are really areas of hyperplasia.
There is a vague association between the prolactin levels and the
tumor size (see Fig 1, p. 259). It is really very unreliable to use an
absolute level; tumors are usually obvious with levels of more than
200 ng/ml although you can get really quite big tumors with much
lower levels than that, so there is not much association.

A word about symptoms. Amenorrhea is much commoner than in
those patients in whom there is no radiologic evidence on routine
radiography of a pituitary tumor. There is a high incidence of irregular cycles, but the important thing is that you can have regular
cycles, absolutely regular menstruation, and never a missed period,
yet a history of infertility with anovulation or defective luteal phase
associated with hyperprolactinemia. This infertility would be completely abolished when the prolactin level is low. So you can have
this deficit luteal phase syndrome with suspected pituitary tumor. It
is a little more common when there is no radiologic abnormality of
the fossa. So what is the incidence of galactorrhea in the high prolactinemic syndrome? The generally reported incidence of galactorrhea
is 30%. In our hands it is 80% because we look for the galactorrhea
with much greater enthusiasm than most people. Let us remember

*See Table 2, p. 258.

the different syndromes: amenorrhea, oligomenorrhea, and regular cycles, with or without galactorrhea.

Hyperprolactinemia is much less common in men, but when it occurs, it much more commonly presents with large tumors and local problems, largely, I suppose, because men take longer to seek medical advice when their major problem is impotence, than girls do when their problem is infertility or menstrual disorders. But impotence, relative or absolute, and no other symptom is the clinical feature of hyperprolactinemia. The patients frequently are completely normal on clinical examination and do not have oligospermia. There is no consistent data to support the view that oligospermia is a way of presentation of hyperprolactinemia. Trials in Europe have shown quite clearly that simple treatment with a prolactin-lowering drug does not actually help oligospermia. The patients are usually impotent but if they can produce a seminal specimen, it has a low volume although a normal sperm concentration. So that is the clinical context.

What about hormone reserve before treatment? Our patients with B3 to B5 fossa that we suspect of having prolactinomas are all thoroughly investigated. We check gonadotropin levels with LH-releasing hormone tests. We look at the progesterone levels of women in the luteal phase of the cycle. The occurrence of menstruation is totally inadequate as an endocrinologic way of assessing the gonadotropin adequacy, because women can present with regular cycles, ovulation, and infertility. You must investigate the adequacy of the second half of the cycle, because if you have a normal luteal phase of progesterone, the whole cycle has been adequate. The progesterone rise must be maintained for an adequate length of time. We find that approximately one third of our prolactinoma patients have impaired gonadotropins before treatment. The remainder are either normal or have excessive gonadotropin responses to the releasing hormone. ACTH and TSH deficiency is unusual; growth hormone deficiency does not really matter, but it occurs in two thirds of patients. We document ACTH and growth hormone deficiency, of course, by doing an insulin hypoglycemia test, thyroid by measuring TSH during the TRH test and thyroxine levels.

Medical treatment of hyperprolactinemia is of course based on the known hypothalamic control mechanisms for prolactin, which nowadays are accepted to be predominantly inhibitory by the prolactin-inhibiting factor dopamine, which passes to the prolactin-secreting cells and directly inhibits the secretion of prolactin by activating dopamine receptors on the anterior pituitary. And so we can use any dopamine-active drug, any dopamine agonist that has a long enough length of action. The ergot alkaloid bromocriptine, developed by Edward Fluckiger in the late 1960s, before we really knew for sure that prolactin existed in man, is the drug that holds the greatest sway as yet. But there are many dopamine agonists that could be used with sufficient length of action. When we started using it, exactly ten years ago (the first patient to take it started to take it in January, 1971), all we knew was that it suppressed prolactin by an action directly on the pituitary gland in the rat. We had no idea how that came about. But around 1973 it became clear that this was a dopamine agonist and also that dopamine could directly inhibit prolactin secretion.

Figure 2 (p. 260) illustrates the mechanism. This is a patient whose prolactin-secreting tumor was removed by transsphenoidal surgery at another hospital and made available to us for study. We dispersed the cells with trypsin and suspended them in a matrix of Biogel beads in what we grandly call a pituitary column so it could be perfused. The pituitary column is a National Health Service 2-ml syringe! We could then correct the effluent from these anterior pituitary cells and measure anything that came out and add anything we liked to it—hypothalamic extract or drugs. The solid bars show the effect on human prolactin secretion from these isolated cells when dopamine is added in a concentration found in the portal capillary blood. You see when dopamine is added prolactin secretion is inhibited. Black columns show when dopamine is removed and prolactin secretion is disinhibited. The cross-hatched area is when we add bromocriptine. You see bromocriptine added here. Once again, just like dopamine, prolactin secretion is directly inhibited. If we added a dopamine receptor blocker, bromocriptine would not work. It is a specific dopamine agonist action. However, there is one big difference between the action of bromocriptine and that of dopamine. When you stop dopamine, the effect begins to wear off within 30 minutes. When you stop bromocriptine, however, the effect is prolonged for many hours afterward, and there are good data suggesting that there is persistent occupancy of the dopaminergic receptors on the pituitary cells. That accounts for the very long action of this compound. It is therefore a long-acting dopamine agonist that is a functional analogue of the natural physiologic prolactin-inhibiting factor. Here is a slide from Mike Thorner, who used to work for us, showing an in vivo situation in a group of hyperprolactinemic women sampled throughout the day. The square symbols show that the control prolactin levels are very high. Bromocriptine is then given. As the bromocriptine level rises, the prolactin levels fall. However, the fall of the prolactin levels continues long after the bromocriptine has begun to fall away, an in vivo reflection of the persisting action of bromocriptine that we saw in vitro; it is a long-acting dopamine agonist which is a functional analogue of the hypothalamic prolactin-inhibiting factor.

I thought it would be of interest to you to see data from the first patient ever treated with bromocriptine in January, 1971. This patient is a man. There are two different sorts of prolactin. One is bioactive prolactin, as measured in the cultured pseudopregnant rabbit breast assay. We kept the samples and subsequently radioimmunoassayed them. As Dr. showed you, the bioactive levels are much higher actually than the immunoreactive. Three out of the first five patients whom we treated before therapy had very much higher bioactive levels than immunoreactive. Dr. Cowden is beginning to show us why that is. This patient had galactorrhea and impotence for two years. We put a breast pump on one of his breasts for three minutes and got 6 ml of milk out of it. Interestingly enough, he also secreted oxytocin and vasopressin during that suckling. I think it is the only recorded case of a man secreting oxytocin and vasopressin during breast-feeding. We did not know what to do for him and we heard about this drug from Switzerland. We asked for some and we gave it to him tentatively. His prolactin level fell precipitously. The milk disappeared in five days. A few days later, his potency returned. The milk returned within a few days and then a few days later he became impotent. We left him on treatment for about 8 months and he was normally potent and without galactorrhea. We then stopped bromocriptine. His prolactin level rose. This man has been receiving bromocriptine therapy for ten years. We take him off it every year or two and the whole thing comes back, so we put him back on treatment. During that time, on his own bromocriptine, his wife has had two children and his potency has remained normal. This is the normal story of bromocriptine treatment in the male with galactorrhea that goes away and potency that returns remarkably quickly.

What about the women? We have now treated about 250 women with hyperprolactinemia. The interval to resumption of menstruation is brief although the first cycle may not be ovulatory. Usually the second cycle is and by the third cycle the progesterone levels are normal, regardless of the length of amenorrhea. We have had some patients who had amenorrhea for 15 years and whose periods returned in a month or two. Notice the interval to resumption of menstruation within 2 months: the overall figure is 60% and then there is a gradual rise to 70% within five months (see Fig 5, p. 263). But we need to break that down into prolactinomas, and people with no evidence of a tumor on conventional screening. In women in whom there is no plain radiologic evidence of a tumor, there is a much faster and much more complete rate of return of menstruation that is ovulatory. The return in suspected pituitary tumors is slower, but it comes back. There is always a residual small group of patients who do not have return of cyclicity because they are gonadotropin-deficient. But even some who are gonadotropin-deficient before treatment may have resumption of menstruation. Some of these patients with tumors had had surgery for large tumors with big suprasellar extensions, so it is not surprising that some of them had gonadotropin deficiency. What matters is that there is a rapid return of ovulatory menstruation irrespective of the length of amenorrhea.

As for pregnancy, the patients are very fertile; there is rarely a problem of conception once they are on treatment. It is our policy to recommend to patients that they take mechanical contraceptive precautions until they have had three regular cycles, and then, if everything else is all right, to tell them that they can get pregnant. Of 80 such patients of ours who have become pregnant, many who had 10, 12, or 15 years of amenorrhea, 30 conceived in less than one month and another 10 in the second month. Thus, 40 of 80 of these chronically infertile patients became pregnant within two months of conception despite many years of infertility (see Fig 6, p. 264). We have had some patients who have had second babies and we have had one patient who has had a third pregnancy while on bromocriptine. The incidence of multiple ovulation is no greater than in the general population, and in neither our figures nor the collected figures throughout the world is there any increased incidence of abortion in those patients. And let us remember that this treatment with dopamine agonist therapy reverses the hyperprolactinemic hypogonadism without any risks whatsoever of the development of hypopituitarism.

Clinicians recommending surgical treatment must remember that the first hormone to go in any pituitary lesion, be it surgical or spontaneous, is LH. You have done a patient no good at all if you have ablated her pituitary gland when she was young and in the fertile age group so that she ends up with normal prolactins but is LH-deficient. She will be estrogen-deficient and infertile. The consequences of that, particularly on her libido, vaginal mucosal integrity, and bones, are considerable up to 20 to 30 years later. That is a very big price to pay, even if the risk is only 18%. You can alternatively treat such patients with tablets and run no risk of inducing deficiency and have an excellent prospect of improving their pituitary function.

There is a major problem, let us not escape it. In patients with big tumors (a B-4 or B-5 fossa in our grading) there is a risk that when they get pregnant the tumor may enlarge. The risk of enlargement of tumors during pregnancy is small if it is a microadenoma, B-3 or less, about 2%. It is one in four as far as we can tell in patients with B-4 or B-5 fossae, as evidenced from the collected series of Gemzell. So it is a real risk. What can we do to prevent that happening? You can (1) do nothing and then treat it if it occurs; (2) give bromocriptine, which will shrink the tumor; or (3) operate. I suggest that we should anticipate the problem. You could do a selective removal of the tumor, but we hear there is an 18% risk of inducing permanent infertility. You could irradiate them before conception. We use a linear accelerator using 4,500 rads, less than 180 rads a day, with a 3-field technique, and that is totally safe. We have never had radiobiologic damage in 250 patients treated with the current technique. We have never seen or encountered a patient treated this way whose tumor has enlarged during pregnancy. We have seen some patients who have not been treated and who have been given bromocriptine elsewhere and who have had tumor enlargement during pregnancy. So I think they should be given radiotherapy at least 3 months before attempted conception.

This is our management. If the prolactin level is over 100 ng/ml and the patient has a B4 or B5 fossa, a macroadenoma, she has some contrast study or a study with the very sensitive new CT scanner. We do not treat such patients if they have partially empty fossa. If they have a suprasellar extension, we get rid of that first. We then irradiate them in the way that we have described. They then get pregnant and we see them monthly to follow their central visual fields. To date, no patient who has had radiotherapy has shown any evidence whatsoever of tumor enlargement in pregnancy, and radiotherapy has not prevented any patient from conceiving. It has not induced hypopituitarism in prolactinoma patients except for growth hormone deficiency—an important biochemical function in adults.

So at this moment, the summary to date is that hyperprolactinemia is a common cause of infertility in women and impotence in men. It is readily and safely treated with bromocriptine. Pituitary tumors must be actively sought and treated before you let a woman get pregnant. The need for exogenous gonadotropin is now very small; only patients who are gonadotropin-deficient need it. And most of the patients we see who are gonadotropin-deficient have had pituitary surgery.

But what about the tumor mass when medical treatment is given? Our attention was drawn to this some time ago by a patient who started with field defects and refused surgery. During bromocriptine therapy her field defects went away completely. This prompted us to review all the plain skull films of our patients with tumors and hyperprolactinemia. The first woman with a pituitary tumor to go on to bromocriptine therapy in 1971 had a B4 fossa, which was abnormal throughout. In 1978 the fossa was virtually normal. Undoubtedly the tumor had shrunk. An acromegalic prolactinemic patient who had not been treated at all between 1957 and 1973 was examined; her fossa was progressively enlarging. In 1973 she began to take bromocriptine. By 1978 it was completely normal. So we began to look at the mass of the tumor when it was actually rather large, but it is difficult to interpret the change in fossa. What we do know is that 20% of 69 prolactinoma patients with or without acromegaly had shown shrinkage of the fossa size on bromocriptine therapy on plain skull x-ray studies. We also know that if a pituitary tumor shrinks, it normally does not result in shrinkage of the fossa; it normally results in a partially empty fossa. So our figure of 20% must have been a gross underestimate of the true incidence of shrinkage of the tumor. So we began to look at the soft tissues. Figure 7, p. 266 shows a CT scan of an acromegalic hyperprolactinemic young man who had complete pituitary deficiency of all the other hormones, visual field defects, and diabetes insipidus. He was gonadotropin and thyroid-deficient, and had no circulating cortisol, either at rest or during insulin-induced hypoglycemia. On bromocriptine therapy his pituitary gland shrank dramatically. Moreover, his pituitary function returned to normal. His insulin tolerance test before bromocriptine therapy shows that he was completely ACTH deficient; during bromocriptine therapy his basal and stress ACTH reserve is completely normal. He was hypothyroid before treatment, euthyroid during treatment. His testosterone level was low before treatment; during treatment it was normal. His diabetes insipidus had completely gone, as had his visual field defect. He now has normal pituitary function.

So we embark on the study of patients with massive extrasellar extensions to their pituitary tumors, patients who normally would go to emergency neurosurgery to decompress their visual pathways. Ours is an ongoing study. The air encephalogram of one such patient showed the front end of the third ventricle to be compressed by the massive suprasellar extension of this patient's prolactinoma before treatment. During treatment, the visual field defect had gone and the tumor shrank right back into the fossa, so that we could now give him external radiotherapy. It is unsafe to give it in the presence of suprasellar extension. As soon as it shrunk back into the fossa, we can give him radiotherapy. In our current study of massive pituitary tumors with extrasellar extensions, we have 15 patients, 14 of whom have prolactinomas; three had acromegaly, one a nonfunctioning tumor. Twelve of these 15 patients have decreased in size in the space of three months. We reevaluate them in three months; we see them frequently in that interim period. Three tumors have not changed. No tumor has enlarged. Field defects that were present before treatment in eight patients improved in seven; three are completely normal; they have deteriorated slightly in one patient. (We have now operated on that patient.) In a number of these patients pituitary function improved in as little as three months as the tumor shrank. It is particularly important that LH comes back. This improvement is not only observed at St. Bartholomews. A patient of Thorner and Rogol's in Virginia had suprasellar extension of a prolactinoma. Two weeks after the patient began to take bromocriptine the tumor looked a shrunken prune. Of course, if you stop the treatment the tumor gets bigger again. There are lots of dopamine agonists available now. There are bromocriptine; Lergotrol, which was withdrawn because it was hepatotoxic; Pergolide, which is given in one dose a day and lasts for more than 24 hours; Lysuride, which is simpler to make and cheaper; and others coming along.

So we can conclude that ergot-related dopamine agonists lower prolactin levels and reverse associated hypogonadism, and in patients with acromegaly, they lower GH levels and improve clinical features. There is no associated risk of hyperpituitarism. On the contrary, pituitary function usually improves, and now we know that small and large functioning tumors often shrink with resolution of neighboring complications.

I will now briefly address myself to the clinical problems of a female patient, age 35, with an apparently normal fossa. Why should we expose this woman who has hyperprolactinemia to surgery? She is single and does not wish to have a pregnancy. It may well be that her hyperprolactinemia has induced an estrogen deficiency. She may well have a dry vagina and a poor libido. Before making a decision I would like to know a lot more about her social life and interests. She has a normal fossa, she may well have a microadenoma. We would fully evaluate her from an endocrinologic point of view, the way I have described. I would suggest there is absolutely no indication to treat this patient surgically. She should be treated medically with bromocriptine because with her history she has a very high probability of complete resolution of her hypogonadism with resolution of any associated depression, improvement in libido, improvement in her estrogen status, reduction in the risks of all the factors that go with estrogen deficiency, and restitution of normal ovulatory cycles. She will be fertile. I agree she will then be a risk at getting pregnant, but then she can complain about that, together with the rest of her normal friends. Girls wish to have an image of being female, and even if not interested in becoming pregnant they hate being amenorrheic. Many of our patients are extraordinarily elated to resume the normal functioning of a woman and the normal hormonal status and social status that go along with that. This can be easily and safely established using medical treatment.

## Rebuttal by George T. Tindall, M.D.

I would like to congratulate Dr. Besser on an excellent talk. There are several points I wish to discuss. While temporary damage to one pituitary-target organ axis may occasionally occur as a result of transsphenoidal surgery, it is very rare for an experienced surgeon to produce panhypopituitarism. While the immediate postoperative incidence of one or more axes being impaired is on the order of 15%–18%, the chance of permanent damage is less than 5%. The next item that I wish to discuss is mainly one of clarification. In Dr. Besser's previous publications, he has recommended that female patients with the amenorrhea-galactorrhea syndrome due to a prolactinoma be treated with bromocriptine and irradiation, the latter therapy for the purpose of preventing the pituitary tumor from sudden enlargement and/or hemorrhage during the pregnancy. In my opinion, this extent of therapy is inappropriate. Also, I was under the impression from some of Dr. Sheline's work, that pituitary irradiation carries a certain risk of producing relative hypopituitarism; perhaps later Dr. Sheline can comment on this issue.

I recently heard Dr. Mike Thorner present his work on treating prolactinomas with bromocriptine. Radiologically, he showed a significant reduction in tumor size during drug therapy, but a relatively quick return in tumor size when the drug was discontinued. This tells me that the drug does not eradicate the tumor, and if you choose the option of treating prolactinomas with this agent, then you are committing a patient to long-term bromocriptine therapy, perhaps indefinitely, and we simply do not know enough about the long-term effects of this drug to accept this recommendation at this time. It may be that bromocriptine may prove to be a valuable preoperative adjunct to surgery for if a very large tumor can be significantly reduced in size, it might make it easier for the surgeon to effect a total removal.

## Argument of George T. Tindall, M.D.

The physician should have clearly defined goals as to what should be accomplished in treating pituitary tumors. The therapeutic goals for prolactinomas should include (1) eradication of the tumor with minimal morbidity and essentially no mortality; (2) relief of symptoms, i.e., restoration of menstrual periods, alleviation of headache, etc.; (3) reduction of elevated levels of prolactin to normal (less than 25 ng/ml); (4) minimal risk of damaging pituitary endocrine function; and (5) restoration of pituitary endocrine function in some cases.

The indications for transsphenoidal surgery in prolactinomas should include (1) desire for fertility in women with the amenorrhea-galactorrhea syndrome; (2) relief of mass effect; (3) small tumors that show definite increase in size on serial CT scan; and (4) small tumors that show definite increase in size on serial CT scans. The operative techniques that I use have been described previously and are very similar to those described by Wilson, Laws and Hardy. Following removal of the tumor, I prefer to use absolute alcohol in the tumor bed provided there is no tear in the diaphragm sellae. I realize the use of alcohol in this manner is controversial. Our results, as well as the recommended diagnostic workup in women with the amenorrhea-galactorrhea syndrome due to suspected prolactinomas, are cited in detail in the chapter by Dr. Faria and myself and need not be repeated here.

I believe that the discussion between Dr. Besser and myself, should not be made on the basis of how good modern transsphenoidal surgery has become, but rather should focus on the shortcomings of bromocriptine. Bromocriptine has produced symptomatic relief and has lowered prolactin levels in patients with prolactinomas. True, documented tumor shrinkage has occurred. However, the drug is not tumoricidal and thus has to be regarded as a method for relieving symptoms, but not for curing disease. In a broad sense, bromocriptine is analogous to Tegretol in the treatment of trigeminal neuralgia in that it provides symptomatic relief but does not cure the disorder. In other words, bromocriptine is not analogous to the use of penicillin in pneumococcal pneumonia. The enthusiasm of some clinicians over the initial results with bromocriptine in prolactinomas has lead to the suggestion that the drug can be used as primary treatment for these lesions, and surgery reserved for patients in whom actual tumor regression fails to occur. In my opinion, this approach is inappropriate because the data currently available to support this suggested therapeutic approach are inadequate. For instance, one of the major gaps is the paucity of pathologic studies on prolactinomas removed from patients who have received either short-term or long-term bromocriptine therapy. In virtually all reported cases of tumor regression caused by bromocriptine, the assessment of the regressive change was based on either clinical data or radiologic evidence. Prolactinomas are relatively unpredictable. Many of them remain small and undergo no significant size increase for indeterminate and long periods of time. A few even regress spontaneously. However, the significant fact is that many of these lesions progress to larger tumors and with each increase in tumor size, the likelihood of complete surgical excision and thus cure; decreases, and I know of no way to predict which ones are going to grow.

As long as a safe operation and surgical expertise are available, why not treat these tumors when they are small and the chance of total excision is highest? When small tumors are removed, the chance of impairing pituitary glandular function permanently is less than 5% and even then it usually involves only one axis. While bromocriptine is generally safe and causes no real serious side effects, it can result in hypotension, particularly if the drug is not started gradually. Many patients experience nausea and some patients simply do not feel generally well while on the drug. Some patients stop taking the medication after several months because they do not want to take long-term therapy without guaranteed cure. It is a relatively expensive drug. At the present time, despite sporadic case reports proclaiming success in bromocriptine, I am reluctant to recommend the use of this drug as primary therapy for prolactinomas. I believe that a more objective attitude on the part of the medical enthusiast is in order. Why not make a studied effort to determine those situations in which the drug will probably have positive benefits rather than proclaim it as a cure-all for this tumor while at the same time condemning surgery? The drug will probably play an important role in preoperative shrinkage, certain recurrent tumors, and in those patients with postoperative persistent hyperprolactinemia but in whom there is no remaining tumor.

## Rebuttal by G. M. Besser, M.D.

Thank you for giving me the opportunity to clarify some points that I obviously did not make entirely clear. The papers of ours that you have read, which discuss the problems relating to the risks of tumor enlargement in pregnancy, and your comments are very relevant. When we started getting these patients pregnant, the true incidence of risk of rapid enlargement of pituitary tumors in pregnancy was not really known. Everybody recognized that these occurred from the days of Pergonal-induced, gonadotropin-induced pregnancies in patients with pituitary tumors. We did not actually understand the risks, however, and initially we decided to give pituitary radiation, which we knew by then to be protective to patients who had large microadenomas, those not quite 1 cm across, in other words, patients with a big B3 fossa and prolactin level of over 100 ng/ml. However, when the very next review of Wang came out, it was quite clear to us that the risks of microadenomas getting bigger in pregnancy was low, about 2%, as you say, and we immediately stopped giving radiotherapy. We do not recommend radiotherapy to patients with microadenomas. We just let them get pregnant and we have not regretted that to date. The radiotherapy that is given, is given to patients with our grading of B4 or B5—the macroadenomas. That is the group that according to Wang has a 25% chance of enlargement. Many asked, why don't we just continue bromocriptine therapy through pregnancy? We do not. We ask the patient to stop taking bromocriptine. Should they miss a period by 48 hours, they are so regular, they get pregnant. They come up for a sensitive HCG test and that is that. Why do we not continue through pregnancy? There is no evidence of teratogenicity. The reason that I will not recommend that as routine is that I think we need 20 to 30 years' follow-up on the babies before we know that there are no delayed effects of continuing bromocriptine through pregnancy. There probably are none. I am worried about the relation between diethylstilbestrol and vaginal carcinoma that did not come up for 20 years and I am frightened that something like that might happen.

So I am not prepared to give bromocriptine throughout pregnancy. We stop it at the first missed period unless there is a positive indication. If any of my acromegalics got pregnant, I would continue it through pregnancy. That has not happened yet, but we have cushingoid patients who are controlled on bromocriptine, which is rather unusual. We have continued their bromocriptine through pregnancy and we certainly treat patients who have developed large tumors with fill defects because they have not had prophylactic radiotherapy. For such a patient I would regard emergency treatment with bromocriptine to be mandatory. So I would only continue bromocriptine through pregnancy if it is a positive indication. We are giving 4,500 rad to prevent the one in four risk of tumor enlargement with macroadenomas. Now we have a much higher incidence of hypopituitarism in radiotherapy given for acromegaly. We have not yet encountered hypopituitarism or impairment of conception in prolactinoma patients irradiated in the manner I mentioned. We probably will because we are not getting past the ten-year follow-up period when we would expect it. But the women have completed families by ten years and so the problems are fewer. It is safe then to give estrogen replacement therapy if they are on bromocriptine because you keep the prolactins down. As for the bouncing back of the patient whose massive tumors we have shrunk, as soon as the tumor gets back into the fossa, we can give radiotherapy. In our unit we have not seen a recurrence after that sort of radiotherapy for a prolactinoma, with one exception. One patient who was operated on for suprasellar extension had radiotherapy. Bromocriptine therapy six weeks later blew up a very big cyst that had to be operated on the second time. But that was very early. Otherwise we have not seen recurrence as yet.

# Panel III: Prolactin-Secreting Tumors

*Moderator:* JAMES R. GIVENS, M.D.
*Panelists:* WILLIAM H. DAUGHADAY, M.D., EDWARD R.
LAWS, M.D., JAMES T. ROBERTSON, M.D., ELIZABETH A.
COWDEN, M.D., ANNE P. FORBES, M.D., GEORGE T.
TINDALL, M.D.

GIVENS: *Since surgery gives best results in small tumors, why not pretreat the large or invasive tumors and then operate?*

TINDALL: Currently, I am treating certain large prolactinomas with bromocriptine. The patients are started on 2.5 mg daily for the first week, 5 mg daily for the second week, and 7.5 mg daily at the beginning of the third week. The latter dosage is maintained for six weeks at which time surgery is performed. A CT scan (GE 8800) before treatment, at three weeks after achieving therapeutic levels of 7.5 mg daily, and immediately before surgery, is obtained to assess the degree of tumor reduction. The study is in a preliminary stage, but I can say that significant reductions in prolactinomas have occurred and this structural change will probably work to the advantage of the surgeon in terms of making the removal easier.

BESSER: We physicians are only too delighted to be able to help the neurosurgeon by making his job simpler. By the way, bromocriptine is not an experimental drug, except in the U.S., under the auspices of the Food and Drug Administration. I would point out to you that in Europe, Asia, even in developing countries, doctors are now routinely using bromocriptine and that it has been used for ten years. It is now clear that the majority of massive or small prolactinomas shrink on bromocriptine therapy. Suppose you have a young patient on bromocriptine who has a massive tumor that is clearly shrinking. You are following the visual fields very carefully, twice a week, because you are worried about them. His or her headache has been

0-8151-3530-0/82/0006-0313-0328-$03.75

relieved in 48 hours and the patient has had her first period for some eight or nine years or the previously impotent man has immediately, in a few days, become potent. Suppose the patient says to you, "I am so much better, Doctor, I don't think I want to have my operation. Do I really need it?" What would you say to him?

TINDALL: I have treated just such a patient. In this patient, shrinkage occurred within three weeks as demonstrated by the CT scan. The patient asked that "since I am better and the tumor has shrunk, why do you have to operate?" I pointed out to him that if we were to stop the drug, the tumor would, in all likelihood, return to its original size and further the drug does not eradicate the tumor. Thus, to cure the lesion, surgery was advised.

DAUGHADAY: I would like to ask Dr. Besser to make a comment and ask him if he has encountered any similar patients. We have had two patients with macroadenoma who have responded with extraordinary sensitivity to bromocriptine. One of them whom Ed Laws and I cared for developed rhinorrhea on bromocriptine. A second patient whom we treated in St. Louis, who had an absolutely incredible collapse of a huge suprasellar tumor, not only developed rhinorrhea but developed spontaneous pneumoencephalogram. To us this indicates that we had pulled the plug out of the bottle. Have you ever had that type of experience?

BESSER: Well no, but I have been waiting for it. I am very interested to hear that you have had that happen. In this last big tumor group we have had one patient who had blockage of the nasal passageways and documented polyps containing pituitary tissue. The polyps shrank away and her nasal passages became unblocked. I was expecting her to get cerebrospinal fluid (CSF) rhinorrhea and we warned her about it, but it has not yet happened. But that is just a more dramatic evidence of shrinkage of the tumor. I guess our neurosurgical colleagues are very good at plugging CSF leaks when necessary.

LAWS: *I think the crucial question is, what is the mechanism by which bromocriptine can affect a shrinkage of the tumor? That it really can is a matter of speculation, but I would be interested to hear what your current thoughts are about that.*

BESSER: Well, it is speculation, of course, and we are all absolutely amazed by the speed with which tumors shrink. The story of bromocriptine has been that there has always been something surprising around the corner. Every time we solve one enigma, we find something new. We were amazed to see the change in the fossa, and we have been even more amazed at how quickly these massive tumors shrink. I obviously don't know why they shrink so quickly. I wonder about the vascularity. We know that during pregnancy, when normal pituitary gland enlarges because it becomes stuffed full of mammotropin, and under estrogen stimulation, where the same thing can occur, the vascularity in and around the pituitary increases. We know that prolactinomas are very vascular tumors, and I suspect that as long as they are secreting prolactin very actively, blood flow through them is very large and as soon as you shut down secretion blood flow falls. But it must clamp down very quickly, because the fields begin to get better in a few days and the headaches go away within a very few days.

In the laboratory animal, at least, there is a tremendous change in the lysosomal pattern of these tumors and the lysosomes get completely blown up. I don't know if Dr. Kovacs would have obtained the human samples right at that time of rapid resolution. I would rather doubt it. But I think there may be a great increase in internal cytolytic activity during bromocriptine.

TINDALL: The time course of shrinkage on the drug, and the return to the original size when the drug is stopped, are too rapid to be explained by cell replication. The relatively rapid changes in size on the tumor are probably due to some mechanism that results in reduction of individual tumor cells.

FORBES: *Is this drug 100% effective or have you encountered any medical failures?*

BESSER: It is certainly not 100% effective. There are patients who show a small fall in very high prolactin levels or, very rarely, no fall at all, but they are very uncommon. It is more common to get a fall toward the normal range and then to get them to stick but even this is unusual. There are rat pituitary prolactin-secreting tumors that do not contain dopamine receptors and I presume that these patients with resistant tumors similarly do not have dopamine receptors. But the group that particularly interests me is the one who comes down and then sticks at a high level but whose periods return. So I think that Dr. Cowden is going to be able to show us in due course that what we have done is to preferentially suppress the biologically active form of the circulatory hormone and that what is left is the immunoactive form without much biologic activity that shows up in the prolactin radioimmunoassay. I would be only too delighted to provide her with as many samples as she likes of patients who are going on to bromocriptine, including a few who are resistant.

COWDEN: Well, I would be delighted to receive them, but I think that I should perhaps tell you about a couple of Michael Thorner's patients whom we have looked at. Their tumors had very massive shrinkage. The first one suppressed from levels of around 3,000 down into the normal range and those levels were borne out very closely by the bioassay. The second patient, who showed a shrinkage within three weeks, had a level that did stick at about 1,000 ng/ml. It had been substantially reduced from 4,000 or 5,000 to 1,000 ng/ml and would go no further. In fact, when we did the bioassay in those samples, biologic activity was stuck at 1,000 ng/ml, so the correlation was really very close.

BESSER: Yes, but did that patient have return of gonadal function? The ones that I would like to see tested are the ones whose immunoreactive prolactin levels stay up, but whose clinical syndrome of hypogonadism seems to partially or completely resolve.

COWDEN: This was a male patient. His clinical syndrome had resolved, but his testosterone had doubled in the three-week period.

QUESTION FROM THE AUDIENCE: *Could I perhaps ask a question of you, Dr. Besser, about the obviously very large number of patients with microadenomas whom you have treated with bromocriptine? Why do you think there seems to be the difference in sensitivity to the apparent tumor or lytic effects of bromocriptine between these patients and the patients who have the very large tumors?*

BESSER: I am not aware that there is any difference. Dr. Nillius in Uppsala arranged for the exploration of the fossa of a patient whom he had treated for a microadenoma for six months and who was operated on. There was a dimple in the gland where the microadenoma had been. They could find no evidence of the microadenoma. Of course, their problem was that they had not explored the fossa before treatment, so they could not be absolutely certain that it was there. All the endocrine and radiologic studies were consistent with the presence of a microadenoma before treatment. But they certainly couldn't find it—all there was after treatment was a hole, so I am not sure there is any difference. Are you convinced by the evidence that there is a difference?

COMMENT: I think that it is fairly convincing that most people's experience with microadenomas and bromocriptine treatment, even for fairly prolonged periods of years, is that when you stop the bromocriptine, the levels in most patients come back up much more smartly than, for instance, in a patient who has a big tumor and has been given bromocriptine when the level tends to stay down for considerably longer.

BESSER: That really is not our experience. In both groups of patients, in our experience, the prolactin does come back in those with apparent microadenomas. It may slow down for two or three days, but then it rapidly rises. It often rebounds to a higher level than one started with initially when you stop therapy and then comes back down into the original range. I have never suggested that I regard the medical treatment as a permanent tumorolytic. I don't think it is. It is for that reason that we would give radiotherapy to patients with massive tumors that we have shrunk away, in order to protect them from rapid enlargement should they stop treatment.

TINDALL: I believe that there is some implication in the literature that large tumors with very high prolactin levels, tend to respond better than the small tumors.

DAUGHADAY: I don't have direct data myself. Von Werder in Munich has been one of the largest contributors to the view that hormonal suppression, at least for a matter of months, is more apt to occur in the macroadenomas than in the microadenomas. But I would agree that the data are not definite at the present time.

ROBERTSON: What I am concerned about is, as you said in your statement, that you don't know the long-term morbidity effects of bromocriptine on the fetus. You have to rely on a patient and drug compliance for an indefinite period of time, and you have not had any x-ray morbidity as yet. I agree with you that you haven't had enough cases followed for a long enough period of time to see it. You give bromocriptine to the group with macroadenomas and I feel that you should use some sort of ablative procedure in the group with microadenomas. Why have you chosen x-ray instead of bromocriptine, particularly if the tumor is small and has an exceedingly low morbidity and mortality? Bromocriptine is quick and efficient and is often a one-step move that ends the whole situation.

BESSER: Speed is not entirely of the essence. Fast cars are more dangerous than the ones that go slowly. We do not irradiate small tumors. I must say again that we only irradiate very big tumors that have had extrasellar extensions or macroadenomas in girls who wish to get pregnant. That irradiation is not associated with hypopituitarism, at least for many years after it is given, when prolactinomas are treated. In other words, patients come to us with gonadal dysfunction. Gonadal dysfunction is resolved and their pituitary function, far from being worsened, is actually improved, with or without radiotherapy. Only the occasional patient who presents with established hypopituitarism may fail to respond, but even then prior hypopituitarism often improves with drug-induced tumor shrinkage. It is most unusual for pituitary function to be impaired in any way in the small tumors provided they have been kept away from the surgical curet.

*Why would you not turn to surgery rather than radiation?*

BESSER: Because of the lack of evidence of hypopituitarism being instituted as a result of the radiotherapy in the time that the patient wishes to get pregnant. I am well aware that when Dr. Tindall told you about hypopituitarism he wasn't speaking of panhypopituitarism. I think that none of us would be discussing it if it were panhypopituitarism in 18% of the patients. But monotrophic hypopituitarism in any ablative lesion or progressive lesion of the pituitary in the great majority of patients affects LH first. That is the hormone of greatest interest to our patient and her partner and it is a major disaster when LH deficiency occurs as a result of therapy, and it is much more likely to occur within the potentially fertile life of the patient after surgical ablation of the lesion than after radiotherapy.

ROBERTSON: George, I think the thing that you ought to tell this group exactly how many of those 18% required any sort of replacement therapy. Was it simply an endocrinologic test that showed a minor deficit for a period of time, as you have implied? How many of that group really require long-term replacement therapy? We just don't have that problem in the small tumor.

TINDALL: Let me clarify that issue. In the immediate postoperative period, e.g., within the first two weeks, approximately 15–18% of our operative patients have some pituitary endocrine deficiency. This usually involves only one axis and involves the pituitary thyroidal axis in about half the cases. Most of these cases recover and our long term incidence of pituitary endocrine insufficiency related to surgery, is less than 5% and as I have indicated earlier, is usually limited to only one axis. Also, I would point that some degree of hypopituitarism may occur after radiotherapy and I wonder if Dr. Sheline would comment on this subject?

BESSER: May I just comment on the question about the hypopituitarism? I think that it is highly unusual and contrary to most people's experience to say that you get hypothyroidism as the first deficiency. We must know the evidence on which the conclusion is based. Are the gonadotropins normal, the progesterone levels adequate throughout the luteal phase? To actually get postural hypotension as the presenting clinical symptom of ACTH deficiency means you are a long way along the line of ACTH deficiency, because the first thing that happens in ACTH deficiency is impairment of the ACTH reserves and the basal levels remain normal for a very long time. You certainly do not get postural hypotension when you have normal basal cortisols, merely an impaired response to stress—a dangerous situation. So you are way down the line by the time that you are getting hypothyroidism and postural hypotension as the cause of cortisol deficiency.

SHELINE: As to the question about conventional radiotherapy inducing hypopituitarism, the figure that you are quoting, which I used yesterday, is strictly for patients with acromegaly. I know of no similar figure for other types of pituitary tumors. I would also add that half of those were not thought significant enough to require replacement therapy.

QUESTION: *How many times did you operate on microadenomas that were not found on the x-ray or CT scan? Have you ever not found a tumor?*

TINDALL: Probably 5 cases, when the polytomes and CT were negative, and yet a tumor (prolactinoma) was found at exploration.

QUESTION: *In New York there are a number of endocrinologists who feel that maybe hypoprolactinemia is not a bad state. Would you say that these women should stay on bromocriptine until, let's say, the age of 55, at the time of menopause, or should they be allowed to continue with their prolactin and be treated with estrogen? How would you manage that?*

BESSER: That has very interesting and, I think, important implications if the patient has a clinically, apparently significant abnormality on the fossa x-ray. In patients with large fossae (grades B4 and B5) and high prolactin levels, to date, whenever we have stopped bromocriptine therapy the hyperprolactinemia has come back. So we now routinely stop therapy six months after the last baby, when they have completed their family to see if they still need bromocriptine. To date, all the ones with clear tumors have had to go back on bromocriptine because of hyperprolactinemia. A significant number amongst the group with absolutely no abnormality of the fossa, do not develop a recurrence of hyperprolactinemia. In our experience, therefore, a significant proportion of the patients with a normal fossa, once they have completed their families, can stop the bromocriptine and have normal menses thereafter. Now that is an interesting group, because we have recently analyzed a series of prolactin observations that bears on this.

We have always advocated that if the prolactin taken by venipuncture from an outpatient seems inconsistent with the clinical situation, for example, a level sometimes high and sometimes normal, and you are not sure if it is stressed or not, you should get the patient up to the ward as an outpatient, put a needle into a vein, leave it in three quarters of an hour, and then sample every 15 minutes for two hours. In such cases the prolactin will often come right down into the normal range. Therefore, it is assumed that the patient must get unduly stressed by venipuncture, accounting for the hyperprolactinemia, and most have assumed that the outpatient prolactin levels are not clinically significant. We have recently found that we have got over 100 sets of patient data. We have compared the results of this rapid sampling procedure with the 2 or 3 outpatient values in the same patient. We have just analyzed them (Moult et al., *Clin. Endocrinol.* 14:387, 1980). We have found that rapid sampling fell into three patterns, one in which the prolactin level remained high and nonpulsatile. Interpretation was clearly no problem. In the second pattern the level was pulsatile below and above the upper limit of normal. Then there is this third group, a substantial number of patients whose prolactin levels on the rapid sampling immediately fall into the normal range, yet when sampled by conventional outpatient venipuncture had consistently high levels. In our desperation to treat these chronically infertile patients we had to give them bromocriptine as if they had persistent hyperprolactinemia. Now we have found that lowering the prolactin level blocked the stress-induced hyperprolactinemia and they rapidly conceive, that is, their response is just as if they had had consistent hyperprolactinemia. In our experience, once those patients have completed their families you can stop the bromocriptine and they will be completely normal and have normal prolactin levels and gonadal function. I believe that is one mechanism of stress infertility. These women are stressed by something in their environment and get a high prolactin level that makes them infertile. You can lower the manifestation of the stress with bromocriptine and let them have families and they no longer have stress hypoprolactinemia. So that is the group in which we can stop bromocriptine therapy. Now we are always asked what we do for this sort of patient, one who perhaps doesn't mind that she has amenorrhea and doesn't want to conceive. Should we treat without any evidence of a tumor? In our institution it is as follows: Some patients have low and others, normal estrogen levels. Those situations with hyperprolactinemic amenorrhea, I think, are potentially dangerous. They are theoretically dangerous anyway. If the estrogen levels are low, they get the estrogen deficiency states, as in the patient with premature menopause. They may get osteoporosis, loss of skin integrity, a dry vagina and atrophic vaginitis. I think they need the kind of protection against hypoestrogenism that Dr. Forbes suggested. We feel that it is dangerous to give estrogens unless you lower their prolactin level first. Their estrogen states will return to normal when you lower their prolactin level with bromocriptine, so you might as well just treat them with the one drug. We know that it is dangerous for those with normal estrogen levels to have unopposed, noncycling estrogens because that is the situation that occurs in the polycystic ovarian disease and there is endometrial hyperplasia and an increased instance of carcinoma of the uterus. The women with hyperprolactinemic amenorrhea, I think, should be treated with bromocriptine. I would not treat the woman who has infrequent cycles, say, every six, eight, or ten weeks, and who does not wish to be treated, because she is stripping her endometrium adequately.

QUESTION: *Given the case of a macroadenoma extending well beyond the sella, regardless of what the ultimate plan of therapy is, you either shrink it down and radiate or shrink it down and perform transsphenoidal surgery. What dosage do you start with? How rapidly do you advance the dosage? And is there any predicting factor for the probability of the tumor shrinking?*

BESSER: I am aware of no report, published or unpublished, of patients whose tumor has gotten bigger on bromocriptine therapy. I think that is the first thing that we have to accept. The question about how you give bromocriptine is very important, because the initial side effects can be unpleasant if therapy is not started properly. There is only one kind of patient to whom you can give a full dose immediately and in whom no one has ever found any side effects, and that is the puerperal woman in whom you wish to suppress lactation. Puerperal women can take a full dose of 7.5 mg a day straightaway, providing you start within 24 hours of delivery. It is strange how they totally tolerate the dopamine side effects. Now in all other patients, you get these side effects if you don't give the drug properly, but they are the same as with L-dopa in parkinsonian patients. These side effects are common to all dopamine agonists. However, they may be completely avoided in the vast majority of patients. I would like to tell you exactly what we do, because it is so effective in avoiding unpleasant side effects as treatment starts. We tell the patients in a written handout that there may be side effects of postural hypotension, nausea, and vomiting. It is terribly important for them to realize that, having taken their tablet they may get short-term postural hypotension so if at night they get out of bed to go to the lavatory, they run the risk of fainting and injuring themselves. It is important to start treatment at night so that they can conveniently lie down for 6–8 hours after the first dose. So the patients ought to get undressed, ready for bed, and pass urine. They then take a sandwich and a glass of milk to bed. They eat half the sandwich and drink half the glass of milk and then they take a half tablet (1.25 mg) and they finish their sandwich and glass of milk and they stay flat until the next morning. They do that every night for two or three nights and then they take a whole tablet in the middle of that snack for a couple of nights and then they move it forward to the middle of their evening meal. Two or three days later, they take half of one tablet in the middle of breakfast. If they tell me they do not have breakfast, they only have a cup of coffee, I tell them they don't get treated, because I have explained to them the problems of side effects. They must have a bulky breakfast, at least until they are established on bromocriptine. In due course they work up to the usual dose of 1 tablet (2.5 mg) three times a day in the middle of a meal. It must be taken with food. If they get very slight symptoms, which they may still, if they are very sensitive, then you tell them to go back one increment and wait one week and then increase it. So if the patient takes it slowly and does not increase it more frequently than every four to eight hours, two per week, depending on the sensitivity of the patient, you will not get those initial side effects. Remember, give it in the middle of the food. We learned the hard way during the early part of our experience with bromocriptine. It really is not a problem if you do it that way.

QUESTION: *How high do you push the dosage?*

BESSER: Enough and not too much. We monitor the prolactin levels and we take it after one to two weeks on a particular dosage. You almost always have to use 5 to 7.5 mg a day, but there is a small group of resistant prolactinoma patients and we go on increasing the dose until the maximum benefit is achieved. For acromegaly, we use between 30 and 60 mg a day. For prolactinoma patients, I don't think we have ever gone above 40 mg a day. It is very, very rare, however, to have to go above 10 mg a day. So it is monitored by the prolactin. Get it into the midnormal range. We don't want to completely suppress it. The same is true for shrinkage of big tumors. We use the prolactin as a tumor marker. By the way, it is not true that in acromegaly you have to have high hyperprolactinemia to shrink the tumor. We have a number of purely GH-secreting acromegalic tumors without hyperprolactinemia that have also shrunk.

QUESTION: *Dr. Besser, with your combination of bromocriptine in macroadenomas and radiation, have you had any cures and subsequently taken them off bromocriptine and not had hypoprolactinemia?*

BESSER: In all honesty, we are just beginning to take them off. We did not let anybody get pregnant until 1974, I think it was, because we did not have the teratogenicity data until then, and I can't answer that question. I can answer it for acromegaly, as I did this morning, but I can not actually, in all honesty, answer it for hyperprolactinemia. We are currently doing just this.

QUESTION: *Dr. Tindall, one of your indications for surgery was an experienced neurosurgeon. How frequently should a surgeon do this procedure to maintain a good surgical technique?*

TINDALL: You probably need to do a minimum of 20–25 operations per year.

BESSER: Are only experienced surgeons allowed to do it? How does one learn?

TINDALL: Neurosurgeons who have a particular interest and committment in learning and performing pituitary surgery should arrange to spend some time with any one of a number of neurosurgeons who are performing relatively large numbers of transsphenoidal operations each year. In addition, some time should be spent in anatomical dissections of both wet and dry sphenoid blocks.

QUESTION: *I have two questions. First, Dr. Besser mentioned that this patient's cure may cost eighty dollars per month. That comes out to about $960 per year, and it takes ten years, so the cure costs about $9,600. I wonder what the cost is for the neurosurgical procedure. Second, on one of your slides, I think, you had four of 12 patients with big tumors that did not respond to bromocriptine. If that was correct then what do you do about this?*

BESSER: This is a joint project with a number of neurosurgeons and because of the ethics of the situation we agreed that we would completely evaluate the patient with contrast radiography and full endocrine evaluation, including an insulin tolerance test and full releasing hormone stimulation and basal hormone measurements. They have their visual fields plotted initially once or twice weekly. At three months they have the complete reevaluation, including contrast radiology, and we have agreed with the neurosurgeons that if they are not better by then, they will go to neurosurgery. So that is what we do. They then go in for decompression, whichever way the surgeon chooses.

QUESTION: *There was a report recently about abnormal chest x-rays with bromocriptine. What has been your experience with this?*

BESSER: There was a report from Rinne,* in Finland, in the *Lancet* that out of some 50 odd patients with parkinsonism, he got fleeting lung shadows and he felt that he should report this. In fact, some of the patients had lung shadows before and one of them got better while receiving bromocriptine. Now there was no controlled group whatsoever, either of patients with or without parkinsonism, and of course, those with the disease are elderly and immobile and very

---

*Pleuropulmonary changes during long-term bromocriptine treatment for Parkinson's disease. *Lancet* 1:44, 1981.

prone to getting chest infections. So there was absolutely no evidence whatsoever that the chest shadows were associated with bromocriptine therapy. I personally felt it premature that that should have been reported without a controlled group. But we were obviously concerned about it. So we randomly pulled x-rays of 47 acromegalic patients who had been treated for more than one year. The duration of treatment was longer than it was for the parkinsonian group and the dosage of bromocriptine they received was about the same. We x-rayed them again and reviewed all the x-rays of this group. Of 47 patients, five had lung shadows; two shadows were present before treatment; two patients had developed tuberculosis, one because of steroid treatment as part of treatment for leukemia, which left us one patient who had a lung shadow that was not diagnosed and that developed while she was taking bromocriptine and disappeared in the space of some six weeks. It was never diagnosed and she remained on bromocriptine for four years afterward and it never reappeared. I don't think there is any evidence that that report provides any basis for us to suppose that lung shadows are associated with bromocriptine therapy.[†] Really, it is up to the people who report it to produce a controlled group of parkinsonian patients.

QUESTION: *Dr. Besser, you mentioned one patient with a nonfunctional pituitary tumor that shrunk with bromocriptine. Do you know of any other data?*

BESSER: You are quite right and that is staggering because we didn't expect it to reduce in size and in fact I was amazed that the neurosurgeon suggested we try medical treatment. We had been longing, of course, to treat a nonfunctioning tumor. We were amazed at three months to find that it had reduced in size too. Now the fact that the prolactin is not outside the normal range doesn't mean that tumor is not secreting a small amount of prolactin, because we don't have tissue to immunoassay. But it did surprise us and I don't know of another case. I do know that not all nonfunctioning tumors respond, because Reginald Hall has had a couple with apparently nonfunctioning tumors that have not shrunk on bromocriptine therapy. So I wouldn't expect them to shrink.

ABBOUD: I am an endocrinologist at Mayo and I wanted to share with you our experience in the management of prolactinomas, particularly the microadenomas. We have had a total experience with about 140 patients with prolactinomas: about 60 to 70 of them have

---

†Besser G. M., Wass, J. A. H.: Pleuropulmonary shadows on bromocriptine. *Lancet* 1:323, 1981.

had microadenomas. Our line of treatment of microadenomas is transsphenoidal surgery with selective adenomectomy. In 80% of the patients, we have had resolution of the problem, in the sense that prolactin dropped down to normal. They resume normal menstrual periods, and their endocrine function in the basal and provoked stages are all normal and the provoked stage for us is an insulin tolerance test with which we can assess GH-ACTH axis, and the thyrotropin-releasing hormone (TRH) test when we assess the prolactin and the TSH axis. We don't have gonadotropin-releasing hormone available in the United States. For now, we have a method of treatment that can cure 80% of the patients. Now we come to the other issue and that is with the use of bromocriptine. We show the figure that Dr. Besser had about the resumption of normal menstrual periods in those who have had bromocriptine. The figure showed that 80% of them resumed normal menstrual function: 20% of them did not show resumption. So, granted that he may be a few percentage points better than transsphenoidal surgery, I don't think that this state of affairs would lead one to opt for bromocriptine just to prevent hypopituitarism.

BESSER: Yes, but you have not yet been able to tell the progesterone levels in these women that are menstruating and you have not yet been able to tell the interval to conception or the conception rate. That is what we want to know.

ABBOUD: In terms of getting progesterone, sure we can get millions of hormones on any patient that really would stand still for a few minutes. But the problem is, why do we need the progesterone? We need it to document ovulation. Why do I need to document ovulation? I would need to document it in all those who are interested in fertility, because when those who are not interested in fertility tell me they are menstruating regularly every four weeks, whether they have short luteal phase or not, it is nice to know, but it is not critical. Now in all the patients who had a microadenoma, whose prolactin level dropped to normal, and who resumed normal periods, there is no one who wished to become pregnant who was not able to do that. I think this is the best progesterone value that I can give you.

BESSER: Well, I certainly agree with that. I was taught by a gynecologist who said that the only true proof of fertility is the patter of tiny feet. I would agree with that absolutely, but I think that we are trying to answer a question for the medical profession at large, and that is why we need to know the progesterone level.

QUESTION: *Would both of you address what would be adequate follow-up?*

TINDALL: I see the patient at 1, 6, and 12 months after surgery. Further follow-up is made by either the patient's endocrinologist or internist or both. Currently, CT scans are proving very useful in followup, particularly in detection of early recurrence, which in my experience with transsphenoidal surgery, has been relatively rare.

BESSER: We see patients usually four weeks after the start of treatment, after we have given them written instructions as to how to start the treatment. We then see them two months later, then three months later, and then once every three months for one year, and then once every six months. But in the middle of that, before they are seen, we arrange for them to come up to the ward as outpatients to have the necessary outpatient tests so that test results are available when they are seen for clinical evaluation and radiologic evaluation. We go on seeing them the rest of the time. We have very close relationships with this very large group of patients. Of course, the socioeconomic situation is quite different in Great Britain and the health service provides a different relationship. So patients are perfectly happy to come. I personally have followed patients now for 20 years.

TINDALL: Dr. Besser, let me ask how you would manage a patient in whom the surgeon tells you he is convinced that the tumor was completely removed. The pituitary gland was saved, but was flattened out against the diaphragm sellae. Postoperatively, the patient has a prolactin level of 120 and still has amenorrhea.

BESSER: The patient receives radiotherapy to prevent the recurrence. We estimate the recurrence eventually at one in ten patients with macroadenomas if they are not irradiated. We would then fully evaluate them in the way that I have described and we would put them on bromocriptine. Now what is going through my mind and has been for sometime is whether we really need to get in the radiotherapy to prevent recurrence if we are going to give them bromocriptine. Now to answer that question, we are probably going to have to do some sort of randomized trial. We have not set that up yet. I think there is a very good possibility that we could avoid the radiotherapy if we were going to treat them with bromocriptine.

COWDEN: In the postoperative assessment a much smaller series of patients from Glasgow (around 50) who have been operated on for prolactinoma in the last $3^{1}/_{2}$ years with regular endocrine follow-up, there has been no patient with a microadenoma who has been operated on who has developed any form of clinical or biochemical endocrine failure as a result of surgery. In addition, there have been a number of patients in whom gonadotropin reserve was diminished preoperatively and returned postoperatively.

QUESTION: *Would you discuss the cost efficiency of bromocriptine versus other forms of therapy?*

BESSER: I am not in a position to do that, because, of course, with the National Health Service, that is not a problem as far as individual patients are concerned. We can choose the form of therapy that we consider to be in the patient's best medical interest. We do pay attention to the potential cost to the nation, of course, because it costs us all in taxes. But that is not our prime consideration. I'm afraid that I am never prepared to discuss the best medical treatment for an individual patient in terms of cost. I am just not brought up to do that and I don't have that mental circuit. I have to decide what is in the best interest of my patient. Then we can arrange to pay for the necessary medicine.

QUESTION: *I would like to bring up the topic of pituitary apoplexy, give two examples, and see how you would treat a girl who presents to you for the first time with a 12-year history of galactorrhea and amenorrhea. She is blind from bleeding into the pituitary fossa. Also take the patient that has a long standing pituitary tumor who two days before had a fresh myocardial infarction. How do you treat the patient?*

BESSER: The first patient I would immediately send to a neurosurgeon. For the second patient, I suppose I would try medical treatment first, and then I don't really know what I would do under those circumstances. I would try and get the patient to the surgeon. I mean, what I would actually do is call the neurosurgeon and ask him to come see the patient with me and between us we would decide.

TINDALL: Both of your patients have pituitary apoplexy and both have acute visual loss. I think that both situations represent true emergencies. In the first case, I would advise immediate surgical decompression by the transsphenoidal approach. The second patient is a bit tricky. One has to decide if it is worth the risk of a second myocardial infarction or life-long blindness. One option, if the facilities are available, is to stereotactically place a large bore needle into the tumor, transnasally, and try to aspirate the necrotic portion of tumor, thus providing some decompression and thus enhancing the chance that vision will not be permanently lost. Afterwards, some type of definitive therapy probably irradiation, could be instituted.

BESSER: I would agree with that absolutely.

QUESTION: *Why does much of the residue of these tumors become invasive?*

BESSER: A lot of them are invasive if by that you mean local invasion, erosion of the bone with perhaps a polyp going into the bone and sometimes the surrounding sinuses.

QUESTION: *I mean, why does it invade the dura mater?*

BESSER: Oh well, I think you have to assume that most of the macroadenomas are invasive. There are good data for that, particularly in the acromegalic tumors. An awful lot of the prolactinomas are invasive as well.

COMMENT: The reason that I asked that, of course, is that it seems to me it makes adenomas generally difficult to remove and, I would assume, may make them more difficult to treat by any means.

# Postoperative Evaluation of Pituitary Status

RAYMOND V. RANDALL, M.D.

*Division of Endocrinology/Metabolism and Internal Medicine, Mayo Clinic and Mayo Medical School, Rochester, Minnesota*


EDWARD R. LAWS, JR., M.D.

*Department of Neurologic Surgery, Mayo Clinic and Mayo Medical School, Rochester, Minnesota*


CHARLES F. ABBOUD, M.D.

*Division of Endocrinology/Metabolism and Internal Medicine, Mayo Clinic and Mayo Medical School, Rochester, Minnesota*

FOLLOWING OPERATION for a pituitary adenoma, we are interested in the function of the anterior pituitary gland, the neurohypophysis, and, if the pituitary adenoma was functioning, whether there is still hyperproduction of a hormone or hormones. Evaluations are made during the immediate postoperative period, approximately three months after operation, one year after operation, and annually thereafter. Because pituitary adenomas may again manifest themselves as long as 20 years or more after the initial treatment, we believe that patients who have been treated for a pituitary adenoma should be followed indefinitely.

Table 1 outlines the steps for postoperative evaluation of pituitary status. Function of the anterior pituitary is evaluated by measuring: (1) the levels in the blood of prolactin and growth hormone; (2) the

329

0-8151-3530-0/82/0006-0329-03-$03.75

TABLE 1.—POSTOPERATIVE EVALUATION OF PITUITARY STATUS

---

Anterior pituitary function
    Measure blood PRL, GH, ACTH, TSH, and FSH, LH and do dynamic studies when
        indicated
    Measure end-organ hormones: blood thyroxine, corticosteroids or cortisol,
        estrogens, testosterone, and urinary 17-ketosteroids and 17-ketogenic steroids or
        17-hydroxycorticosteroids
Posterior pituitary function
    ADH measured indirectly by measuring urinary volume and osmolality
    Oxytocin not measured
CT scan of sellar area with contrast enhancement, axial and coronal views
Standard x-ray views of head and polycycloidal tomograms of sella turcica
Visual fields

---

levels in the blood of the tropic hormones—adrenocorticotropic hormone (ACTH), thyroid stimulating hormone (TSH), follicle-stimulating hormone (FSH), and luteinizing hormone (LH), which stimulate the endocrine end-organs, namely, the adrenal cortex, thyroid, and gonads; (3) the levels in the blood of the hormones produced by the endocrine end-organs; and (4) the response of the anterior pituitary hormones to stimulation or suppression tests. Measuring the hormones secreted by the endocrine end-organs is usually more informative than measuring the tropic hormones, because the distinction between low normal values of tropic hormones and abnormally low values is imprecise.

Evaluation of neurohypophyseal function is done indirectly by measuring the ability of the kidney to conserve water and to make a concentrated urine. The function of the neurohypophysis in regards to oxytocin is rarely investigated because there is no practical, clinical assay for oxytocin, and the secretion of oxytocin is probably not essential for well-being even though it has many known physiologic effects.

The presence of residual hyperfunctioning pituitary adenoma cells is detected by measuring the blood levels of hormone or hormones produced in excess by the tumor prior to operation. It is, of course, entirely possible for hyperfunctioning adenomatous tissue to be present but not make its presence known because its secretion of hormone(s) is not enough to raise above normal the levels of that (those) hormone(s) in the blood. Unfortunately, no such markers in the blood exist for nonfunctioning pituitary adenomas, but one can search for the postoperative presence of residual adenomatous tissue by doing a contrast-enhanced computed tomographic (CT) scan with one of the newer scanners.

## Immediate Postoperative Evaluation

The immediate postoperative period is defined for our purposes as the time, usually five to seven days, the patient is in the hospital immediately following operation. The only function of the anterior pituitary that is evaluated during this period is that in relation to the adrenal glands, since lack of function of the thyroid or gonads will not usually lead to serious problems between the immediate postoperative period and reevaluation of the patient approximately three months later. However, if there has been definite failure of the thyroid gland prior to the operation, we have the patient start to use a thyroid preparation, usually L-thyroxine, after the operation and discontinue it eight weeks before the next evaluation three months after the operation. Likewise, impaired production of prolactin or GH will not lead to problems prior to the evaluation three months after operation.

### Adrenal Function

The immediate postoperative evaluation of adrenal function and interpretation of tests of adrenal function vary depending on whether the pituitary adenoma was producing ACTH in excess. All patients who undergo attempted removal of a pituitary adenoma, regardless of whether the adenoma is hyperfunctioning, are prepared with large doses of a short-acting adrenocortical steroid. Each patient is given 40 mg of prednisolone sodium phosphate (Hydeltrasol, made by MSD) intramuscularly one hour preoperatively and every eight hours on the day of surgery, followed by 20 mg intramuscularly every eight hours on the second postoperative day. If the patient is doing well, the administration of prednisolone sodium phosphate is stopped on the third or fourth postoperative day and blood for corticosteroids and ACTH is drawn that afternoon and the next morning. The patient is watched carefully for possible adrenocortical failure during this period. If the patient had a non-ACTH-producing adenoma and the blood corticosteroids are normal, no additional adrenocortical steroid is given unless the patient should have signs or symptoms of adrenocortical insufficiency prior to the next endocrine evaluation three months after the operation. If the blood corticosteroid values are below the normal range or in the borderline portion of the normal range, the patient is given adrenocortical steroid replacement therapy. We usually have the patient take 20 mg of hydrocortisone orally each morning around breakfast time and another 10 mg orally in the late afternoon or early evening around the time of the patient's supper or dinner. It is perfectly feasible to use the less expensive preparation, prednisone, giving 2.5 mg or 5.0 mg each morning and 2.5 mg in the late afternoon or early evening.

Patients are advised to triple their doses of adrenocortical steroid in the event of a minor illness with fever, or minor surgical or dental procedures. They are also told that in the event of a major illness, severe trauma, or operation they should be given large doses of parenteral adrenocortical steroid. If an acute situation arises, they will need to be given rapid-acting adrenocortical steroids in the form of prednisolone sodium phosphate, given intramuscularly, as noted before, or 100 mg of hydrocortisone sodium succinate (Solu-Cortef, made by Upjohn), given intravenously each six-to eight-hour period. Patients are also advised that they need to receive parenteral adrenocortical steroids should they have vomiting and not be able to take the oral medication. We ask our patients to have with them at home or when they travel a rapid-acting adrenocortical steroid that they can give intramuscularly or subcutaneously in the event of vomiting or severe illness when they are unable to obtain medical help *at once*. Probably the most convenient form is dexamethasone sodium phosphate (Decatron Phosphate, made by MSD) which comes as a 1-ml solution of 4 mg of dexamethasone sodium phosphate in a disposable syringe, which is packaged with a needle suitable for intramuscular (IM), subcutaneous, or intravenous (IV) use. The patients and members of their family are instructed how to administer this material by the IM route. The patients are also asked to wear a necklace or bracelet with a Medic Alert emblem that states that they have had pituitary surgery and should be given adrenocortical steroids. Other pertinent information such as the need for antidiuretic hormone, drug allergies, bleeding tendencies, etc. can be imprinted on the emblem. Application blanks can be obtained by writing to Medic Alert Foundation, P.O. Box 1009, Turlock, CA 95380.

If the patient had an ACTH-producing adenoma causing Cushing's disease, and the blood corticosteroids are found to be low or absent, the patient is given continuous oral replacement therapy and advised about the need for additional adrenocortical steroids. If the blood corticosteroids are normal, replacement adrenocortical steroids are not given. Most patients in the latter category will ultimately prove to have had incomplete removal of the ACTH-producing pituitary adenoma and frequently will have a return of Cushing's disease requiring further treatment. If the blood corticosteroids are increased above the normal range, some decision should be made about additional treatment for the still active Cushing's disease. A second operative approach to the pituitary is unlikely to relieve the Cushing's disease, if an experienced surgeon carefully explored the pituitary during the initial procedure. If the patient has severe, life-threatening Cushing's disease, a bilateral total adrenalectomy is performed as soon as it has been determined that the Cushing's disease was not relieved by the operation on the pituitary. If the Cushing's disease is not life-threatening the use of radiotherapy can be considered with the realization that it may be months or several years before maximal effects of the radiotherapy become manifest. If it is thought that the patient's condition is such that one cannot wait for radiotherapy to take effect, but bilateral adrenalectomy is not warranted, then, in addition to radiotherapy, the patient can be given the antiserotonin agent cyproheptadine hydrochloride (Periactin Hydrochloride, made by MSD),[3] or the 11-β-hydroxylase blocking agent, metyrapone (Metopirone, made by Ciba).[2]

Because of the lag in getting reports on plasma ACTH, these values do not play a role in the immediate decision about treating a patient after an operation for an ACTH-producing adenoma causing Cushing's disease. Rather, the determinations are used later for comparison with preoperative and subsequent postoperative results.

## NELSON'S SYNDROME

The term "Nelson's syndrome" is used to denote a patient who has been successfully treated for Cushing's disease by bilateral total or radical subtotal adrenalectomy and subsequently develops manifestations of an ACTH-producing pituitary tumor. Because these patients have had total or radical subtotal removal of their adrenal glands, they take daily maintenance therapy consisting of an adrenocortical steroid, such as hydrocortisone or prednisone, and a mineralocorticoid, such as fludrocortisone acetate (Florinef Acetate, made by Squibb). Following attempted removal of the ACTH-producing pituitary tumor and tapering of the prednisolone sodium phosphate given immediately before and after operation, these patients continue their usual replacement therapy. Blood for ACTH determinations is obtained at 8:00 A.M. and 4:00 P.M. about three or four days after operation. If the values for ACTH are normal, low, or undetectable, then the patient is followed carefully. If the values are still above normal, then additional treatment such as radiotherapy, cyproheptadine, or a combination of the two is considered.

## Postoperative Diabetes Insipidus

Postoperative diabetes insipidus is less frequent following transsphenoidal removal of pituitary adenomas than when the adenomas are approached by the transfrontal route, because there is less likely to be damage to the hypothalamiconeurohypophyseal system. Nonetheless, any of the three classic patterns of postoperative diabetes insipidus may be seen (Fig 1): (1) transient diabetes insipidus; (2) permanent diabetes insipidus with an interphase, the so-called triphasic pattern; or (3) permanent diabetes insipidus without an interphase. These patterns were first noted by Fischer et al.[1] in their classic studies on animals, and were subsequently confirmed in patients who had been operated on for lesions in and around the pituitary and hypothalamus.[5]

In humans, transient polyuria begins a few hours to four days following operation, lasts one to six days and is followed by a return of normal urinary volumes and normal or near normal ability to concentrate the urine.

In the triphasic pattern of diabetes insipidus, the transient phase of polyuria and polydipsia begins a few hours to two days after operation and may last one to five days. The transient phase is followed by a period known as the interphase during which there is essentially normal intake of water and normal urinary output—indeed, the urinary volume may fall to less than normal. The polyuria and polydipsia return some time between the fourth and ninth days after operation and last indefinitely. In some instances the polyuria and polydipsia may diminish after several months and return to normal

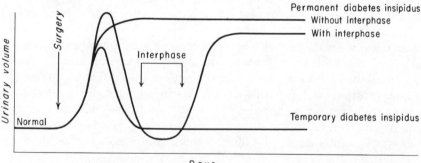

Fig 1.—Schematic curves showing patterns of onset of postoperative diabetes insipidus in man. (From Randall R.V.: Medical problems associated with pituitary operations. *Med. Clin. N. Am.* 46:1037, 1962. Used by permission of W.B. Saunders Co.)

or near normal volumes, and the need for treatment of the diabetes insipidus may disappear. In some patients, there may be only a partial interphase during which the urinary volume and intake of water decrease only slightly following the initial, transient diabetes insipidus. Then after two or three days, the polyuria and polydipsia return and reach levels similar to those during the transient phase.

Permanent diabetes insipidus begins a few hours to four days after operation and may last indefinitely. In some instances, however, the polyuria and polydipsia may decrease after a few months, even though the patient does not develop anterior pituitary failure, and the need for treatment of the diabetes insipidus may disappear.

In order to detect the onset of diabetes insipidus following operation, the fluid intake and the volume and specific gravity or osmolality of *each* urinary voiding are measured. Serum electrolytes are monitored frequently in all patients who develop diabetes insipidus. Since it is not possible to tell which pattern of diabetes insipidus is developing when polyuria and polydipsia first start, patients are treated with short-acting aqueous vasopressin (Pitressin, made by Parke-Davis), which has an effect lasting four to seven hours. One can also use 0.3 to 0.5 ml of vasopressin tannate in oil (Pitressin Tannate, made by Parke-Davis), which will have an effect lasting 12 to 15 hours. When treating a patient during the onset of postoperative diabetes insipidus, one should not give the next dose of antidiuretic hormone (ADH), be it short-acting aqueous vasopressin or the long-acting vasopressin tannate in oil, until the effects of the previous injection of ADH are beginning to wear off, as signaled by an increase in urinary volume and a fall in the urinary specific gravity or osmolality. One can then discontinue the use of antidiuretic hormone at the appropriate time should the diabetes insipidus be transient, or should the patient be entering the interphase of the triphasic pattern. During the interphase the patient is under the influence of excessive amounts of antidiuretic hormone being released without control by the damaged hypothalamiconeurohypophyseal system, is unable to excrete a waterload rapidly, and is thereby subject to water intoxication, particularly if excessive fluids are given intravenously. Under these circumstances, the administration of exogenous antidiuretic hormone only adds to the problem.

If the patient develops permanent diabetes insipidus, then appropriate treatment with the intranasal insufflation of lysine-8-vasopressin (Diapid nasal spray, made by Sandoz) or desmopressin acetate (dDAVP, made by Armour) or one of the oral, non-ADH forms of treatment, such as chlorothiazide, chlorpropamide, etc., can be started.[4] Patients who have been operated by the transsphenoidal route, can usually absorb lysine-8-vasopressin or desmopressin acetate through the nasal mucosa without difficulty within several days after the nasal packs have been removed.

In evaluating a patient with postoperative diabetes insipidus, it should be remembered that what seems to be transient diabetes insipidus followed by a return of urinary output and fluid intake to normal amounts may actually be transient diabetes insipidus followed by an interphase with permanent diabetes insipidus in the offing. There is no way during the onset to distinguish between the two patterns. Hence, if the hospital stay is only four to six days after the operation, the physician should be aware and the patient warned that the diabetes insipidus might return after the patient leaves the hospital.

## Diabetes Insipidus Without Thirst Drive

Some patients, following operations in and around the pituitary, may develop diabetes insipidus without an adequate thirst drive, and, hence, have neither polydipsia nor polyuria to draw attention to the underlying diabetes insipidus. This is when measuring the specific gravity or osmolality of the urine and serum electrolytes during the postoperative period is helpful. Such patients will have a normal fluid intake and urinary volume, but the urine will have a low specific gravity or osmolality. If the condition is unrecognized and not treated with antidiuretic hormone, the patients may develop increased serum osmolality, sodium and chloride, and hypovolemia. Should the condition persist, and not be treated, patients may become progressively drowsy, comatose, and die. It is not unusual under these circumstances to see the serum sodium level go as high as 180 to 190 mEq/L. Unfortunately, the diabetes insipidus may persist indefinitely, as may the lack of thirst drive. Such patients should be treated with antidiuretic hormone and must be instructed to drink adequate amounts of fluid. If they do not, they are constantly at risk for developing hyperosmolality of the serum, hypovolemia, and ultimately unconsciousness.

## Syndrome of Inappropriate Secretion of Antidiabetic Hormone

Patients who have operative procedures in and around the pituitary may develop the syndrome of inappropriate secretion of antidiuretic hormone. This syndrome is characterized by (1) a decrease in serum osmolality and serum sodium; (2) an extracellular fluid volume that is normal or only slightly increased, without edema; (3) a urinary osmolality greater than the serum osmolality; (4) the urinary excretion of sodium equal to or greater than the intake of sodium; and (5) ultimately convulsions, unconsciousness, and even death, should the condition persist and go untreated.

## POSTOPERATIVE CT SCAN AND PLOTTING OF VISUAL FIELDS

When feasible, a CT scan of the head, with contrast medium, is obtained during the immediate postoperative period. The scan is helpful, particularly when dealing with a large pituitary adenoma, in determining whether all of the adenoma has been removed. It is important to obtain a scan, particularly if, during transsphenoidal removal of the pituitary tumor, the sella turcica was packed with a muscle plug. Muscle plugs may subsequently be mistaken for a persistent or recurrent pituitary adenoma; a postoperative CT scan is useful for future comparisons. When dealing with nonfunctioning pituitary adenomas, which, of course, do not have a tumor marker such as prolactin, GH, etc., scans with one of the newer CT scanners are the only practical way to detect failure to resect totally the adenomas or to detect their early regrowth. In places where it is not possible to obtain scans with one of the newer CT scanners, visual fields should be plotted during the periodic evaluations subsequent to the operation. It is our policy to plot the visual fields before and a few days after the operation. On subsequent examinations the visual fields are plotted regardless of whether a CT scan is performed, if the patient had a visual field defect before or after operation, if the patient had an adenoma greater than 10 mm in diameter, or if radiotherapy was given, because visual field abnormalities can occur not only with regrowth of the tumor but also with development of a secondary empty sella.

## HEAD X-RAYS AND SELLAR TOMOGRAMS

The standard x-ray views of the head (anterior-posterior, posterioanterior (PA), and lateral stereoscopic views) and PA and lateral polycycloidal tomograms of the sella turcica are taken during the examination at three months. They are used to determine whether the bony operative changes have repaired themselves; whether the sella has grown smaller and recalcified, if enlargement and decalcification were present preoperatively; whether intrasellar or suprasellar calcification is still present, if either was present before operation; and as a basis for future comparison, if similar roentgenograms are taken later.

Before the new CT scanners became available, standard x-ray views of the head and tomograms of the sella turcica were obtained at each examination following operation. Enlargement and/or decalcification of the sella turcica are frequently present, with persistence or recurrence of a pituitary adenoma. However, recent experience with well over 100 follow-up examinations, during which standard x-ray views of the head and tomograms of the sella turcica as well as CT scans of the sella were obtained, has convinced us that we get more information from the CT scans, when taken with one of the new scanners, such as the General Electric 8800, than from the standard x-ray views and tomograms combined. Our CT scans are taken with axial and coronal views through the sella turcica both without and during the infusion of contrast medium. Currently, on examinations following the one at three months, we no longer routinely obtain

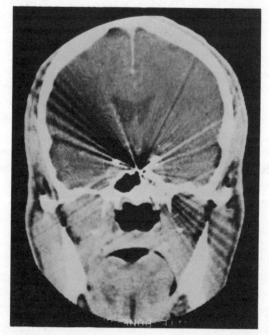

**Fig 2.**—CT coronal view of head showing artifacts from tantalum vascular clip placed in sella turcica as a marker during operation for a pituitary tumor causing acromegaly.

standard x-ray views of the head or tomograms of the sella but rely on CT scans.

It formerly was our practice to place one or two tantalum vascular clips in the sella turcica as a marker at the time of operation. The rationale was that movement of the clips subsequent to the immediate postoperative period was usually indicative of regrowth of the tumor. Unfortunately, these clips cause artifacts on the CT scan and obscure the interpretation of scans taken in the same plane as the clip (Fig 2). For this reason, we no longer use these clips as markers.

## FUNCTIONING PITUITARY ADENOMAS

If the patient had a functioning pituitary adenoma prior to operation, measurements of the hormone or hormones that were produced in excess are made at least once, or preferably twice, during the immediate postoperative period. In most instances, finding normal values for such hormones usually means that the hyperfunctioning adenoma has been sucessfully removed, while increased values indicate that hyperfunctioning tumor tissue still remains. Unfortunately, at times, when a hyperfunctioning adenoma has not been totally resected, there may be normal postoperative blood values for the hormone in question that will later be supplanted by increased values as the residual adenomatous tissue grows larger.

## Evaluation at Three Months and Annually

Extensive evaluation of the patient is planned about three months following operation because by then the inability of the anterior pituitary to elaborate some or all of its hormones, if such takes place, is usually firmly established. A decision can then be made as to whether replacement therapy is warranted.

How extensively patients are studied during evaluations subsequent to operation depends on the facilities available, whether patients are being studied under a protocol calling for extensive studies, and whether one wants to do the minimum amount of study necessary to provide information adequate for proper care and treatment of the patient. We will review first the steps that are followed in an intensive investigation and then those that are followed during an adequate workup with minimal laboratory studies. Specific details about each of the various tests are not given because they are adequately covered in standard texts.

## ADRENAL TESTING

Tests done at three months in reference to the hypothalamic-pituitary-adrenal axis depend on whether the patient, prior to operation, had a pituitary adenoma that was producing ACTH in excess.

If the pituitary adenoma was not producing ACTH prior to the operation, when the patient returns in three months, replacement treatment with hydrocortisone or other adrenocortical steroid, if the patient is taking such, is stopped two or three days before testing, and the patient is watched carefully. It has been our experience that 30 mg of cortisone or hydrocortisone, divided into two or three doses a day, is unlikely to suppress the hypothalamic-pituitary-adrenal axis of patients who are capable of functioning normally in this regard. We measure the 24-hour urinary excretion of 17-ketosteroids and 17-ketogenic steroids (or 17-hydroxycorticosteroids) and blood corticosteroids or cortisol level at 8:00 A.M. and 4:00 P.M. Further testing of the axis can be done, if desired, by measuring the adrenal response to insulin-induced hypoglycemia or the response to the administration of metyrapone. Additional information can be obtained by measuring plasma ACTH along with the blood corticosteroids or cortisol at 8:00 A.M. and 4:00 P.M., and during insulin-induced hypoglycemia or the administration of metyrapone. We usually reserve such testing for patients of unusual interest or when we are involved in special studies. While a normal response to hypoglycemia generally indicates that the patient will respond satisfactorily to physical stress, we still advise that such patients be given large doses of parenteral adrenocortical steroids in the event of surgery, severe illness, or other undue physical stress. If a patient has abnormally low or low normal values for urinary and blood adrenal steroids, the patient is advised to take replacement dose of hydrocortisone, cortisone, or prednisone indefinitely and, of course, to use additional adrenocortical steroids in times of illness, operation, undue physical stress, etc., as outlined above.

Our experience has been that patients who have definite adrenal insufficiency prior to operation for their pituitary adenoma are unlikely to recover normal adrenal function following the operation. Likewise, patients who have normal adrenal function prior to operation but impaired adrenal function three months after operation are subsequently unlikely to develop normal adrenal function. For this reason, we do not stop replacement therapy with adrenocortical steroids, and test the adrenal function of such patients at examinations subsequent to that done at three months after operation.

Patients who have excess production of ACTH causing Cushing's disease prior to operation on their pituitary adenoma are usually adrenally insufficient following the operation if there has been successful removal of the pituitary adenoma. An attempt is made to reduce gradually and ultimately to stop the dosage of daily adrenocortical steroids prior to reevaluation three months after operation. If this is possible and if the patient has normal urinary excretion and blood levels of adrenocortical steroids, then dexamethasone suppression and metyrapone testing is done at three months to determine whether the hypothalamic-pituitary-adrenal axis responds normally. If, at three months, the patient is on larger than physiologic amounts of adrenocortical steroids, adrenal testing is postponed. It should be realized that some patients cannot be weaned from replacement therapy for as long as a year after operation, and an occasional patient will require an even longer time.

If the patient had Nelson's syndrome prior to operation on the pituitary adenoma, replacement therapy with adrenocortical steroids is not stopped because such patients by definition have had a total or radical subtotal bilateral adrenalectomy. Plasma ACTH is measured at 8:00 A.M. and 4:00 P.M..

## THYROID TESTING

Intactness of the hypothalamic-pituitary-thyroid axis is determined by measuring the amount of circulating thyroxine in the blood. If the level is low, the patient is given replacement therapy with L-thyroxine, which is continued indefinitely. The axis can be tested further by the administration of TRH and measuring the TSH response. We usually do this when testing the pituitary's ability to secrete prolactin when the patient is given TRH. Blood TSH alone (that is not followed by TRH testing) is usually not measured because, as pointed out earlier, the dividing line between low normal and abnormally low TSH values is ill-defined because of the nature of the assay.

It has been our experience that if thyroid function is low prior to removal of a pituitary adenoma, it is likely to be so three months after operation. However, since there are occasional exceptions, we do not usually give patients replacement therapy immediately following operation if their thyroid function was low before operation, unless they are actually myxedematous. When replacement therapy is given, it is stopped approximately eight weeks before the examination at three months after operation, so thyroid function can be reevaluated.

## GONADAL TESTING

The return of menses in a woman in the menstrual age group who had amenorrhea prior to the removal of a pituitary tumor is evidence that the ovaries are functioning but not necessarily ovulating. If the patient has midcycle cramping or spotting, or has a midcycle rise in morning rectal basal temperatures, then ovulation is almost certainly taking place. The return of menses following the removal of a pituitary adenoma is most commonly seen when patients have had a prolactin-producing pituitary adenoma. However, it occasionally may be seen in patients who had a nonfunctioning pituitary adenoma or a pituitary adenoma producing GH in excess. The resumption of menses and ovulation in a patient who had hyperprolactinemia preoperatively is no assurance that the blood prolactin level has returned to normal, because some patients may resume normal ovarian function if there has been only partial but not complete return of prolactin values to normal.

In men, a return of libido and potentia is good evidence that gonadal function has been restored. If the patient had azoospermia or oligospermia, the return of a normal sperm count is confirmatory evidence that testicular function has returned to normal. The palpation of a normal-feeling prostate on rectal examination is good evidence that the male patient is making normal or essentially normal amounts of testosterone, since the prostate is a sensitive biologic indicator of testosterone production. Again, in patients who have prolactin-producing pituitary tumors, these findings do not necessarily mean that the prolactin level in the blood has returned to normal.

In testing patients at three months, in addition to the findings noted above, we usually measure FSH and LH in the blood of both sexes, estrogen in females and testosterone in males. Although it is not available for clinical use in the United States, gonadotropin-releasing hormone (GnRH) is useful in testing the ability of the pituitary gland to produce normal amounts of FSH and LH. Testing with clomiphene citrate can also be done, but we do not do this routinely.

## GROWTH HORMONE

We do not usually measure GH in adult patients following removal of a pituitary adenoma unless the adenoma was producing GH. However, in adolescents and preadolescents it becomes important to know whether adequate amounts of GH are being made. We use one of the standard tests, such as the insulin hypoglycemia test or propranolol-glucagon test, to determine GH responsiveness.

When patients have had a pituitary adenoma producing excess GH, the ability of hyperglycemia to suppress the secretion of GH is determined by doing a glucose tolerance test and obtaining blood for GH values at the same time blood is drawn to measure the glucose values.

## PROLACTIN

Prolactin in the blood is measured at three months following operation regardless of whether the patient had a prolactin-producing adenoma. Some patients during the removal of a pituitary adenoma not producing prolactin may have damage to the hypothalamus or portal blood system and develop hyperprolactinemia. If the patient had a prolactin-producing pituitary adenoma, then in addition to obtaining

| | | |
|---|---|---|
| O | Female ⎫ Position on chart denotes | **CRANIAL NERVE DEFECTS** |
| ▲ | Male ⎭ preoperative prolactin value | VFD — Visual field defect |
| ⊚ | Number = diameter, in mm, | VFDI — Visual field defect improved |
| | of microadenoma | VFN — Visual fields returned to normal |
| ☐ | Postoperative prolactin value | EOMW — Extraocular motor weakness |
| **ENDOCRINE DEFICIENCIES** | | EOMI — Extraocular motor weakness, improved |
| Ø | Bar = partial anterior pituitary failure | EOMN — Extraocular motor weakness returned |
| ● | Solid symbol = complete anterior pituitary | to normal |
| | failure | **TUMOR INVASION** |
| SXR | Sexual retardation | ♂ — Invasion of diaphragm or suprasellar region |
| SMR | Somatic retardation | O→ — Invasion of right lateral dura or cavernous |
| TDI | Transient diabetes insipidus | sinus |
| PDI | Permanent diabetes insipidus | →O — Invasion of left lateral dura or cavernous |
| MEN | Multiple endocrine neoplasia, Type I | sinus |
| **MENSES** | | ♀ — Invasion of sphenoid dura or sellar floor |
| A | Secondary amenorrhea | **TREATMENT** |
| A° | Primary amenorrhea | C — Craniotomy |
| O | Oligomenorrhea | S — Shunt |
| M̲ | Irregular menses | TS — Transsphenoidal operation |
| M | Return of menses | RF — Transsphenoidal radiofrequency |
| **LACTATION** | | thermocoagulation |
| G | Galactorrhea | XRT — Radiation therapy |
| G̶ | Transient galactorrhea | BR — Bromocriptine |
| G̶/̶ | Cessation of or no galactorrhea | **MISCELLANEOUS** |
| **PREGNANCY** | | CSF — CSF leak |
| P | Pregnancy (not completed) | CSFT — Transient CSF leak |
| TP | Term pregnancy | CSFR — CSF leak repaired |
| (TP) | Wife had term pregnancy | PAp — Pituitary apoplexy |
| SB | Stillborn | ESS — Empty sella syndrome (CT = diagnosed by |
| SAb | Spontaneous abortion | CT scan) |
| IAb | Induced abortion | ⌐ — Course after patient left our care |
| | | ? — Subsequent course unknown |

**Fig 3.**—Key to symbols used in charting data from patients with prolactin-producing pituitary adenomas (prolactinomas) (From Randall R.V. et al.: Transphenoidal microsurgical treatment of prolactin-producing pituitary adenomas: findings and results in 100 patients. Submitted for publication to Mayo Clinic Proc., 1982. Reproduced with permission.)

one or more baseline values for prolactin we usually do a TRH stimulation test. Most patients who have had complete removal of a prolactin-producing pituitary tumor will have an increase in the secretion of prolactin following the administration of TRH, as opposed to the usual failure of TRH to stimulate the secretion of prolactin in those patients who have residual pituitary adenoma and hyperprolactinemia.

## HYPERFUNCTIONING PITUITARY ADENOMAS

The most commonly occurring hyperfunctioning pituitary adenomas are those producing prolactin, GH, or ACTH, or the combination of GH and prolactin. The methods we use for testing are given under the appropriate headings above.

Tumors that produce excessive TSH or FSH and LH, or prolactin in combination with TSH or FSH and LH, are rare. Testing consists of measuring the blood levels of the appropriate hormone or hormones.

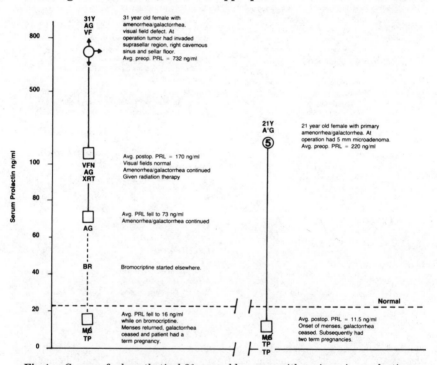

**Fig 4.**—Course of a hypothetical 31-year-old woman with an invasive prolactinoma *(left)*, and that of a hypothetical 21-year-old woman with a microprolactinoma (prolactinoma ≤ 10 mm in diameter) *(right)*.

We have had occasion to study only one patient whose pituitary tumor produced TSH. He was studied before and following operation by attempting to stimulate the release of TSH by the administration of TRH. We did not test the patient's response to attempted suppression by the administration of triiodothyronine but plan to do so if we see a similar patient in the future. Likewise, it would be interesting to know the uptake of radioiodine by the thyroid both before and after operation on the pituitary adenoma. If we saw a patient with an adenoma producing excessive FSH and LH, we would be interested in knowing the response to GnRH before and after operation and whether the administration of large doses of estrogens would suppress the secretion of excessive FSH and LH.

## CT Scans

Although CT scanning of the pituitary area is not an endocrine test, we consider this to be as essential for the evaluation of patients at intervals following operation for pituitary adenoma as we do prior to operation. Scanning provides valuable information as to whether there is persistent or recurrent pituitary tumor, particularly in those patients with nonfunctioning adenomas. Scanning also provides information as to whether the patient is developing a secondary empty sella, which is particularly apt to happen following the removal of large pituitary adenomas or when the patient has been given radiotherapy following operation.

It is not unusual for a patient to develop a visual field defect a few years following operation for a pituitary adenoma. The question immediately arises as to whether the patient has a persistent or recurrent tumor, or whether there is an empty sella with prolapse of the chiasm into the sella causing the visual field defect. If the patient is known to have a secondary empty sella, it is likely that the visual field defect is due to this. The question of tumor vs empty sella can usually be settled rapidly by obtaining a CT scan with contrast enhancement. It should be remembered, however, that a persistent or recurrent pituitary adenoma can coexist with a secondary empty sella. Again, a CT scan with contrast enhancement should readily show this.

## Visual Fields

Visual fields are plotted at the time of the examination, three months after operation. This is true regardless of whether the patient had a visual field defect prior to operation. At subsequent annual examinations, visual fields are plotted in any patient who had a visual field deficit prior to operation or who had a pituitary macroadenoma (diameter greater than 10 mm) even though a visual field deficit was not present prior to operation. If the patient had a microadenoma (≤10 mm in diameter), and did not have a visual field deficit prior to or immediately after operation or at the three month's recheck, then the visual fields are not replotted at subsequent examinations unless there are symptoms of visual dysfunction, evidence of recurrent tumor on the CT scan, or the patient has a secondary empty sella.

## MINIMAL TESTING

If one is interested in doing the minimal testing that will give adequate information at three months following operation for a pituitary adenoma, one can do the following: (1) Adrenal glands: measure

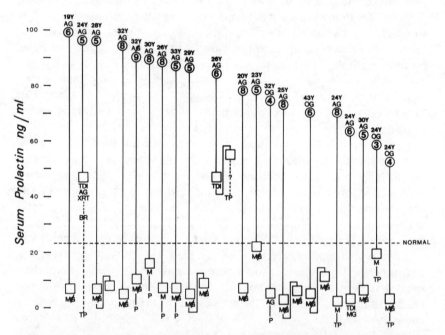

Fig 5.—A chart with data from 20 females with prolactin-producing microadenomas and average, basal, preoperative serum prolactin values between 50 and 100 ng/ml. P denotes pregnancy in progress at the time the chart was drawn. (From Randall R.V., et al.: Neurosurgical management of 100 patients with prolactin-producing pituitary adenomas: findings and results in 100 patients. Submitted to Mayo Clin. Proc., 1982. Reproduced with permission.)

24-hour urinary 17-ketosteroids and 17-ketogenic steroids (or hydroxycorticosteroids), and plasma corticosteroids or cortisol at 8:00 A.M. and 4:00 P.M. (2) Thyroid gland: measure serum thyroxine. (3) Gonads: in females who are in the menstruating age group, inquire as to whether menses have returned and, if galactorrhea was present prior to operation, whether it has disappeared. In patients who are either younger or older than the menstrual period of their lives, measure blood FSH, LH, and estrogens. In males, palpate the prostate and inquire as to libido and potentia; if in doubt, obtain semen analysis. If still in doubt, measure blood FSH, LH, and testosterone. (4) Growth hormone: insulin hypoglycemia tests in adolescents or preadolescents. In patients who are operated on because of acromegaly, gigantism, or a combination of the two: glucose tolerance test with GH measurements. GH tests are not done in adults without acromegaly, gigantism, or a combination of the two. (5) Prolactin: measure basal prolactin levels regardless of whether the patient had a prolactin-producing pituitary adenoma. (6) CT scan of head and visual fields: obtain in all patients, but omit visual fields in patients who had a microadenoma if visual fields were normal both before and immediately following the operation.

## Annual Examination

The testing done at annual examinations is the same as that outlined for examination at three months following operation for a pituitary adenoma.

We firmly believe that patients should be followed indefinitely. Although our experience with patients following transsphenoidal surgery is limited to nine years, we know from 30 years of experience with patients who were operated on by the transfrontal route that pituitary adenomas can make their reappearance as long as 15 to 20 years or more following the initial operation. It will be at least another 15 to 20 years before we will have adequate information concerning the course of an adequate number of patients who have been operated on by the transsphenoidal route. Until this information is available, it behooves us to follow all patients carefully.

## Graphic Displays of Data From Patients With Pituitary Adenomas

We (Raymond V. Randall, M.D., Division of Endocrinology/Metabolism and Internal Medicine; Edward R. Laws, Jr., M.D., Department

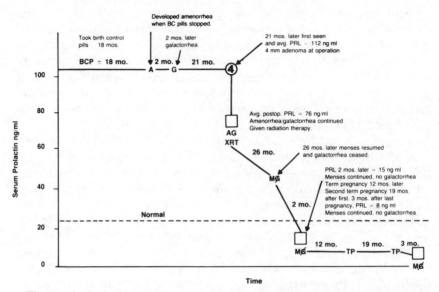

**Fig 6.**—A chart showing the sequence of events in a hypothetical 24-year-old woman with an invasive prolactinoma. The dimension of time has been added.

of Neurologic Surgery; and Marvin L. Ellingson, Section of Medical Graphics, Mayo Clinic and Mayo Medical School) have devised a set of symbols that permits us to chart the preoperative and postoperative findings, treatments, endocrine status, and other data from a number of patients with pituitary adenomas. The same method can be used to display, in a temporal fashion, similar information for individual patients (Figs 3–6). Although it takes a short time to become familiar with the various symbols, we have found this method to be useful for displaying, in a relatively small space, large amounts of data from a number of patients with pituitary adenomas.

## BIBLIOGRAPHY

1. Fischer C., Ingram W.R., Ranson S.W.: *Diabetes Insipidus and the Neurohormonal Control of Water Balance: A Contribution to the Structure and Function of the Hypothalamico-Hypophyseal System.* Ann Arbor: Edwards Brothers, 1938.
2. Jeffcoate W.J., Ress L.H., Tomlin S., et al.: Metyrapone in long-term management of Cushing's disease. *Br. Med. J.* 2:215, 1977.
3. Krieger D.T., Amorosa L., Linick F.: Cyproheptadine-induced remission of Cushing's disease. *N. Engl. J. Med.* 293:893, 1975.
4. Nussbaum P.B.: Diabetes insipidus, in Conn H.F. (ed): *Current Therapy 1980.* Philadephia: W.B. Saunders Co., 1980, pp 485–488.
5. Randall R.V., Clark E.C., Dodge H.W. Jr., et al.: Polyuria after operation for tumors in the region of the hypophysis and hypothalamus. *J. Clin. Endocrinol. Metab.* 20:1614, 1960.

# Pituitary and Parapituitary Tumors of Childhood and Adolescence

ALAN D. ROGOL, M.D., PH.D.

*Departments of Pediatrics and Pharmacology*
*The University of Virginia School of Medicine*
*Charlottesville, Virginia*

To INTRODUCE THE TOPIC of pituitary and parapituitary tumors in children it is crucial to realize that the growth pattern is a dynamic statement of any individual's development that in turn reflects his or her anterior pituitary function. It is important to know how the child arrived at a particular point on the chart. Thus, the growth chart represents a dynamic pattern rather than a static point. In this first section I shall review the concepts necessary to define growth and development before presenting data on specific tumors and hormonal therapy.

## Growth and Development

There are a number of charts available that represent the statural growth of normal children over the past several decades. Perhaps the most universal are those adapted from the data obtained by the National Center for Health Statistics.* 

Accurately plotted growth parameters are perhaps the most important statements that can be made for each child's statural growth. Each chart has a number of percentile lines to indicate how one child

---

*Monthly Vital Statistics Report, vol 25, no 3, Suppl. (HRA) 76–1120. Health Resources Administration, Rockville, Maryland, June, 1976. Data from the Fels Research Institute, Yellow Springs, Ohio.

0-8151-3530-0/82/0006-0349-0375-$03.75

compares to the mean for the entire population. It should become apparent (see the discussion on growth patterns below) whether the individual child demonstrates normal statural growth, a variant of normal growth, or pathologic growth.

The particular point where an individual is placed at any time may be related to a "height age" that is representative of how an individual child relates to other children in terms of linear growth. The height age is obtained by drawing a line perpendicular to the height axis from the patient's plotted point to the 50th percentile (darkest line) irrespective of whether the plotted point is above or below the 50th percentile line. Most of the patients in whom one is considering a pituitary or parapituitary tumor have a retarded height age compared to chronological age (slow growth), although a few will demonstrate accelerated growth (e.g., childhood acromegaly and gigantism).

The growth charts also contain graphs for plotting weight and, importantly, on the reverse, a chart with percentiles of weight for attained linear stature. This portion may be quite helpful in defining, for instance, hypopituitarism (or growth hormone deficiency), for which most children are relatively overweight for height. For young children an added feature is the head circumference chart, an invaluable aid in defining intracranial pathology and response to therapy in children whose fontanelles have not anatomically fused.

Throughout development the child's body proportions change—one has a relatively long trunk (compared to extremity length) at birth, but becomes relatively long-limbed by the end of puberty. The upper-to-lower-body segment ratio is determined (lower segment: pubis to feet; upper segment: crown to pubis) and compared to that obtained in normal children.[1] At birth this ratio is approximately 1.7:1 and reaches 1:1 by age eight to ten. The body proportions are very sensitive to the effects of thyroid hormone and may be an early clue to pituitary or thyroid dysfunction. Finally, the bone age or dental age may be used to assess developmental status. There have been a number of methods of obtaining this measure (for a discussion see reference 2), but as a screening procedure the method of Greulich and Pyle[3] has proved to be the most practical. A single radiograph of the left hand and wrist is obtained and the epiphyseal developmental maturation compared to that of children (girls and boys separately) of various ages by using an atlas.[3] These data allow one to determine the child's growth pattern and development and should then help to determine which children (usually short ones) should be considered "at risk" for endocrine (pituitary) dysfunction.

The growth patterns of these children and of the rare tall-for-age patient should provide an important and very often first clue to intra-cranial pathology. Four growth patterns for shorter-than-average children may be seen. The first is growth in a channel at, or slightly below, the third percentile with normal growth velocity and the bone age commensurate with the chronological age. This pattern is characteristic of genetic short stature and limited growth potential and implies that there is neither a nutritional, metabolic, nor endocrinologic abnormality that prevents the patient from attaining full growth potential, since maturation will occur at the appropriate chronological age.

The second pattern is growth in a channel, slightly below but parallel to, the third percentile. The growth velocity is within the low normal range, and the bone age approximates the height age rather than the chronological age. In early childhood this pattern is characteristic of constitutional delay of growth. Less commonly, the growth pattern can be significantly below the first percentile and still be compatible with this diagnosis. Minimal normal growth velocity, however, is 5 cm or 2 inches per year from ages three to 12 years. The vast majority of these children will not undergo adolescence at the usual age and are considered to have constitutional delay of adolescence. These patterns imply that the growth potential is adequate, but that ultimate height and sexual maturation will be achieved later than usual. However, it should be kept in mind that the mildly malnourished or mildly systemically ill child may show the same growth pattern, although such children will often be underweight for height.

The third pattern is growth in a channel relatively parallel to, but far below, the third percentile. The growth velocity is at the lowest limits or slightly below the normal range, and the bone age is significantly retarded, more closely approximating the height age rather than the chronological age. This pattern is characteristic of a child with an extreme degree of constitutional delay in growth and adolescence or, commonly, malnutrition and mild systemic illness. However, early mild pituitary insufficiency may present with this growth pattern.

The final growth pattern and the one seen most commonly in congenital or acquired pituitary insufficiency, is growth in a channel that progressively deviates from the third percentile or from a previously recorded growth channel. The growth velocity is abnormally low and the bone age is markedly retarded. This pattern is characteristic of moderate to severe chronic systemic illness or endocrinologic disease. The last pattern does not indicate which endocrine gland is affected, but usually implies thyroid or pituitary dysfunction.

## Pituitary and Parapituitary Tumors in Children

Endocrine dysfunction associated with tumors in the hypothalamic-pituitary region may be manifest by at least three distinct mechanisms. First, the tumor may directly interfere with pituitary function. Second, it may disrupt the normal anatomical relationship of the hypothalamus to the pituitary. Third, the tumor may disturb the hypothalamic nuclei that synthesize the releasing factors or the releasing inhibiting factors for the anterior pituitary, or disturb those that synthesize the posterior pituitary hormones. The tumors that most frequently cause endocrine disturbances in children include craniopharyngioma, glioma (of the optic nerve, optic chiasm, and hypothalamus), hypothalamic hamartoma, pineal tumors, and pituitary adenoma.

### CRANIOPHARYNGIOMA

Craniopharyngiomas are the most common tumors of childhood in the area of the pituitary and hypothalamus and account for nearly 10% of all intracranial tumors of children and adolescents.[4] These most often present in childhood between the ages of six and 14 years, predominantly among boys. The classical triad includes manifestations of increased intracranial pressure, endocrine dysfunction, and visual system disturbance. Headache and vomiting are the most common manifestations of increased intracranial pressure. Decreased growth rate, diabetes insipidus, and delayed sexual maturation constitute the more common endocrine symptoms. The visual system dysfunction may include loss of acuity, field deficits, and papilledema.

The most prominent symptom of increased intracranial pressure in children with closed fontanelles is a throbbing frontal or dull aching headache, especially when awakening. It may occur as often as daily or only several times a year. Vomiting is less often severe and projectile and often is attributed to gastroenteritis or other childhood infection. Most of the endocrine abnormalities are subtle except for the occasional explosive onset of diabetes insipidus. The growth chart (especially growth velocity) may point to intracranial pathology only retrospectively. In the adolescent, delayed pubertal development may be the presenting sign, although in rare instances precocious sexual development can occur with craniopharyngiomas. "Hypothalamic" symptomatology of extreme obesity or emaciation, poor temperature regulation, or somnolence may occasionally be noted at presentation.

Visual disturbance is very common, but many of the younger children do not complain of decreased acuity or diplopia (e.g., VI nerve palsy). The objective findings depend upon the precise location of the tumor and of the anatomic variant of the optic chiasm (e.g., prefixed or postfixed). Symptoms are present in as many as 90% of patients with an asymmetrical bitemporal hemianopsia, the most common visual disturbance.[4] Since the majority of tumors begin above the chiasm, the bitemporal defect often begins in the inferior rather than the superior quadrants. Papilledema may be a prominent ophthalmologic sign of increased intracranial pressure.

Less commonly, craniopharyngiomas may present with signs and symptoms of muscle incoordination and decreased power (monoplegia, hemiplegia) or psychological disorders and decreased level of consciousness.[5] Although an unusual tumor in infants, craniopharyngioma must be considered in this group of children, since it is a congenital tumor arising from squamous remnants in the region of the upper portion of the anterior lobe and the pituitary stalk (remnants of the craniopharyngeal duct).[6]

From the radiologic perspective, childhood craniopharyngiomas are associated with suprasellar or intrasellar calcification, often most easily defined by computerized tomographic (CAT) scan, although it may be noted on skull radiographs and may be accompanied by ventricular dilatation. Several unusual characteristics may allow CAT scanning to differentiate this tumor from others in the same anatomic region. The craniopharyngioma is usually calcified and may contain multiple cystic areas within the tumor mass. Since the fluid often is composed of cholesterol, these cystic areas may appear as low density areas on the CAT scan. Differentiation from pituitary adenomas may be considered if there is little sellar enlargement or if the extension from the sella is posterior and superior rather than anterior and lateral, as is more common for the pituitary adenoma. In addition, craniopharyngiomas are much more prevalent tumors than pituitary adenomas during childhood and adolescence.

Relatively few children have had complete endocrinologic assessment prior to surgery. Most data point to deficiencies in GH and antidiuretic hormone, although there are reports of deficiencies of most of the remaining anterior pituitary hormones.[7] Virtually none of the deficiencies is reversed by surgery and a number of new ones are encountered that require adequate replacement of thyroxine, cortisol, and GH for the patient to grow optimally. It should be pointed out that some children do show an adequate growth response postoperatively, although there are apparently inadequate GH responses to physiologic and pharmacologic stimuli. These patients underscore the complexities of the hormonal regulation of growth and indicate that other substances termed growth factors (e.g., somatomedins) or insulin itself may be able to sustain longitudinal growth for some time in the absence of adequate GH secretion.[8, 9]

*Case report.*—The patient, a white boy four years ten months old, was referred in 1975 for evaluation of polyuria, polydipsia, and an enlarged sella with a suprasellar calcification (Fig 1). No abnormalities were noted until the patient was 12 months of age. Since that time, the parents noted that he drank often and urinated frequently. In the preceding year the patient increased his frequency of drinking to every hour, woke up three times each night to urinate and drink, and seemed clumsier than before. In the preceding three months, he began to complain of intermittent frontal headaches at the end of the day that were relieved by aspirin and rest. The patient had one to two hard stools per week, a pattern present from birth. There were no complaints referable to the visual system, no vomiting and no loss of gross motor or language milestones. Previous growth points were unavailable.

**Fig 1.**—Growth chart of a child with hypothalamic hypothyroidism before and after surgery *(lower arrow)* and administration of hGH *(upper arrow)*. See text for a description of this patient's clinical course.

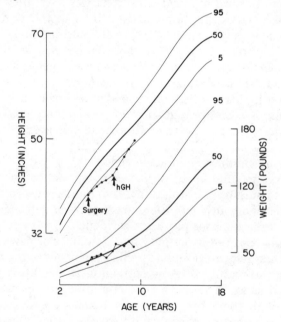

Physical examination was normal except for a height of 100 cm (height age at three and a half years) and a left inferior temporal visual field defect. The bone age was two years four months. Laboratory investigation revealed an abnormal water deprivation test, no GH response, but adequate cortisol response to hypoglycemia, a normal serum thyroxine concentration, and a normal TSH response to thyrotropin-releasing hormone (TRH) stimulation. Arteriography and pneumoencephalography demonstrated a well-localized and calcified suprasellar mass, and the presumptive diagnosis of craniopharyngioma was made. The patient received glucocorticoids prior to and during surgery. The tumor was exposed by a frontal approach and was dissected free from the optic nerve, right carotid artery, hypothalamus, and the infundibulum. The patient's fluid status was initially maintained by volume replacement and then antidiuretic hormone therapy. Postoperatively, the patient was maintained on Pitressin tannate-in-oil and volume replacement. A low serum thyroxine determination was noted and the patient was begun on thyroid replacement as well as 10 mg of cortisone acetate per day.

Upon reevaluation at five years two months, he was noted to be 102 cm tall and to have a normal visual field examination. Laboratory evaluation revealed prepubertal gonadotropin concentrations, a normal TSH response to TRH (the patient had not received thyroid replacement for six weeks), and normal GH responses to arginine and glucagon stimulation. A diagnosis of hypothalamic hypothyroidism was made and the patient was maintained on thyroxine replacement and 10 mg of cortisone acetate per day.

At six years one month of age he was admitted for study of the adrenal axis. Physical examination was unremarkable except for a height of 106 cm. He had not received glucocorticoids for the two months preceding his admission. Following metyrapone, the urinary 17-ketogenic steroids rose from a baseline of 2 mg to 10.7 mg per day.

At seven years four months of age he was evaluated for poor growth (height, 110 cm; growth velocity, 4 cm per year after surgery). Growth hormone levels were less than 1 ng per ml despite stimulation with arginine and insulin or following the onset of deep sleep. The plasma cortisol level responded appropriately to hypoglycemia.

At age seven years ten months the patient was begun on GH, two units intramuscular (IM) three times a week. Since the initiation of GH therapy, the patient has grown 15 cm in one and one half years (growth velocity, 10 cm per year). His present medications include

GH, two units IM three times a week, Desmopressin acetate (dDAVP) 10 μg bid by nasal insufflation, and L-thyroxine, 150 μg per day.

## GLIOMAS OF THE OPTIC NERVES AND OPTIC CHIASM

Gliomas of the optic nerve represent approximately 3% to 4% of all intracranial tumors during childhood. They probably are congenital tumors, since more than 80% of them are found in children less than ten years old and since they present relatively late in their course.[10] At the time the diagnosis is initially made, there may be involvement of the chiasm, one or both of the optic nerves, and adjacent brain tissue. The earliest signs and symptoms are most often referable to the visual apparatus and include two major patterns. The first, the intraorbital optic nerve glioma, presents with intraorbital proptosis, ipsilateral visual loss, papilledema, and strabismus and/or nystagmus. The latter two signs are especially prominent in children who have lost significant vision before age five.[10-12] The second, or intradural, type presents most often with bilateral visual loss (more than 90%), obstructive hydrocephalus, and hypothalamic dysfunction. A significant number (about 35%) of patients with gliomas of the optic nerves or chiasm are sexually precocious or have associated neurofibromatosis.[4] Visual loss occurs in more than 90% of patients, but the visual field deficits are extremely variable and often nonspecific.

Radiographic studies often show enlarged optic foramina and, less commonly, sellar alterations, evidence of increased intracranial pressure, and, rarely, calcification. CAT scans may be the best tool for defining the exact nature and extent of disease, since the optic nerves, chiasm, and sellar and suprasellar regions can be visualized.[13]

In the absence of hypothalamic involvement (see below) dysfunction of the hypothalamic-pituitary axes is uncommon. There are no specific endocrinologic syndromes that uniquely point to the diagnosis of gliomas of the optic nerves or optic chiasm. Therapy for these disorders remains controversial. The tumors are considered by some to be astrocytomas of low grade malignancy,[14] but others believe them to be congenital nonneoplastic and self-limited.[11] The natural history is uncertain and variable.

At present the conservative approach is to plan therapy for each patient based upon the location of the lateral borders of the tumor and whether it extends into the chiasm or shows greater posterior involvement. The therapeutic approaches have included the entire spectrum, from no specific therapy to limited surgical or radiation therapy to radical surgical excision.

## GLIOMAS OF THE HYPOTHALAMUS

Hypothalamic gliomas occur primarily in early infancy and arise from the floor or walls of the third ventricle. They are likely to infiltrate downward to involve the optic chiasm or upward to involve the thalamus. However, it is often difficult to decide whether the process actually began in the hypothalamus or reached those anatomical structures as a direct extension from the optic chiasm (e.g., glioma of the optic chiasm as the primary tumor). The presenting signs and symptoms depend upon the precise location of the tumor in this area, but may include diabetes insipidus, obesity, emaciation, hypogonadotropism, and precocious puberty, in addition to the eye signs referable to involvement of the optic chiasm. Signs and symptoms of increased intracranial pressure may predominate and are caused by occlusion of the foramina of Monro or by a tumor filling the anterior portion of the third ventricle. The most common cell type is a low-grade astrocytoma that causes symptoms by its direct mass effect rather than by metastases. It is often called a juvenile astrocytoma of the hypothalamus and grows slowly, either as a solid mass or with multiple cysts. If it is cystic, the fluid more closely resembles the protein-rich coagulating fluid of malignant tumors than the machinery oil, cholesterol-rich fluid of cystic craniopharyngiomas.

These infants may present with increased intracranial pressure or signs and symptoms related to the visual system, but quite commonly they present with the diencephalic syndrome of extreme emaciation with relatively normal length, vomiting, hyperkinesis, alert appearance, inappropriate euphoria, and pallor without anemia. They lack subcutaneous fat and are distinctly underweight for their length. Their failure to thrive most often begins within the first six months of life. Clues to its etiology may include irritability, optic atrophy, nystagmus (especially rotatory nystagmus), and hydrocephalus. Both the eye signs and the complete syndrome are more likely to occur if the tumor is more anteriorly than posteriorly located within the hypothalamus.[15, 16]

The diencephalic syndrome is almost exclusively seen in infancy. Some believe that it is related to the age of onset of compression of the hypothalamus, since it is not seen in patients with craniopharyngiomas or other tumors within this anatomical area that present later in childhood, despite the fact that such tumors displace the third ventricle in a manner similar to that of opticochiasmatic gliomas.[17] Patients with hypothalamic gliomas are less likely to have neurofibromatosis than those with more anteriorly placed opticochiasmatic gliomas.[18] The cerebrospinal fluid (CSF) protein concentration is often elevated. In patients with the characteristic clinical presentation the differential diagnosis is not complex. However, patients in the same age group with tumors of the posterior fossa and brain stem may also present with failure to thrive and vomiting. Distinction from the diencephalic syndrome is most often made by the accompanying neurologic findings referable to the posterior fossa and the lack of anterior visual system dysfunction.

Some of the newer diagnostic modalities may be quite helpful since CAT scanning allows an excellent definition of the orbits, optic nerves, chiasm, and suprasellar area.[13] A helpful finding even on the plain skull radiograph may be the backward reclining J-shaped sella indicative of flattening of the tuberculum sellae with an increased sellar opening, spreading of the clinoid processes, and atrophy of the dorsum sellae.

The endocrinologic deficits depend upon the precise location of the tumor and may include diabetes insipidus and anterior pituitary failure. In a subset of patients there may be a syndrome of hypersecretion of GH, i.e., the patients may present with large hands, feet, and genitalia. There are high basal GH levels and paradoxical GH responses to hyperglycemia and hypoglycemia. A possible explanation for this phenomenon could be a decrease in GH-release inhibiting factor (somatostatin), as GH-releasing factor secretion (most posteriorly placed neurosecretory cells) continues.

Treatment for these often slow-growing tumors varies from no specific therapy to surgical excision to radiation therapy to a combination of surgery and radiation therapy. Since most series are small and since a variety of tumors and locations is involved, it is not difficult to see why no single modality of therapy is clearly superior.

## HAMARTOMAS OF THE HYPOTHALAMUS

Diencephalic hamartomas are most often located in the interpeduncular fossa and may be contiguous with the median eminence. Since the cellular content resembles that of the small ganglion cells of the tuber cinereum and since these tumors secrete gonadotropin-releasing factor (GnRH), they are often called accessory hypothalami. The hamartomas are thus circumscribed normal hypothalamic tissue found in an abnormal location in or near the posterior hypothalamus. The lesions may be nondestructive or invasive and destructive; in the latter case they cause neurologic signs and symptoms. They occur almost exclusively in boys, often within the first two years of life.[19]

Clinically, the patient is characterized by rapidly progressive pubertal development, markedly increased growth velocity, and extremely advanced skeletal development.[20] The degree of neurodevelopmental impairment is quite variable, but neurologic deficits are often minimal. Physical examination reveals the rapidly progressive pubertal changes that are accompanied by a bilateral testicular enlargement not seen with sexual precocity caused by gonadal steroid-secreting tumors.

## TUMORS OF THE PINEAL REGION

Although tumors in this region have been called dysgerminomas, ectopic pinealomas, and teratoid or atypical teratomas, it may be best to consider them as suprasellar germinomas to emphasize their histologic similarity to the seminoma of the testis or dysgerminoma of the ovary.[6] Tumors in this region may present in three relatively distinct patterns.[21] (1) The mass may reach the pituitary stalk and optic pathways after arising in the pineal region and metastasize anteriorly, giving rise to Parinaud's syndrome, chiasmatic compression, hydrocephalus, and hypopituitarism; (2) the tumor may arise within the anterior portion of the third ventricle and spread to involve the optic nerves, optic chiasm, hypothalamus, and pituitary; ventricular obstruction occurs early, but visual failure, hypopituitarism, and diabetes insipidus are delayed in onset; (3) the tumor is located mainly beneath the cerebral hemispheres in the region of the optic chiasm and may extend into the pituitary fossa. Signs and symptoms of chiasmatic compression and hypopituitarism occur early, but ventricular dilatation is a later phenomenon.

The onset is often at the end of the first and beginning of the second decade of life. It may be rapid and include the classical triad of visual disturbance, diabetes insipidus, and evidence of anterior hypopituitarism, or as noted above, it may be delayed and include signs and symptoms of increased intracranial pressure or vague symptoms of dizziness, lightheadedness, fatigue, weakness, and mild visual disturbance. Upon examination, however, papilledema, impaired light reflex, and accommodation and paralysis of upward gaze (Parinaud's syndrome) are very common.[22]

The differential diagnosis includes most of the preceding tumors, histiocytosis X, and metastatic disease. Helpful diagnostic studies are lumbar puncture, since malignant cells may appear in the CSF, and computerized tomography, with special emphasis on the optic nerves, chiasm, and suprasellar region. These scans are most helpful in children in differentiating this tumor and craniopharyngioma, both of which occur at a similar age. Craniopharyngioma is more likely to be cystic and show the low or negative attenuation constants indicative of cholesterol. The craniopharyngioma is also more likely to be densely calcified. Since tumors in the pineal region are more likely to be associated with precocious sexual development, obtaining a serum or CSF sample for the β-subunit of hCG may be very helpful and have therapeutic implications, since the germinoma-type tumors that secrete hCG are very sensitive to radiation therapy.

As noted for the tumors described previously, a number of therapeutic modalities have been attempted. It is apparent that therapy for each patient should be individualized based upon the exact location of the tumor, its size as well as its type (β-subunit hCG assay; biopsy), before definitive therapy (surgery, radiation, or a combination of both) is attempted.

*Case report.*—The patient, a white girl eight years four months old, presented with persistent headaches for two weeks and an acute decrease in visual acuity (Fig 2). She had been growing at the 90th percentile; her developmental milestones were within normal limits and she had no complaints of polyuria or polydipsia. Maternal and paternal heights were 5'9" and 6'0" respectively. Physical examination revealed a height of 135 cm (height age, nine and one half years), no sight in the right eye, a left temporal hemianopsia, cool extremities, mottled skin, and prepubertal sexual development. The serum prolactin level was 23 ng/ml, FSH was less than 2 mIU/ml, LH was 4 mIU/ml, TSH was 2.7 μU/ml, and 8:00 A.M. cortisol concentration was 5.2 μg/dl. Skull film showed sellar erosion with loss of the posterior clinoid processes. The CAT scan demonstrated a suprasellar mass without calcification. Angiography revealed a 3-cm mass above the anterior clinoid processes. The patient was treated with L-thyroxine and dexamethasone.

At surgery, a solid suprasellar mass was found by means of a bifrontal approach. The mass surrounded the right optic nerve but did not invade it and extended across the optic chiasm to the left optic nerve and into the sella. Removal of the tumor resulted in destruction of the pituitary stalk. The intrasellar extension of the tumor could not be removed and was cauterized.

After surgery the patient developed diabetes insipidus that was treated with fluid replacement and aqueous vasopressin. The ophthalmologic examination returned to normal and the patient was discharged. She received L-thyroxine, 100 μg/day; cortisone acetate, 25 mg/day in divided doses; and Pitressin tannate-in-oil, 2 units IM every other day.

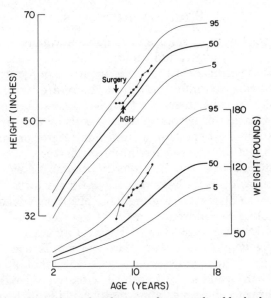

**Fig 2.**—Growth chart of a girl eight years four months old who had a suprasellar mass. At surgery *(upper arrow)* tumor was removed and eight months later she began to receive hGH *(lower arrow)*. For details see text.

The histologic diagnosis of the tumor was uncertain, but a germinoma was considered the most likely diagnosis. Radiation therapy was begun and 5,000 rad were delivered to the sella and pineal regions over a five-week period.

At 8 eight years eight months of age the patient was mildly obese, but had not grown since surgery. Cortisone acetate was decreased to 20 mg/day and she continued to require antidiuretic hormone replacement. At nine years of age, she still had not grown. Neither arginine nor insulin-induced hypoglycemia raised the serum growth hormone level above 1 ng/ml. Serum FSH and LH levels after gonadotropin-releasing hormone (GnRH) did not rise above 4 mIU/ml. TRH administration (200 μg IV) failed to raise the TSH level above 2.1 μU/ml or the prolactin level above 5.5 ng/ml. In addition to ADH deficiency, growth hormone and TSH deficiencies were documented. Deficiencies of ACTH and gonadotropins were presumed. Human growth hormone (hGH), 2 units IM three times a week, was added to the patient's medications. Having received hGH for the past 34 months, the patient has grown 10 cm per year and has shown no evidence of residual or recurrent tumor. Her present daily replacement medications include: dDAVP, 5 to 10 μg per nasum; hydrocortisone, 20 mg; L-thyroxine, 100 μg; and hGH, 2 units IM three times a week.

## PITUITARY ADENOMAS

Pituitary adenomas in children are quite uncommon, representing less than 1% of all intracranial tumors. Since the hypothalamus controls the rate of secretion of the anterior pituitary hormones through releasing and release-inhibiting factors, there are two possible etiologies for pituitary adenomas. First, these tumors may arise de novo from transformation of normal pituitary cells or may arise from excessive secretion of a hypothalamic releasing factor or inadequate secretion of a hypothalamic release-inhibiting factor.

The pathophysiology, symptomatology, diagnostic evaluation, and therapy for these diseases have recently been reviewed.[23] In this section I shall try to review the highlights of pituitary adenomas as they specifically relate to children.

GIGANTISM AND ACROMEGALY.—GH-secreting tumors are very uncommon before epiphyseal closure. The major difference between the disease in children and adolescents as opposed to that of adults is that excessive growth occurs usually with the crossing of height percentile lines on the growth chart, i.e., abnormally rapid growth velocity. This factor along with a family history will help to differentiate the growth pattern from constitutional tall stature. In addition to the excessive growth velocity, there may be signs and symptoms of the tumor itself, e.g., headache, visual disturbance, and increased sellar volume as well as those referable to the excessive hormonal secretion—acral enlargement, excessive sweating, soft tissue overgrowth, and visceromegaly.[24] Laboratory diagnosis can be made by noting increased concentrations of GH and/or somatomedin C in the blood, by excessive variability in GH concentration during the day, by a paradoxical increment in GH concentration following a glucose load or a paradoxical decrement following a dopaminergic agent, or by a rise in GH concentration after administration of TRH or, more rarely, GnRH.

The differential diagnosis is often not difficult. Constitutional tall stature, cerebral gigantism (Soto's syndrome),[25] Marfan's syndrome, and multiple endocrine neoplasia, type 1, should be considered.[26] The therapeutic considerations are similar to those in the adult, except that preservation of gonadotropin secretion may be more critical than in patients who are beyond their reproductive years. Surgery by the transsphenoidal route may be optimal if a small adenoma can be removed. The other modalities—conventional and heavy particle radiation therapy and medical therapy with dopamine agonists—are reviewed in greater detail elsewhere in this symposium.

*Case report.*—The patient, a girl four years one month old, presented with vaginal bleeding (Fig 3). She was the 2.2-kg product of a normal full-term pregnancy. No physical, social, or developmental abnormalities were noted in her first four years of life. Physical examination revealed a height of 110 cm (height age, five years four months), a weight of 20 kg, 3 cm of breast tissue bilaterally, evidence of estrogenization of the vaginal mucosa, and a large café-au-lait spot that covered parts of the anterior and posterior thoracic wall and the lateral aspect of the left neck. Rectal examination was normal and the uterus was judged to be prepubertal in size. Her bone age was four years two months. X-rays of her femur, humerus, hand, fibula, and skull revealed multiple lesions of polyostotic fibrous dysplasia. Her serum FSH and LH concentrations were less than 1 mIU/ml. The diagnosis of McCune-Albright syndrome was made and the patient was begun on medroxyprogesterone (MPA); at first she was given 5 mg per day and then increased to 10 mg per day to stop menses. At age five years six months, while she was receiving MPA, her plasma estrone level was 200 pg/ml and her plasma estradiol level was 50 pg/ml.

**Fig 3.**—Growth chart of a girl with gigantism and acromegaly. At age seven years four months *(arrow)* she began to receive bromocriptine. For details see text.

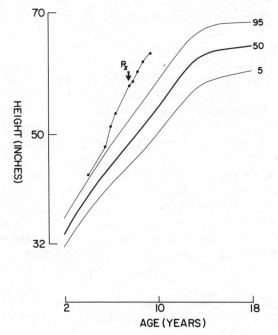

At six years of age, the patient was noted to have accelerated growth velocity, rotatory nystagmus, galactorrhea, an enlarged thyroid, and thoracic scoliosis. Her height was 132 cm (an increase of 7.5 cm in the past six months). Serum prolactin concentration was 200 ng/ml. In the next four months, the patient grew 3.5 cm. A lateral skull film revealed no abnormalities of the floor of the sella, but a thickening of the supraorbital rim, base of the skull, mandible, and obliteration of the ethmoid and sphenoid sinuses were noted. GH values ranged from 10 to 30 ng/ml. There was no suppression of the elevated GH values by hyperglycemia. Serum prolactin levels ranged from 100 to 150 ng/ml. The prolactin level did not change following TRH administration. GnRH stimulation test (100 µg IV bolus) resulted in prepubertal FSH and LH responses. Over the next three years, the patient underwent four LHRH tests. One of these tests resulted in prepubertal FSH and LH responses, the other three in pubertal FSH and LH responses. Serum TSH level failed to rise after TRH administration. The T4 concentration was 9.1 µg/ml at the time of the TRH test. Radioactive uptake at six and at 24 hours were normal both prior to and after the administration of 30 days of 200 µg of L-thyroxine. Thyroid antibodies, long-acting thyroid stimulator (LATS), and LATS protector assays were negative. All subsequent serum T4 levels were normal.

At seven years four months of age, the patient was evaluated prior to bromocriptine therapy, since transsphenoidal hypophysectomy would have been difficult due to the skull changes. She was 144 cm tall (growth velocity, 8.75 cm per year). Her bone age was ten. No abnormalities of the sellar area were noted on pneumoencephalography. Serum growth hormone ranged from 7.5 to 16.9 ng/ml and did not change following bromocriptine administration. The prolactin concentrations did not fully suppress after bromocriptine. The patient was discharged and received bromocriptine, 10 mg per day, and MPA, 10 mg per day.

At eight years eight months of age, she was 156 cm tall (growth velocity, 8.5 cm per year). Her facial features had become more coarse with prominence of the left orbit. Bone age was 11 years. Multiple GH concentrations were elevated, but prolactin levels were fully suppressed by bromocriptine therapy. To suppress the GH concentrations bromocriptine therapy was increased to 20 mg per day.

At nine years four months of age she had not resumed menses despite eight months without progestational therapy. The patient's height was 160 cm (growth velocity, 6.25 cm per year). On physical examination the left ocular ridge remained prominent. On sexual examination her breasts were Tanner stage IV, and her pubic hair, Tanner stage III. She had a normal pelvic examination, and no decrease in thoracic scoliosis. Her bone age was 13 years six months. Skull film showed a normal sella but progression was noted of the hyperostotic process. GH values during the course of the day ranged from 7.7 ng/ml to 40.6 ng/ml. The patient underwent a laparoscopic examination that revealed dormant ovaries with two small paraovarian cysts adjacent to the left ovary. At present, she is receiving 20 mg of bromocriptine per day.

CUSHING'S DISEASE.—Cushing's disease results from excessive ACTH secretion by the pituitary and leads to bilateral adrenal hyperplasia and excessive cortisol secretion. It is relatively rare in children, but one of the first manifestations of hypercortisolism is growth failure. The disease may be so mild that the presenting complaint is growth failure or, when plotted on a growth chart, abnormally slow growth velocity.[27] In addition to growth failure, there is cutaneous atrophy with the formation of striae, central obesity, easy bruising, facial plethora, proximal myopathy and glucose intolerance (but rarely is there frank diabetes mellitus). Occasionally psychologic symptoms may predominate and range from depression to overt psychosis.

The laboratory diagnostic scheme to differentiate Cushing's disease from other causes of Cushing's syndrome is similar to that of the adult and is discussed in detail elsewhere in this symposium. The therapy in children may differ slightly from that in adults. Transsphenoidal hypophysectomy is preferred if an adenoma is found on neuroradiologic investigation, and in some patients even if an adenoma cannot be anatomically defined.[28, 29] Radiation therapy to the pituitary fossa is apparently more efficacious than in adult subjects. Jennings et al.[30] have noted that 12 of 15 children were "cured" by conventional radiation therapy as defined by normal growth and sexual development and normal cortisol levels. Bilateral adrenalectomy certainly is successful in curing Cushing's disease, but may be followed by Nelson's syndrome (sellar expansion and hyperpigmentation) in 25% of children[31]; in addition, lifelong complete adrenocortical replacement, including mineralocorticoids is necessary.

*Case report.*—The patient is an 11-year-old white girl referred for evaluation of obesity (Fig 4). Her early growth pattern was along the 50th percentile for stature and the 75th percentile for weight. Her motor and intellectual development was considered within normal limits, her school performance in the A range. At age eight she began to gain weight excessively as her rate of statural growth declined (see

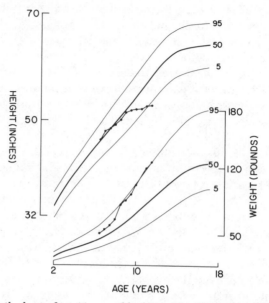

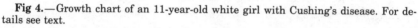

**Fig 4.**—Growth chart of an 11-year-old white girl with Cushing's disease. For details see text.

Fig 4) and she became grossly overweight for her attained length. Thelarche began approximately two years prior to referral. Although she subsequently developed pubic and axillary hair, she had not begun to menstruate.

On physical examination she was obese with rounded facies. Her blood pressure was 116/68. Except for her obesity, bilateral, striae on the flanks and excessive fat tissue over the posterior neck, the physical examination was within normal limits. Sexual development had reached Tanner stage II to III for breasts and stage III for pubic hair. Her clitoris was of normal size.

Laboratory examination revealed a hematocrit level of 49% and normal electrolyte concentrations and liver function tests. Her morning and afternoon cortisol concentrations were elevated (38 and 33 mg/dl), as were her urinary free cortisol and 17-ketogenic steroid values. Although tomography of the sella turcica showed a small focal area of thinning of the lamina dura, CAT scan of the head after the administration of contrast material showed no intrasellar or suprasellar mass. Serum cortisol remained elevated following dexamethasone (20 µg/kg), although the baseline plasma ACTH concentration was within the normal range except on a single occasion.

She underwent transsphenoidal microsurgery where necrotic soft tissue was removed by aspiration. The cavity was packed with alcohol impregnated gelfoam. Postoperatively she has required continued hydrocortisone replacement therapy, since her baseline cortisol values are consistently in the 1 μg per dl range.

HYPERPROLACTINEMIA.—Hyperprolactinemia due to a pituitary adenoma is very rarely diagnosed in childhood, but may occur during adolescence. Its presentation is similar to the very common syndromes in women, but may also present with delayed or arrested puberty in males or primary or secondary amenorrhea in females. As noted for adults, galactorrhea may occur in both sexes, but is not a particularly discriminating sign for hyperprolactinemia.

Diagnostic evaluation and the controversy concerning therapy do not differ from those concerning the adult and are discussed in greater data elsewhere in this symposium.

THYROTROPIN AND GONADOTROPIN-SECRETING TUMORS.—These uncommon tumors are extremely rare in children and do not differ from tumors of the few adult patients previously noted.[32] However, precocious puberty may develop in children with intracranial tumors either from the early activation of the hypothalamic-pituitary-gonadal axis or by the secretion of chorionic gonadotropin (hCG), which stimulates gonadal steroid secretion.

## DIFFERENTIAL DIAGNOSIS

The differential diagnosis among the intracranial tumors in children may be difficult to make; however, there are some features of specific tumors that may aid in exact diagnosis. Many of the neoplasms mentioned above have peak incidences in relatively narrow age ranges. The diencephalic syndrome and tuber cinereum hamartomas occur almost exclusively in patients less than two years old, and craniopharyngiomas most often first present in children older than six. Some tumors are apparently sex selective such that neoplasms of the pineal region and tuber cinereum hamartomas are found more commonly in boys.

Some intracranial neoplasms occur with very prominent endocrinologic or metabolic features, e.g., the diencephalic syndrome and precocious sexual development. Others may be discovered because of ophthalmologic or neurologic signs and symptoms, for example gliomas of the optic nerves or optic chiasm. Some tumors may present with endocrinologic deficits—the poor growth and delayed sexual development with craniopharyngiomas. On the other hand, a rare tumor will be discovered by pituitary hyperfunction—pituitary adenoma and gigantism.

In addition to the tumor neoplasms noted above, a number of non-neoplastic conditions must be considered, including benign intracranial hypertension (pseudotumor cerebri), chronic subdural hematoma, nontumorous hydrocephalus, intracerebral hematoma, brain abscess, cysts, and miscellaneous masses. However, many of these can be dismissed by using the historical data, physical examination, growth data, and neurodiagnostic tests, especially CAT scanning.[13, 33] Benign intracranial hypertension usually presents without focal neurologic findings. A history of otitis media, glucocorticoid withdrawal, or hypervitaminosis A may be helpful, as is the setting of a very obese, iron-deficient adolescent young woman.

Chronic subdural hematomas occasionally may be confused with intracranial tumors. A history of meningitis, trauma, or blood coagulation defect is often helpful. Focal neurologic signs and seizures may point to the correct diagnosis. The CAT scan is often diagnostic of subdural fluid collections.

Similarly, the presenting signs and symptoms of nontumorous hydrocephalus associated with congenital malformations, meningitis, encephalitis, aqueductal stenosis, or subarachnoid hemorrhage may be confusing, but the history, spinal fluid analysis, and computed tomography of the head may point to a correct diagnosis. Space-occupying, nonneoplastic lesions such as intracerebral abscesses or hematomas and cystic lesions may present in a manner identical to intracranial neoplasms, but the patient's history and neuroradiologic examination often lead to a correct diagnosis.

A number of granulomatous and neoplastic diseases of the hypothalamus can present in children with endocrinologic deficits, for example, poor growth, delayed sexual maturation, and diabetes insipidus without or with only a few neurologic signs or symptoms. The outstanding example is histiocytosis X, although very rarely tuberculosis, sarcoidosis, and metastic lesions can cause the disordered pituitary function.

Finally, idiopathic hypopituitarism must be considered; here, however, neurologic deficits are distinctly uncommon, except when the hypothalamic dysfunction is part of a more complex syndrome, e.g., septo-optic dysplasia[34] or other defined syndromes.[35]

## ENDOCRINOLOGIC ASSESSMENT AND THERAPY

The preneurologic and postneurologic therapy (surgery and radiation therapy) assessment in children differs little from that for adults and is discussed in greater detail in other chapters of this book. It would perhaps be prudent to emphasize some of those areas that are more relevant to the pediatric patient.

GROWTH HORMONE.—Linear growth is critically dependent upon hypothalamic and anterior pituitary function, so that evaluation of GH secretory dynamics may be more relevant to the child or adolescent than to the adult. The growth chart and especially the recent growth velocity may be the first clue to insufficiency of anterior pituitary function; if the growth velocity falls within the normal range, it is likely that anterior pituitary function is adequate. Several physiologic factors, including sleep and exercise, are important to the release of GH, and obtaining blood samples after sleep or exercise for concentrations of GH can define the status of GH function. These "screening" tests may be negative in some normal children as well; therefore, pharmacologic testing with arginine monohydrochloride and/or insulin-induced hypoglycemia, both strong stimuli to GH release, is indicated in those patients with inadequate GH responses to the physiologic stimuli. Lack of adequate growth and inadequate GH reserve in the presence of adequate adrenocortical and thyroid hormone function indicate a need for GH replacement therapy. GH is available from the National Pituitary Agency for those patients who are documented to have insufficient reserve or secretion, especially if they are prone to hypoglycemia. At present, patients must be entered into a research protocol (mainly at major medical centers) to be eligible for free hormone. The usual dose is 1 to 2 international units three times a week. GH is now available commercially though at great cost. Recent technological developments employing recombinant DNA technology will, however, rapidly decrease this cost. As noted above, one must adequately restore thyroid (and adrenal) function before valid testing for GH sufficiency can be accomplished.

THYROID STIMULATING HORMONE.—Since an undetectable TSH concentration (in most assays) cannot distinguish between normal and inadequate TSH reserve and secretion, it is necessary to use tests of TSH concentration and hormonal binding (e.g., the serum $T_4$ by radioimmunoassay and the $T_3$ resin uptake test) to adequately evaluate TSH status. It should be remembered that adequacy of adrenal function (or replacement therapy) should be assured before treating potentially hypopituitary (inadequate ACTH reserve) individuals with TSH. TSH may be adequately replaced using 2.5 to 5 µg/kg/day in children more than three years old and up to 10 µg/kg/day in younger children.[36, 37]

ADRENOCORTICAL HORMONES.—Adrenocortical hormonal status reflects adequacy of pituitary ACTH function, since ACTH determinations are not readily available. The normal diurnal pattern of cortisol (high in the morning, lower in the evening) reflects adequacy of baseline ACTH function, but does not guarantee adequate ACTH reserve for stressful situations. Since the site of glucocorticoid insufficiency is either the pituitary or hypothalamus, the cortisol response to insulin-induced hypoglycemia or the urinary or plasma steroid response to metyropone should be tested. Replacement therapy in children is most easily accomplished with hydrocortisone, since small dosage changes can be more readily made. It is important to remember that very slight overreplacement of glucocorticoid, just as with very mild Cushing's disease or syndrome, can cause growth retardation.[27] Therefore, the patient walks the tightrope between underreplacement and adrenocortical insufficiency on the one hand and overreplacement with growth retardation and other signs and symptoms of Cushing's syndrome on the other. The oral replacement dosage is approximately 20 to 25 mg/per sq m of body surface/day of hydrocortisone with a wide individual variation.[38] Usually two thirds of the dose is given in the morning and one third in the evening to mimic the normal diurnal variation of ACTH and cortisol secretion. During stressful situations (e.g., fever, accidents, and surgery) the quantity of glucocorticoid replacement must be increased twofold to fivefold and administered intramuscularly or intravenously, if oral medication cannot be tolerated. In older patients more potent glucocorticoids (e.g., prednisone and prednisolone) may be given in doses equivalent to those for hydrocortisone.

Patients recovering from transsphenoidal surgery for Cushing's disease often present several therapeutic dilemmas. First, they often show signs and symptoms of adrenocortical insufficiency despite seemingly adequate amounts of glucocorticoid replacement. Apparently, their tissues have become accustomed to rather large cortisol concentrations and it takes time to acclimate to "normal" glucocorticoid levels. Second, the hypothalamic pituitary axis remains suppressed for long periods (up to one year, but three months is more usual). The basal cortisol level returns to normal before the response to stress is adequate. Therefore, a rational plan is to gradually taper the dose of glucocorticoid until it is less than physiologic replacement and await the return of normal baseline function, which is indicated by a morning (8 A.M.) cortisol level of more than 10 μg/dl. Once this has been achieved the glucocorticoid replacement may be discontinued except for stressful situations. Pituitary ACTH secretion returns before the adrenal response to it; therefore glucocorticoid and not ACTH should be given for stressful situations. Adequacy of adrenal response can be tested after return of baseline function by measuring plasma cortisol concentrations before and after the administration of synthetic ACTH.[39]

It is especially important that patients who are at risk of adrenal insufficiency wear a Medic Alert necklace or bracelet.

GONADAL STEROID HORMONES.—The gonadotropic hormones are usually not replaced directly, but patients are treated with gonadal steroid analogues. Although the interpretation of the results of testing the hypothalamic-pituitary axis for gonadotropin function can be difficult, those patients who have not undergone spontaneous puberty at an appropriate time should receive gonadal steroid replacement. Prepubertal gonadotropin concentrations with prepubertal gonadal steroid values in an adolescent with hypothalamic pituitary dysfunction probably are indicative of the need for therapy. For young men, monthly (every three to five weeks) injections of long-acting testosterone esters, beginning with 50 mg and reaching 150 to 200 mg per month in one to two years, should be adequate for the initiation and maintenance of male secondary sexual characteristics. Testicular size will not increase unless chorionic gonadotropin is also administered. Oral and buccal therapy is also available and doses of these agents should be gradually raised as puberty progresses until full adult male dose levels are attained (e.g., 2 to 10 mg fluoxymesterone per day or 5 to 20 mg testosterone propionate buccal tablets per day). The 17-methylated derivatives of testosterone are associated with an increased incidence of cholestatic jaundice, and if they are used, this untoward effect must be recognized and liver function tests followed periodically.

For women the development of secondary sexual characteristics and monthly withdrawal bleeding can be accomplished with estrogen and progesterone therapy. Multiple varieties of birth control pills are available, as are conjugated estrogens and progestational agents. One should prescribe the smallest amount of estrogen compatible with the development and maintenance of secondary sexual characteristics (often in the range of 20 to 30 µg/day of ethinylestradiol or 0.625 mg/day of conjugated estrogens). Monthly shedding of the endometrium is important to prevent endometrial hyperplasia, so a progestational agent (e.g., medroxyprogesterone acetate 5 to 10 mg/day) should be given. A usual schedule is to give the estrogen for 25 days of each month and combine it with the progestational agent for days 21 to 25. After menses the regimen may be restarted.

ANTIDIURETIC HORMONE.—Posterior pituitary dysfunction may be diagnosed by failure to concentrate the urine in the face of plasma

TABLE 1.—REPLACEMENT THERAPY FOR PITUTARY HORMONAL DEFICITS*

| HORMONE | SIGNS AND/OR LABORATORY FINDINGS | PHARMACOLOGIC AGENT AND DOSE |
|---|---|---|
| Growth hormone | Short stature; poor growth velocity, lack of GH rise to physiologic and pharmacologic stimuli | hGH 1–2 units intramuscularly three times a week |
| Thyroid-stimulating hormone | Short stature; poor growth, clinical hypothyroidism; low serum TSH, thyroxine ($T_4$), and tri-iodothyronine ($T_3$) concentrations | L-thyroxine 2.5 to 5 µg/kg/day orally, ages 3 to 12; may need up to 10 µg/kg/day in younger children |
| Adrenocorticotropic hormone | Anorexia, hypotension, dehydration, weight loss; low plasma ACTH and cortisol concentrations, inadequate response to stress and pharmacologic stimuli | Hydrocortisone 20 to 25 mg/day orally or its equivalent with the more potent glucocorticoids |
| Luteinizing hormone, follicle-stimulating hormone | Lack of pubertal progression; partial regression of secondary sexual characteristics; eunuchoid habitus; low serum concentrations of LH, FSH, estradiol, and testosterone | Men: Testosterone heptanoate 100–200 mg intramuscularly every 3–5 weeks; fluoxymesterone 2–10 mg per day orally. Women: Ethinyl estradiol 20–50 µg per day orally, days 1 to 25; or conjugated estrogens, 0.3 to 1.2 mg per day orally, days 1 to 25, plus medroxy progesterone acetate, 5–10 mg per day orally, days 21 to 25 |
| Antidiuretic hormone | Polyuria, polydipsia; elevated serum and low urinary osmolarity; low serum ADH concentration | dDAVP 5 to 20 µg/day intranasally, Pitressin tannate-in oil 5 units intramuscularly every 36 to 48 hrs, lysine vasopressin nasal spray 4 to 6 times a day |

*Adapted from Costin G.: Endocrine disorders associated with tumors of the pituitary and hypothalamus. *Pediatr. Clin. N. Am.* 26:15, 1979.

hypertonicity. The increased urinary volume and plasma tonicity should respond to vasopressin or its analogues. Although aqueous vasopressin spray and pitressin tannate-in-oil are available, it is apparent that a synthetic analogue, dDAVP, is preferred. Five to 10 μg are administered intranasally through a rhynyle that accompanies the drug. The exact amount and duration for each dose should be determined individually (this is often done at home by the patient, who monitors the urine volume). After stabilization patients usually receive the drug once or twice a day and should be able to sleep through the night without having to arise to urinate.

These general drug dose recommendations have been summarized in Table 1.

## Acknowledgments

The author thanks Dr. Larry Dolan for preparing the case reports and Dr. Robert P. Schwartz of Charlotte, North Carolina, for permission to include information about one of his patients in this chapter. Mrs. Barbara Helton expertly prepared the manuscript.

Research for this chapter was supported in part by Research Career Development Award 5 K04-AM00153 from the National Institute of Arthritis, Metabolism and Digestive Diseases.

### REFERENCES

1. Wilkins L.: *The Diagnosis and Treatment of Endocrine Disorders in Childhood and Adolescence.* Springfield, Ill.: Charles C Thomas, Publisher, 1965.
2. Roche A.F., Warner H., Thissen D.: The RWT method for the prediction of adult stature. *Pediatrics* 56:1026, 1975.
3. Greulich W.W., Pyle S.I.: *Radiographic Atlas of Skeletal Development of the Hand-Wrist,* ed 2. Stanford, Calif.: Stanford University Press, 1959.
4. Post K.D., Kasdon D.L.: Sellar and parasellar lesions mimicking adenoma, in Post K.D., et al. (eds): *The Pituitary Adenoma.* New York: Plenum Medical Book Co., 1980, pp 159–216.
5. Banna M., Hoare R.D., Stanley P., et al.: Craniopharyngioma in children. *J. Pediatr.* 93:781, 1973.
6. Hankinson J., Banna M.: *Pituitary and Parapituitary Tumors.* Philadelphia: W. B. Saunders Co., 1976.
7. Jenkins J.S., Gilbert C.J., Ang V.: Hypothalamic-pituitary function in patients with craniopharyngiomas. *J. Clin. Endocrinol. Metab.* 43:394, 1976.
8. Kenny F.M., Guyda G.J., Wright J.C., et al.: Prolactin and somatomedin in hypopituitary patients with "catch-up" growth following operations for craniopharyngioma. *J. Clin. Endocrinol. Metab.* 36:378, 1973.
9. Costin G., Kogut M.D., Phillips L.S., et al.: Craniopharyngioma: The role of insulin in promoting postoperative growth. *J. Clin. Endocrinol. Metab.* 42:370, 1976.

10. Oxenhandler D.C., Sayers M.P.: The dilemma of childhood optic gliomas. *J. Neurosurg.* 48:34, 1978.
11. Hoyt W.F., Baghdassarian S.A.: Optic glioma of childhood. *Br. J. Ophthalmol.* 53:793, 1969.
12. Dodge H.W. Jr., Love J.G., Craig W.M., et al.: Gliomas of the optic nerve. *Arch. Neurol. Psychol.* 79:607, 1958.
13. Byrd S.E., Harwood-Nash D.C., Fits C.R., et al.: Computed tomography of infraorbital optic nerve gliomas in children. *Radiology* 129:73, 1978.
14. Marshall D.: Glioma of the optic nerve. *Am. J. Ophthalmol.* 37:15, 1954.
15. Burr I.M., Slonim A.E., Danish R.K., et al.: Diencephalic syndrome revisited. *J. Pediatr.* 88:939, 1976.
16. Addy D.P., Hudson F.P.: Diencephalic syndrome of infantile emaciation: Analysis of literature and report of further 3 cases. *Arch. Dis. Child.* 47:338, 1972.
17. De Sousa A.L., Kalsbeck J.E., Mealey J. Jr., et al.: Diencephalic syndrome and its relationship to opticochiasmatic glioma: Review of 12 cases. *Neurosurgery* 4:207, 1979.
18. Roberson C., Till K.: Hypothalamic gliomas in children. *J. Neurol. Neurosurg. Psychiatr.* 37:1047, 1974.
19. Hochman H.I., Judge D.M., Reichlin S.: Precocious puberty and hypothalamic hamartoma. *Pediatrics* 67:236, 1981.
20. Bierich J.R.: Sexual precocity. *Clin. Endocrinol. Metab.* 4:107, 1975.
21. Camins M.B., Mount L.A.: Primary suprasellar atypical teratoma. *Brain* 97:447, 1974.
22. Donat J.F., Okazaki H., Gomez M.R., et al.: Pineal tumors: A 53-year experience. *Arch. Neurol.* 35:736, 1978.
23. Post K.D., Jackson I.M.D., Reichlin S. (eds): *The Pituitary Adenoma.* New York: Plenum Medical Book Co., 1980.
24. Costin G.: Endocrine disorders associated with tumors of the pituitary and hypothalamus. *Pediatr. Clin. N. Am.* 26:15, 1979.
25. Sotos J.F., Cutler E.A., Dodge P.: Cerebral gigantism. *Am. J. Dis. Child.* 131:625, 1977.
26. Baylin S.: The multiple endocrine neoplasia syndromes: Implications for the study of inherited tumors. *Semin. Oncol.* 5:35, 1978.
27. Solomon I.L., Schoen E.J.: Juvenile Cushing's syndrome manifested primarily by growth failure. *Am. J. Dis. Child.* 130:200, 1976.
28. Tyrell J.B., Brooks R.M., Fitzgerald P.A., et al.: Cushing's disease selective transsphenoidal resection of pituitary microadenomas. *N. Engl. J. Med.* 298:754, 1978.
29. Salassa R.M., Laws E.R. Jr., Carpenter P.C., et al.: Transsphenoidal removal of pituitary microadenoma in Cushing's disease. *Mayo Clin. Proc.* 53:24, 1978.
30. Jennings A.S., Liddle G.W., Orth D.N.: Results of treating childhood Cushing's disease with pituitary irradiation. *N. Engl. J. Med.* 297:957, 1977.
31. Hopwood N.J., Kenny F.M.: Incidence of Nelson's syndrome after adrenalectomy for Cushing's disease in childhood. *Am. J. Dis. Child.* 131:1353, 1977.
32. Jackson I.M.D.: Thyrotropin- and gonadotropin-secreting pituitary adenomas, in Post K.D., et al. (eds): *The Pituitary Adenoma.* New York: Plenum Medical Book Co., 1980, pp 141–149.

33. Naidich T.P., Pinto R.S., Krishner M.J., et al.: Evaluation of sellar and parasellar masses by computed tomography. *Radiology* 120:91, 1976.
34. Hoyt W.F., Kaplan S.L, Grumbach M.M., et al.: Septo-optic dysplasia and pituitary dwarfism. *Lancet* 1:893, 1970.
35. Stelling M.W., Goldstein D.E., Johanson A.J. et al.: Hypopituitarism and Dysmorphology in La Cauza C., et al. (eds): *Problems in Pediatric Endocrinology*. London: Academic Press, 1980, pp 101–112.
36. Abbasi V., Aldige C.: Evaluation of sodium L-thyroxine (T$_4$) requirement in replacement therapy of hypothyroidism. *J. Pediatr.* 90:298, 1977.
37. Rezvani I., Di George A.M.: Reassessment of the daily dose of oral thyroxine for replacement therapy in hypothyroid children. *J. Pediatr.* 90:291, 1977.
38. Migeon C.J.: Updating the treatment of congenital adrenal hyperplasia. *J. Pediatr.* 73:805, 1968.
39. Chamberlain P., Meyer W.J. III: Management of pituitary-adrenal suppression secondary to corticosteroid therapy. *Pediatrics* 67:245, 1981.

# Surgical Failure and Tumor Recurrence with Functioning Pituitary Tumor Following the Transsphenoidal Approach

JAMES T. ROBERTSON, M.D.*
AND
JOHN J. DUSSEAU, M.D.†

*Professor and Chairman Department of Neurosurgery
†The University of Tennessee Center for the Health
Sciences, Memphis, Tennessee

TRANSSPHENOIDAL SURGERY of the pituitary gland was introduced by Schlofer in 1907.[1] The technique was modified and used extensively by Cushing and Hirsch.[2-3, 6-8] Within the technical limitations of these earlier years, the procedure was well tolerated. The major problems consisted in failure to remove the entire tumor and infection. The use of the procedure waned, however, as transfrontal craniotomy became more popular. The argument for the transfrontal approach was based on the ability to prevent visual loss and the reduced risk of serious complications, mainly spinal fluid rhinorrhea and infection. Dott learned the procedure from Cushing and continued to use it with enthusiasm. Guiot of France revived our interest in transsphenoidal surgery, and his excellent results led one of his pupils, Jules Hardy, to describe the microsurgical transsphenoidal approach and refine the technique.[4-6] Presently, it is the procedure of choice for the surgical treatment of most tumors of the pituitary gland.

Concomitant with the striking advances in surgical technique were

377

0-8151-3530-0/82/0006-0377-0392-$03.75

the outstanding contributions to endocrinology that led to a better understanding of the clinical syndromes of functioning pituitary tumors and, more importantly, the widespread use of hormonal assays allowing earlier and easier diagnosis of functioning tumors. Striking advances in x-ray diagnosis illustrated by tomography and the widespread use of computerized scanning techniques have served as major complements to clinical diagnosis. These technical achievements have made possible the detection of functioning pituitary tumors in all stages of their evolution, and condemned the previous textbook descriptions of pituitary tumors presenting with grossly enlarged sella turcicas, marked visual impairment and severe endocrine dysfunction as examples of late disease.

Surgical experience has accumulated rapidly during the past fifteen years. Given the recognition that generally the size of the tumor is inversely proportional with the surgical success and the realization of the extremely low mortality and morbidity associated with surgery, endocrinologists have tended to place surgery as the major initial treatment of functioning tumors. Although a superb modality of treatment, surgery is not always curative. In the failed surgical cases, x-ray and medical therapy are definite adjuncts in treatment.

In reviewing surgical experience, it is clear that the stage of a given pituitary tumor correlates with the ultimate result with all forms of therapy. Tumors may be categorized according to neuroradiologic study into four types according to Vezina and Maltais' classification: type 1—a sella of normal shape and size with a limited monolateral bulging of the floor within the sphenoidal cavity; type 2—a slightly enlarged sella with normal outlines; type 3—enlargement of the pituitary fossa with destructive changes strictly localized to a limited portion of the sella floor, and type 4—extensive sella destruction.[40] They may be classified surgically into microadenomas, which are adenomas located entirely within the sella and do not involve more than one half of the sella; macroadenomas, which are still contained in the sella but occupy more than one half of it; and tumors with extension either above or below the sella or growing laterally into the cavernous sinus.[5, 6] In all classifications, the more extensive the tumor the worse the surgical results. On the other hand, surgical decompression of the chiasm and optic nerves has generally led to excellent visual results in most reported transsphenoidal series.

## Rationale for Surgical Treatment

Since it is believed that most pituitary tumors are histologically benign and tend to grow at an unpredictable rate, it is easy to argue that the growth of the tumor, whether it is secreting or not, may otherwise compress and threaten remaining pituitary function, ultimately compress the optic nerves of chiasm, and eventually threaten the life of the patient. Early surgical removal of the tumor is therefore recommended. The case for surgery is strongest with tumors confined to the sella turcica. When successful, surgical therapy is more definitive and much quicker than x-ray or drug therapy. Furthermore, radiotherapy has the drawback of late effects of radiation on the cranial nerves and brain.

The life span of a patient with untreated acromegaly is reduced by approximately 50%.[9, 10] Approximately one half of the patients will die before the age of 50, usually from the ravages of cerebrovascular disease complicated by diabetes mellitus and chronic lung disease. Cushing's disease is much more lethal, leading to death in five years, usually from progressive debility, vascular disease secondary to hypertension and diabetes mellitus.[9, 10] Prolactin-secreting tumors on the other hand are generally not life-threatening. In most cases, female patients have amenorrhea and galactorrhea, and male patients, impotence, gynecomastia and galactorrhea. These tumors can be surgically excised with acceptable results, but available medical therapy, mainly with bromocriptine, is gaining popularity.[9, 10]

Regardless of the tumor type, surgical therapy continues to deserve priority consideration in the treatment regimen; however, since it is not always curative, other forms of therapy must also be considered. Simultaneously, criteria must be delineated for patient selection for surgery or other means. Combination regimens have naturally evolved.

One way to evaluate the role of surgery is to consider surgical failures and tumor recurrences with functioning pituitary tumors. A case is defined surgical failure when the patient with a hypersecreting pituitary tumor continues to have hypersecretion after an attempt at tumor removal. A tumor recurrence is diagnosed when the hormone hypersecretion, discontinued after surgery for a variable period, is resumed later, and active tumor tissue is proved to be responsible for it.

## Prolactin-Secreting Pituitary Tumors

For the purpose of this discussion, cure, tumor recurrence or failure will be considered only in terms of the serum prolactin level. If the prolactin level becomes normal after surgical or medical treatment, a cure is declared. If the level does not become normal, a surgical failure is declared. If the level becomes normal and subsequently returns to high values, a tumor recurrence is declared. Four hundred and forty-two cases have been collected from 29 publications reporting from 1 to 68 patients.[11-39] The number of patients undergoing transsphenoidal surgery with resulting normal serum prolactin level was 292 (66%). The number of patients in whom surgery brought about a decrease in the prolactin level but not to a normal value was 150 (34%). The number of patients receiving postoperative irradiation for a persistently elevated prolactin level was 29 (6%). Of these, the ultimate result is unknown in 11; 17 had decreasing prolactin levels subsequent to conventional radiation but not to normal; and only one was reported as being cured or having a normal prolactin level (Table 1). Thirty-two patients (7%) received bromocriptine therapy for persistently elevated prolactin levels following transsphenoidal surgery. Thirty (94%) achieved normal levels and were considered cured. Two had slight increase in the prolactin level. Eight (1.8%) patients underwent repeat surgery for persistently elevated prolactin levels following the initial surgery. One was considered cured. Three had a decrease in the prolactin level but not to normal. Two had a negative exploration, and the results from two are unknown. Only one true recurrent tumor was proved by operation. Four were suspected because of an increase in the postoperative prolactin assay. The surgical mortality in this collection of patients was zero. The surgical morbidity consisted of the following: transient diabetes insipidus—34; nasal septal perforation—5; hypopituitarism—2; postoperative sellar hematoma—2; spinal fluid rhinorrhea—2; complicating hydrocephalus—1; and unilateral proptosis—1.

Combination treatments that were emphasized consisted of surgery followed by radiotherapy, followed by bromocriptine administration (which resulted in a cure in two patients); and surgery followed by a repeat operation combined with bromocriptine therapy (which lead to cure in one patient). In general, in patients with the amen-

TABLE 1.—PROLACTIN-SECRETING ADENOMAS
REPORTED IN THE LITERATURE

| | |
|---|---|
| Postoperative normal prolactin level | 292 (66%) |
| Postoperative abnormal prolactin level | 150 (34%) |
| Postoperative radiation therapy | 29 ( 6%) |
| 11 Unknown | |
| 17 Decreased level but not normal prolactin | |
| 1 Cure | |
| Total no. of cases | 442 |

orrhea-galactorrhea syndrome, the duration of amenorrhea as well as the prolactin value were generally indicative of the size of the tumor. The greatly elevated prolactin levels, particularly those above 200 ng/ml, were less likely to achieve a cure. True tumor recurrence, proved by reoperation, appears rare (only one case reported). However, five patients were strongly suspected of having a true recurrent tumor, which is an incidence of only 1.1%.

I have operated on 60 patients with histologically proved tumors who had hyperprolactinemia and the appropriate clinical syndrome; four were male. Six were ages 20 or less; 40 age 30 or less; 11 age 40 or less; and 2 were over 50 years of age. Fifteen of 60 (25%) failed to achieve normal prolactin levels after the initial surgery. In two of 60 prolactin reached normal levels and then increased (recurrences). Seven (11.6%) were ultimately reoperated on. Four of the seven were found to have tumor present (57%). One (14%) developed hypopituitarism after the second surgery, and one (14%) subsequently became pregnant. Reoperation was performed 6–53 months between the first and second surgery. Two had absolutely normal postoperative prolactin levels but only one was found to have a tumor at reoperation. One had a postoperative prolactin level of 22 ng/ml (essentially normal) and at reoperation, a tumor was found. After reoperation, one developed hypopituitarism with a postoperative prolactin level of 1.2 ng/ml. One had a higher postoperative prolactin level but clinically no longer has the amenorrhea-galactorrhea syndrome, and one other had no tumor, but a persistently elevated prolactin level and is presently receiving bromocriptine. Of the remaining four patients who had reoperations, one had a lower prolactin level after the second procedure, a tumor was found, and the patient clinically no longer has the amenorrhea-galactorrhea syndrome. One had a slightly lower prolactin level postoperatively, no tumor was found, and the patient is presently being treated with bromocriptine. One had a perfectly normal postoperative prolactin level, a tumor was found. This patient is now normal and has had a normal pregnancy. One had a normal postoperative prolactin level, a tumor was found, and the patient is normal (Table 2). The ten (16.6%) who had persistent hyperprolactinemia but who were never operated on have been treated with bromocriptine (60%). One subsequently became pregnant and is totally asymptomatic (10%). One was given radiation therapy and the present level of prolactin is unknown, and a follow-up on the last patient has not been possible (Table 3).

The preoperative prolactin levels in the 17 patients in whom initial surgery failed were less than 100 ng/ml in six, less than 200 ng/ml

TABLE 2.—SURGICAL RESULTS IN PATIENTS WITH PROLACTIN-SECRETING TUMORS*

| | 1st SURGERY | | | | | | 2d SURGERY | | | |
| AGE | PREOP. PROLACTIN LEVEL | POSTOP. PROLACTIN LEVEL | COMPLICATIONS | TIME UNTIL 2D SURGERY | PREGNANCY BETWEEN 1ST AND 2D SURGERY | BROMOCRIPTINE | PREOP. PROLACTIN LEVEL | POSTOP. PROLACTIN LEVEL | COMPLICATIONS | NORMAL OR PREGNANCY |
|---|---|---|---|---|---|---|---|---|---|---|
| 29 | 58 | 13 | Diabetes Insipidus | 6 mos | No | No | 19.9 (recurrence) | 1.2 | No tumor | |
| 30 | 93 | 97 | No | 19 mos | No | No | 68.9 | 45 | Hypopituitary Tumor | Normal |
| 30 | 865 | 138 | No | 22 mos | No | Yes | 92 | 71 | No tumor | |
| 25 | 56.4 | 22 | No | 22 mos | No | No | 77 | 94 | Bromocriptine Tumor | Normal |
| 28 | 52 | 29.4 | No | 11 mos | No | No | 105 | 1.1 | Tumor | NL pregnancy |
| 25 | 78 | 5.5 | No | 36 mos | Yes | No | 60 (recurrence) | 87 | No tumor | Normal |
| 20 | 125 | 50 | No | 53 mos | Yes | Yes | 91 | 12 | Bromocriptine Tumor | Normal |

*Five failures and two recurrences.
NOTE: Prolactin levels are given in nanograms per milliliter.

TABLE 3.—RESULTS OF BROMOCRIPTINE THERAPY FOR PERSISTENT HYPERPROLACTINEMIA*

| AGE | PREOP. PROLACTIN LEVEL | POSTOP. PROLACTIN LEVEL | COMPLICATION | PREGNANCY | BROMOCRIPTINE | STATUS |
|---|---|---|---|---|---|---|
| 30 | 159 | 74 | No | No | Yes | On bromocriptine (no symptoms) |
| 36 | 119 | 45 | No | No | Yes | On bromocriptine (galactorrhea-amenorrhea) |
| 21 | 620 | 78 | No | No | No | Unknown |
| 31 | 75 | 30 | No | Yes (abnormal child) | Yes | On bromocriptine (not related to pregnancy) |
| 26 | 400 | 45 | No | No | Yes | On bromocriptine |
| 21 (male) | 128 | 70 | No | No | No | Normal pituitary function (?) Residual tumor TRH stimulation No increase in prolactin |
| 30 | 2,000 | 2,000 | Transient diabetes insipidus | No | No | Diabetes insipidus resolved X-ray therapy |
| 36 | 249 | 34.3 | No | Yes | No | Asymptomatic and pregnant 20 mos postop. |
| 31 | 1,200 | 665 | No | No | Yes | Failed on bromocriptine (8 mos of therapy) |
| 25 | 465 | 76 | No | No | Yes | On bromocriptine |

*Ten failures with no reoperation
NOTE: Prolactin levels are given in nanograms per milliliter.

in four, and greater than 200 ng/ml in seven. Surprisingly, only two of the six with prolactin levels less than 100 ng/ml had normal postoperative levels. However, as suspected, only one of four of those patients whose prolactin was less than 200 ng/ml had a normal postoperative level, and only one of six whose preoperative prolactin level was greater than 200 ng per ml had a normal postoperative level (Table 4).

Of the 43 patients who were cured by the initial surgery, 58% had a prolactin level of 100 or less, 29% had a prolactin level of 200 or less, and only 13% had a prolactin level greater than 200 ng/ml. The complications in this series of 60 patients were diabetes insipidus (transient)—6 (10%); diabetes insipidus (permanent)—6 (10%); postoperative hypopituitarism—1 (1.6%); abducens nerve palsy (transient)—1 (1.6%); and delayed epistaxis—2 (3%).

This series is very similar to the literature review, with 72% of patients achieving normal prolactin levels after the initial surgery. Of those reoperated on, only four were found to have tumor present. The absence of tumor in the remaining three is unexplained. In only one of those found to have a tumor could the tumor be considered a true recurrence. The remaining cases are all surgical failures. On the other hand, of the four found to have tumor present at the second operation, all are clinically without symptoms of amenorrhea and galactorrhea and none has a pituitary deficit. The only patient with true tumor recurrence described in the literature also was normal after the second operation. Therefore, if the patient is reoperated on and a tumor is found and removed the prognosis is good. Hypopituitarism was the complication of reoperation in one of the seven patients. There were no other complications. Reoperation was generally not technically difficult and was well tolerated.

In cases of surgical failure or tumor recurrence, alternative treatment methods must be employed. Bromocriptine, an ergot derivative,

TABLE 4.—PREOPERATIVE
PROLACTIN LEVELS IN PATIENTS
WITH FAILURE/RECURRENCES

| Age | <100 | <200 | >200 |
|---|---|---|---|
| 20 or less | | 1 | |
| 30 or less | 4 | 2 | 5 |
| 40 or less | 2 | 1 | 2 |

NOTE: Prolactin levels are given in nanograms per milliliter.

and dopamine agonist are the best drugs for treatment of prolactin-secreting tumors.[9, 10] Since prolactin-inhibitory factor is probably dopamine, this drug offers a new method for handling these tumors. Prolactin levels can be reduced in all cases and normal levels can be achieved in 80–90% of patients. Pregnancy can occur after the drug is initiated and will be maintained even though the drug is withdrawn. Congenital malformations may occur in the fetuses of patients so treated. Approximately 25% of the pregnant patients in whom drug therapy was discontinued developed enlargement of the sella turcica leading to compromise of the visual axis. It is believed that this drug can reduce the tumor size but as to whether or not it will effect a cure is unknown.

Conventional radiation therapy requires considerable time (1–6 years) to affect tumor growth, and probably cannot effect a cure.

In summary, in cases of surgical failure or tumor recurrence, reoperation, bromocriptine therapy and radiation therapy are adjuncts to be considered. Presently, it is our policy in these cases to initiate bromocriptine therapy for at least six months and not to use radiation. After six months, the drug is stopped and the patient kept under observation. If the symptoms return and the prolactin level begins to rise steadily, reoperation is recommended. With further refinement of resolution, computerized tomographic scanning of the sella turcica will allow detection of tumor thus obviating the need for routine reexploration. I agree with Brodkey that with tumors that are obviously invasive an initial treatment regimen with bromocriptine to shrink the tumor followed by surgery may be the best way to promote a permanent cure.[9, 10]

## Hypersecreting Growth Hormone Tumors (Acromegaly)

The same trend toward surgical success with the smaller tumors can be noted in therapy of acromegaly. Indeed, the large invasive tumors are probably incurable by conventional surgical treatment. Many authors who fail to find a discreet adenoma or who find an invasive tumor or tumor with supra- or infrasellar extension recommend radical surgery followed by radiation therapy. A selected review of 122 cases from the literature reveals normal growth hormone levels eventually achieved postoperatively in 77% of the cases[9, 40–42] (Table 5). Generally, in patients with advanced acromegaly who have cardiovascular disease and diabetes mellitus, surgical risks are less than optimal; however, the immediate mortality of surgery remains

TABLE 5.—SELECTED RESULTS OF
POSTOPERATIVE GROWTH HORMONE LEVELS IN
ACROMEGALY

| AUTHOR | NO. CASES | HUMAN GROWTH HORMONE LEVELS | |
|---|---|---|---|
| | | NORMAL | ABNORMAL |
| Wilson | 25 | 23 | 2 |
| Garcia-Uria | 41 | 31 | 10 |
| Giovanelli | 29 | 17 | 12 |
| Brodkey | 27 | 23 | 4 |
| TOTAL | 122 | 94 (77%) | 28 (23%) |

quite low, and the morbidity is very similar to that described for prolactin-secreting tumors. Reoperation is occasionally reported. Of
seven patients reoperated on for surgical failure, six achieved normal
or satisfactory growth hormone levels and one remained abnormal.
The latter was reoperated on the third time; radical excision of the
sella turcica did not effect any change in the growth hormone levels.
Cases of true tumor recurrence do occur when only the growth hormone levels are considered; for example, Brodkey describes three of
27 patients whose postoperative growth hormone levels were less
than 5 ng/ml but who relapsed at one year and required further therapy.[9, 10]

Conventional radiation therapy (4,500–5,000 rad) given over a five
to six week period will eventually produce a reduction in the growth
hormone levels, but up to five or six years may be required for this
effect to occur. It has been reported that 75% of the patients will
eventually have a growth hormone level reduced to 10 ng/ml and
50% to 5 ng/ml or less. Proton beam therapy delivering 12,000–
15,000 rad to the pituitary produces a more rapid fall in the human
growth hormone level in two years, with 90% having levels of less
than 10 ng/ml at 5 years. However, this modality carries the morbidity of hypopituitarism and cranial nerve injuries. Implantation with
yttrium is not recommended because of the high incidence of necrosis
of the floor of the skull with spinal fluid leak in meningitis. Cryosur-
gery is effective but is best in the tumors confined to the sella and is
no better than transsphenoidal hypophysectomy.

It is clear that surgical failures can be reduced by early diagnosis
and by prompt resection of small tumors. If surgery—the modality of
choice initially—fails, conventional radiation therapy with or without bromocriptine is recommended.

## Cushing's Disease

Cushing's disease is a particularly lethal form of pituitary dysfunction. First described by Harvey Cushing in 1932 and for years treated by adrenalectomy, this is now clearly a disease absolutely within the purview of the neurosurgeon.[9, 43] Wilson has stated that "until a superior form of treatment evolves, microsurgical removal of these remarkably occult adenomas offers the highest probability of restoring normal pituitary function to patients affected with the disease."[43] With the appropriate laboratory testing now available and the increasing education of the lay and medical profession, these tumors are recognized very early with increasing frequency. Advances in endocrinology deserve the highest accolades for making this possible. Accordingly, most of the tumors are microadenomas and, not surprisingly, the sellar x-ray findings are usually normal or nearly so. Adenomas are present in almost 100% of the cases. It is occasionally necessary to perform an anterior hypophysectomy when gross tumor tissue cannot be identified in order to effect a cure. Rare cases are reported where diffuse changes in the gland occur, but the clinician must assume that there is always a pituitary adenoma present and seek its removal. The microadenomas may be difficult to find during surgery because they are frequently very small. However, 90% cures are possible with removal of the microadenoma. The results are quite satisfactory with larger tumors, although surgical failure and/or recurrence is more likely to occur with the larger tumors.

In our small series (12 patients) all were cured by the initial surgery. However, one had a true recurrence one year later and when reoperated, an additional adenoma was found and removed with subsequent surgical cure. The successful results of this surgery are among the most astounding clinical events.

Conventional radiation therapy can cause a remission rate in these tumors of 30% in adults and 80% in children. Radiation therapy does not restore a normal diurnal rhythm in the plasma cortisol or normal responses to dexamethasone suppression tests, but patients so treated rarely develop hypopituitarism or infertility. Radiation therapy has the advantage that about half of the patients will need further treatment to control the hypercortisolism.[9, 10] Proton irradiation is also effective but also takes considerable time to effect a remission, and often these patients are so ill as to make an earlier and more rapid form of treatment as surgery the best choice.

Drug therapy is available to treat Cushing's disease.[9, 10] Cyprohep-tadine, a serotonin antagonist, may be effective in reducing the se-cretion of ACTH and may deserve trial in very ill patients preopera-tively or in the occasional surgical failure. Other drugs, e.g., metyrapone and aminoglutethimide, block the production of cortisol from the adrenal cortex. They have no use in long-term therapy but again might be used initially in very ill patients in order to control the ravages of hypercortisolism temporarily prior to surgery.

Nelson's syndrome occurs in patients who have been treated by adrenalectomy for Cushing's disease in about 10% of the cases.[9, 43] The syndrome can be largely prevented if adrenalectomy is combined with simultaneous radiation therapy to the pituitary gland. The syn-drome is delayed in occurrence and is characterized by hyperpigmen-tation and enlargement of the sella. These tumors are said to be very invasive and are extremely difficult to cure. In Wilson's group of 18 patients with Nelson's syndrome, only two achieved normal postop-erative values of ACTH. He recommends cessation of adrenalectomy for the treatment of Cushing's disease as one way to prevent this syndrome and, in the presence of Nelson's syndrome, a total hypo-physectomy is recommended when the tumor is confined to the sella. The problem occurs when tumor extension is present, which is not uncommon, but then one must rely on radical surgery followed by drug and/or radiation therapy. Our limited experience would support this opinion.

## Summary

Regardless of the controversy surrounding the treatment of certain functioning pituitary tumors, several facts are known. Surgical cures as manifested by normal prolactin levels postoperatively occur after the initial surgery in two thirds of the patients. Of the subsets of the clinical syndromes of hyperprolactinemia, the worst results are achieved in those patients whose prolactin levels are in excess of 200 ng/ml and those whose tumor is invasive. Brodkey has suggested that since bromocriptine reduces the size of prolactin-secreting tu-mors, the surgical results might be improved if pretreatment with bromocriptine is administered to patients who are known to be poor responders to surgery alone. The patients with microadenomas with prolactin levels of less than 100 ng/ml are the best surgical candi-dates.

Surgical and medical publications should clearly differentiate be-tween failure of treatment manifested by persistent abnormal hormone levels regardless of the type of tumor and true recurrence of tumor manifested by normal posttreatment hormone levels followed by delayed reappearance of abnormal levels.

From every report, the stage of the disease manifested by neuro-radiologic changes in the sella turcica or by findings at surgery will clearly influence the result of the treatment. Early diagnosis, therefore, is mandatory as is immediate institution of treatment thereafter. Based on the experience with Cushing's disease, there is every reason to believe that if the prolactin- and growth hormone-secreting tumors were diagnosed and operated early, the surgical results would be far superior to those reported. Indeed, microadenoma surgery results are quite good, with virtually no mortality and a low, acceptable morbidity.

The present role of medical therapy alone has not been proved. Clear criteria for this form of therapy must be developed. For the present it is reasonable to expect that combination therapy will continue to be used. Although effective in the treatment of prolactin-secreting tumors, bromocriptine has not been as successful in the therapy of acromegaly. In one series the reduction of growth hormone values to less than 5 ng/ml was noted in only 25% of the patients. The surgical results in the treatment of Cushing's disease with initial medical therapy in the very ill patients is clearly the method of choice. Diagnosis must not be delayed and adrenalectomy should be abandoned. Long-term radiologic and medical therapy of Cushing's disease is not recommended because of delay and predictable lack of effect.

Although surgery remains the most widely used treatment for most pituitary tumors of the secreting variety, the future of medical treatment is most promising, and more clinical trials, particularly with the invasive tumors, are indicated.

The establishment of a medical registry of patients with pituitary tumors, presently underway by The Pituitary Foundation of America, is an excellent beginning toward the solving of many remaining problems in the treatment of functioning pituitary tumors. This step establishes a pituitary task force to allow initiation of rapid new treatment trials and, through cooperative efforts, delineate targets for intense effort to find a reliable curative treatment for pituitary tumors.

## REFERENCES

1. Johnson H.C.: Surgery of the Hypophysis, in Walker A.E. (ed.): *A History of Neurological Surgery*. Baltimore: Williams and Wilkins Co., 1951, p. 152.

2. Cushing H.: Partial hypophysectomy for acromegaly: with remarks on the function of the hypophysis. *Ann. Surg.* 50:1002, 1909.
3. Cushing H.: Operative experiences with lesions of the pituitary body. *Trans. Am. Surg. Assoc.* 31:467, 1913.
4. Dott W.M., Bailey D.: A consideration of the hypophysial adenomata. *Br. J. Surg.* 13:314, 1925.
5. Guiot G.: *Transsphenoidal approach in surgical treatment of pituitary adenomas: general principles and solutions in non-functioning adenomas.* Excerpta Medicus International Congress Series No. 303, 1973, p. 159.
6. Hardy J.: Transsphenoidal neurosurgery of the normal and pathological pituitary. *Clin. Neurosurg.* 16:185, 1969.
7. Hirsch O. Endonasal method of removal of hypophysial tumors: with report of two successful cases. *J.A.M.A.* 55:772, 1910.
8. Hirsch O.: Life-long cures and improvements after transsphenoidal operation of pituitary tumors. *Acta. Ophthalmol. (suppl.) (KBH)* 56:1, 1959.
9. Brodkey J.S.: Hypersecreting Pituitary Tumors. Part I: *Contemporary Neurosurgery, Issue 18.*
10. Brodkey J.S.: Hypersecreting Pituitary Tumors. Part II: *Contemporary Neurosurgery, Issue 19.*
11. Tolis G: Prolactin: physiology and pathology. *Hosp. Pract.* 15:85, 1980.
12. Serri, O., Somma M., Rasio E., Beauregard H., Hardy J: Prolactin secreting pituitary adenomas in males: Transsphenoidal microsurgical treatment. *Can. Med. Assoc. J.* 122:1007, 1980.
13. Leavens M.E., Samann N.A., Jesse R.H., Byers R.M., Larson D.L.: Prolactin secreting microadenomas in women. *Tex. Med.* 76:51, 1980.
14. Casper R.F., Rakoff J.S., Quigley M.E., Gilliland B., Alksne J., Yen S.S.C.: Changes in pituitary hormones during and following transsphenoidal removal of prolactinomas. *Am. J. Obstet. Gynecol.* 136:518, 1980.
15. Veldhuis J.D., Santen R.J.: Pituitary Pseudotumor. Mimicry of recurrent prolactinoma by a chronic intrasellar hematoma. *Arch. Intern. Med.* 139:1309, 1979.
16. Fayez J.A., Sowers J.R., Blanchard S., Finnie B.Y., Morris T.: Update on the diagnosis and management of prolactin-secreting pituitary adenomas. *Mod. Med.* 76:492, 1979.
17. Barbarino A., de Marinis L., Menini E., Anile C., Maira G.: Prolactin-secreting adenomas: prolactin dynamics before and after transsphenoidal surgery. *Acta. Endocrinol. (Copenh.)* 91:397, 1979.
18. Prosser P.R., Karam J.H., Townsend J.J., Forsham P.H.: Prolactin-secreting pituitary adenomas in multiple endocrine adenomatosis, Type I. *Ann. Intern. Med.* 91:41, 1979.
19. Pont A., Shelton P., Odell W.D., Wilson C.B.: Prolactin-secreting tumors in men: surgical cure. *Ann. Intern. Med.* 91:211, 1979.
20. Levine J.H., Sagel J., Rosebrock G., Gonzalez J.J., Nair R., Rawe S., Powers J.M.: Prolactin-secreting adenoma as part of the multiple endocrine neoplasia - Type I (Men - 1) syndrome. *Cancer* 43:2492, 1979.
21. Favre L., Roberts L.M., Cobb C.A., Rabin D.: Gigantism associated with a pituitary tumor secreting growth hormone and prolactin and cured by transsphenoidal hypophysectomy. *Acta. Endocrinol. (Copenh.)* 91:193, 1979.

22. Keye W.R., Jr., Chang R.J., Monroe S.E., Wilson C.B., Jaffe R.B.: Prolactin-secreting adenomas in women. II. Menstrual function pituitary reserves, and prolactin production following microsurgical removal. *Am. J. Obstet. Gynecol.* 134:360, 1979.
23. Murray F.T., Osterman J., Sulewski J., Page R., Bergland R., Hammond J.M.: Pituitary function following surgery for prolactinomas. *Obstet. Gynecol.* 54:65, 1979.
24. Post K.D., Biller B.J., Adelman L.S., Molitch M.E., Wolpert S.M., Reichlin, S.: Selective transsphenoidal adenomectomy in women with galactorrhea-amenorrhea. *J.A.M.A.* 242:158, 1979.
25. Weibe R.H., Kramer R.S., Hammond C.B.: Surgical treatment of prolactin secreting microadenomas. *Am. J. Obstet. Gynecol.* 134:49, 1979.
26. Cowden E.A., Ratcliffe J.G., Thompson J.A., Macpherson P., Doyle D., Teasdale G.M.: Test of prolactin secretion in the diagnosis of prolactinomas. *Lancet* 8127:1155, 1979.
27. Bergh T., Nillius S.J., Wise L.: Bromocriptine treatment of seven women with primary amenorrhea and prolactin secreting pituitary tumors. *Clin. Endocrinol. (Oxf.)* 10:145, 1979.
28. Swanson J.A., Sherman B.M., VanGilder J.C., Chapler F.K.: Coexistent empty sella and prolactin secreting microadenoma. *Obstet. Gynecol.* 53:258, 1979.
29. Jaquet P., Grisoli F., Guibout M., Lissitzky J.C., Carayon P.: Prolactin-secreting tumors. Endocrine status before and after surgery in 33 women. *J. Clin. Endocrinol. Metab.* 46:459, 1979.
30. Sherman B.M., Harris C.E., Schlechte J., Duello T.M., Halmi N.S., Van Gilder J., Chapler F.K., Granner D.K.: Pathogenesis of prolactin secreting pituitary adenomas. *Lancet* 8098:1019, 1978.
31. Carter J.N., Tyson J.E., Tolis G., Van Vliet S., Faiman C., Friesen H.G.: Prolactin secreting tumors and hypogonadism in 22 men, *N. Engl. J. Med.* 299:847, 1978.
32. Dolman L.I., Roberts T.S., Poulson M. Jr., Tyler F.H.: Infertility in patients with hyperprolactinemia from a pituitary adenoma. Effect of transsphenoidal pituitary adenectomy. *Arch. Intern. Med.* 137:1161, 1978.
33. Tindall G.T., McLanahan C.S., Christy J.H.: Transsphenoidal microsurgery for pituitary tumors associated with prolactinemia. *J. Neurosurg.* 48:849, 1978.
34. Gomez F., Reyes F.I., Faiman C.: Nonpuerperal galactorrhea and hyperprolactinemia. Clinical findings, endocrine features, and therapeutic responses in 56 cases. *Am. J. Med.* 62:648, 1977.
35. Schroffner W.G.: Prolactin secreting pituitary tumor in early adolescence. Hormonal and electron microscopical studies. *Arch. Intern. Med.* 136:1164, 1976.
36. Franks S., Jacobs H.S., Hull M.G.R., Steele, S.J., Nabarro J.D.: Management of hyperprolactinaemic amenorrhoea. *Br. J. Obstet. Gynecol.* 84:241, 1977.
37. Horn K., Erharot F., Fahlbusch R., Pickarot C.R., Werder K.V., Scriba P.C.: Recurrent goiter, hyperthyroidism, galactorrhea, and amenorrhea due to a thyrotropin and prolactin producing pituitary tumor. *J. Clin. Endocrinol. Metab.* 43:137, 1976.

38. Chang R.J., Keye W.R., Young J.R., Wilson C.B., Jaffe R.B.: Detection, evaluation, and treatment of pituitary microadenomas in patients with galactorrhea and amenorrhea. *Am. J. Obstet. Gynecol.* 128:356, 1977.
39. Boyd A.E., III, Reichlin S., Turksoy, N.: Galactorrhea-amenorrhea syndrome: diagnosis and therapy. *Ann. Intern. Med.* 87:165, 1977.
40. Garcia-Uria J., et al.: Functional treatment of acromegaly by transsphenoidal microsurgery. *J. Neurosurg.* 49:36, 1978.
41. Giovanelli M.A., et al: Treatment of acromegaly by transsphenoidal microsurgery. *J. Neurosurg.* 44:677, 1976.
42. Wilson C.B., Dempsey L.C.: Transsphenoidal microsurgical removal of 250 pituitary adenomas. *J. Neurosurg.* 48:13, 1978.
43. Wilson C.G., Tyrrell J.G., Fitzgerald P.: Cushing's Disease Revisited. *Am. J. Surg.* 138:77, 1979.

# Pituitary Tumors: Epidemiology

## J.F. ANNEGERS, Ph.D.

*Associate Professor, Department of Epidemiology, The University of Texas School of Public Health, Houston, Texas*

## CAROLYN B. COULAM, M.D.

*Consultant, Department of Obstetrics and Gynecology, Mayo Clinic, Rochester, Minnesota*

AND

## EDWARD R. LAWS, JR., M.D.

*Consultant, Department of Neurologic Surgery, Mayo Clinic, Rochester, Minnesota*

### Introduction

TWO OF THE MAJOR GOALS OF EPIDEMIOLOGY are to (1) describe the frequencies of disease in human populations and (2) to evaluate potential or suspected risk factors. This chapter will review our knowledge concerning the frequency of occurrence of pituitary tumors and analytic studies of possible etiologic factors.

### DESCRIPTIVE EPIDEMIOLOGY

In order to compare the occurrence of pituitary tumors within or between populations or over time it is necessary to have age and sex specific incidence and/or mortality rates. Much of the information on the occurrence of pituitary tumors comes from neurosurgical series that provide only the proportionate morbidity of patients with intracranial tumors. Table 1 presents five series in which the proportion of

393

0-8151-3530-0/82/0006-0393-0403-$03.75
© 1982, Year Book Medical Publishers, Inc.

TABLE 1.—PITUITARY ADENOMAS
AS A PROPORTION OF ALL
INTRACRANIAL NEOPLASIA

| AUTHORS | NO. | PERCENT |
|---|---|---|
| Cushing (1939) | 395 | 14.0 |
| Oliverome (1952) | 368 | 9.4 |
| Ito (1958) | 49 | 4.8 |
| Zulch (1965) | 478 | 8.9 |
| Pastur (1967) | 67 | 9.3 |

TABLE 2.—PITUITARY ADENOMAS AS A
PROPORTION OF ALL INTRACRANIAL TUMORS

| DATA BASE | NO. | PERCENT |
|---|---|---|
| Washington, D.C., S.M.S.A. | | |
| White | 41 | 5.4 |
| Black | 48 | 22.2 |
| West African Composite Series | 36 | 14.2 |

pituitary tumors among all intracranial tumors ranged from 5% to 14%. Such reports reveal something of a given neurosurgical practice but do not provide the desired incidence rates of pituitary tumors in populations. In addition to providing only numerator data, proportionate morbidity reports obviously reflect the nature of each practice. Nevertheless, proportionate morbidity is sometimes the only information available. Heshmat et al.[1] compared the proportionate morbidity among West African blacks with the proportionate incidence of pituitary tumors among the white and nonwhite populations in the Washington, D.C., area (Table 2).

## Mortality Rates

Mortality rates are of limited value in the descriptive epidemiology of pituitary tumors as deaths are rarely attributed to this condition. In the United States in 1976 there were 237 deaths classified as diseases of the pituitary gland. Of these, 24 were classified as pituitary hyperfunction, 53 as pituitary hypofunction, 54 as chromophobe adenomas, and 106 as other or unspecified. The crude death rate for pituitary adenomas in the United States is about one per million population per year (Table 3). In the white population the death rate of one per million is the same in males and females, the rate is slightly higher in black males and considerably higher among black females (2.0 per million).

TABLE 3.—DISEASE OF THE
PITUITARY GLAND MORTALITY
RATE—UNITED STATES 1976
CRUDE DEATH RATE/1,000,000
POPULATION

| SEX | TOTAL | WHITE | BLACK |
|---|---|---|---|
| Male | 1.1 | 1.0 | 1.2 |
| Female | 1.2 | 1.0 | 2.0 |
| Total | 1.1 | 1.0 | 1.6 |

## INCIDENCE RATES

There are only a few reports of incidence rates of pituitary tumors
because these tumors have generally not been classified separately
in tumor registries. Table 4 shows the very low incidence rates of
pituitary adenomas reported in population studies before 1970. The
Connecticut tumor registry reported an incidence rate of 0.45 per
100,000 population per year from 1935 through 1964.[17] A standard
statistical survey of all intracranial neoplasms in the Washington,
D.C., metropolitan area from 1960 to 1969 reported an incidence in
the white population of only 0.23 per 100,000 per year. The nonwhite
population had considerably higher incidence rates, but still only
1.02 per 100,000 in males and 0.76 in females. The higher incidence
in nonwhites is similar to the mortality data, but nonwhite males
rather than females had the higher incidence rate. The study of the
Rochester, Minnesota, population for the period 1935 through 1968
indicated a higher incidence rate of 1.9 per 100,000 per year. The
difference is presumably due to more complete case ascertainment
because of the availability of medical services and the higher autopsy

TABLE 4.—AGE-ADJUSTED INCIDENCE RATES PER
100,000 POPULATION

| DATA BASE | MALES | FEMALES |
|---|---|---|
| Washington, D.C., S.M.S.A.*<br>1960–1969[1] | | |
| White | 0.23 | 0.22 |
| Nonwhite | 1.02 | 0.76 |
| Connecticut 1935–1964†[17] | 0.43 | 0.46 |
| Rochester, Minnesota<br>1935–1968†[10] | | 1.9 |
| Carlisle, England[2] | | 0.8 |

*Standard metropolitan statistical area.
†Includes craniopharyngiomas.

rate in that population. Five of the 19 cases were incidentally discovered at autopsy and were included in the calculation of the incidence rates. An investigation of neurologic diseases in Carlisle, England, disclosed an incidence rate of 0.8 per 100,000 per year but this rate was based on only four incidence cases.[2]

The age-specific incidence rates of pituitary tumors as reported from the Connecticut tumor registry and a survey of intracranial tumors in the Washington, D.C., area are presented on Figure 1. In the white population the age-specific rates rose slowly with age, reaching approximately 0.5 per 100,000 per year by age 40 and approximately 1 per 100,000 per year in the elderly. Among the nonwhite population of Washington, D.C., the incidence rate rose sharply between 40 and 50 years of age to about 3.0 per 100,000 and remained at that level throughout the remainder of the age range.

The lifetime cumulative incidence is a measurement of the effect of age-specific incidence rates over the lifespan. If the 1935 to 1964 Connecticut age-specific rates were experienced over a lifespan of 75

**Fig 1.**—Age-specific incidence rates of pituitary tumors as reported by the Connecticut tumor registry *(solid line)* and a survey of intracranial tumors in the Washington, D.C., area *(dotted lines).*

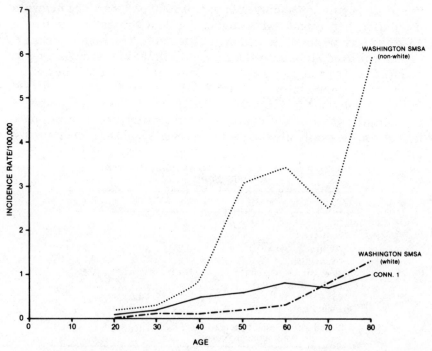

years, the cumulative incidence rate to that age would be 31 per 100,000 or a lifetime risk of 1 in 3,226. Thus, available data on the incidence of pituitary tumors in 1970 showed pituitary tumors to be very rare, occurring mostly in the middle-aged or elderly populations and affecting the sexes equally.

## Prevalence At Autopsy

In contrast to the rarity of the diagnosis of pituitary tumors during life, autopsy studies have long been known to reveal a high prevalence of asymptomatic microadenomas. In 1936 Costello[3] reported that 225 of 1,000 autopsies at the Mayo Clinic revealed pituitary tumors. The prevalence was 22.5% in both sexes, and the ages ranged from two to 86. The age-specific prevalence rates reached 20% by ages 15 to 19 and remained at about that level with increasing age. In 1981 Burrow et al.[4] reported an autopsy series of 120. Pituitary adenomas were found in 27% through the age range of 16 to 86. There was no sex difference and 41% of the tumors had prolactin-containing cells. The authors concluded: "If these results can be generalized, more than one in 10 persons in the general population dies with a prolactinoma." These and other[5, 6] autopsy series show a prevalence of microadenomas at death of 8.5% to 27%. The prevalence reaches this level by adolescence or early adult life and thereafter remains constant. The prevalence at autopsy is similar in both sexes.

### THE RECENT EPIDEMIC OF PITUITARY ADENOMAS

During the late 1970s reports of clinical series[8, 9] and the experience of gynecologists and endocrinologists suggested an increasing frequency of pituitary adenomas in women of childbearing age. However, since no population-based study had come to our attention, we undertook to determine whether, and to what extent, the incidence rates of pituitary adenomas had changed from the previous study. This report contains the results of our earlier study of cases through 1977,[10] and an update of cases in Olmsted County from 1978, 1979, and 1980. The medical index for the population of Olmsted County, Minnesota, was searched for patients with a diagnosis of pituitary tumors from 1935 through 1980. A total of 37 cases symptomatic during the patient's life met the diagnostic and residency criteria. The diagnosis was confirmed by tissue from surgery in 29 and the remainder were accepted as probable cases on radiologic evidence (plain skull films, tomograms, and angiograms). The incidence rates for the periods 1935 to 1969 and 1970 to 1980 are presented in Table 5. Among males the incidence increased with age but did not change after 1970. The rates among females aged 15 and under and those aged 45 and older were similar in the years 1935–1969 and 1970–1980. During the years 1970 through 1980 there was a dramatic increase in the rate among females in the childbearing age group.

The 17 diagnoses made since 1970 among women aged 15 through 44 consisted of 14 confirmed surgically, one based on angiographic evidence and two based on tomograms. The diagnoses in the latter two were uncertain at the time of the earlier study and have not been confirmed. The endocrinologic manifestations of the tumors varied in the 14 patients with histological confirmation. Ten were prolactin-secreting, two had signs of acromegaly, one was considered nonfunctional, and one was the cause of Cushing's disease.

Among the 15 cases that can be considered definite, the onset of symptoms (amenorrhea, galactorrhea, acromegaly, visual disturbance) ranged from five to 24 months prior to diagnosis. In three patients the onset of amenorrhea occurred after the discontinuation of oral contraceptives and in one the onset was postpartum.

If the 1970 to 1980 Olmsted County incidence rates were applied to the 1978 United States population, we would estimate that 5730 pituitary tumors were diagnosed in that year. Two thirds of these would be found in women of childbearing age.

## Risk Factors—Oral Contraceptives

The apparent epidemic of pituitary tumors in women of childbearing age has prompted the suspicion that new etiologic factors in ad-

TABLE 5.—INCIDENCE OF PITUITARY
ADENOMAS IN OLMSTED COUNTY,
MINNESOTA*

| SEX AND AGE | 1935–1969 | | 1970–1980 | |
|---|---|---|---|---|
| | NO. | RATE | NO. | RATE |
| Males | | | | |
| 0–14 | 0 | — | 2 | 1.2 |
| 15–44 | 2 | 0.5 | 1 | 0.5 |
| 45+ | 6 | 2.8 | 2 | 1.8 |
| Females | | | | |
| 0–14 | 0 | — | 0 | — |
| 15–44 | 3 | 0.7 | 17 | 7.4 |
| 45+ | 1 | 0.4 | 3 | 2.2 |

*Mean annual rate per 100,000 persons.

dition to advances in diagnostic and surgical technology may be responsible. The age and sex specificity of the increase makes the oral contraceptive a logical candidate. Oral contraceptives may promote excessive secretion of prolactin, which if uncontrolled would lead to the development of prolactin-secreting adenomas. It has been recognized that the cessation of oral contraceptives results in postpill amenorrhea in at least a small percentage of women.[11] The prevalence of prior use of oral contraceptives by patients with pituitary tumors has been reported by Chang et al.[8] as 84% (21 of 25), Davajan et al.[9] as 70% (59 of 84), Sherman et al.[12] at 70% (30 of 42), and by Hardy et al.[13] at 75% (60 of 80); however, not all case series have reported as high a proportion. Reichlin[14] reported 18 (60%) pill takers in a series of 30 patients, and Thorner and Besser[15] reported a history of oral contraceptive usage in only 7 (10%) of 70 patients. Sherman et al.[12] noted the high prevalence of silent microadenomas as reported in autopsy series and the high frequency of oral contraceptive use reported in most series of patients with pituitary adenomas, and suggested that the inducement of growth of otherwise silent pituitary lesions should be considered a risk of oral contraceptive use. They concluded: "If our estimate of the prevalence of micro-adenomas is correct, the potential for the development of amenorrhea, galactorrhea, infertility, and the complications of pituitary tumor growth may equal or exceed that of other risks attributable to oral contraceptives."

In discussing this issue, Reichlin[14] and Davajan et al.[9] have stated the need for case-control studies to establish the role of prior estrogen use in the pathogenesis of clinically noteworthy prolactinomas. However, to date we are aware of only a small case-control study of patients in Olmsted County, Minnesota.[16]

## Olmsted County Case-Control Study

Our previous case-control study of pituitary adenomas in women of childbearing age from 1970 to 1977 has been updated to include cases diagnosed in 1978, 1979, and 1980. This series now includes a total of 15 patients aged 15 through 44 with a confirmed diagnosis of pituitary adenoma. Fourteen had surgical confirmation and one was diagnosed by angiography and received radiotherapy. The two patients who had been classified as probable on the basis of symptoms and radiologic evidence in the incidence study have not been included in the case-control study.

Each of the 15 patients was matched to four controls to determine whether oral contraceptives or other factors were associated with the development of pituitary adenomas. Controls were obtained from lists of all Mayo Clinic registrations of Olmsted County residents of the same age during the same year in which pituitary adenomas were diagnosed in the patients. These registrations include all women seen by all specialties for any medical contact, including general and preemployment examinations, dental work, blood donors, visits for acute illnesses, house calls, and emergency room visits. The number of potential controls for each case ranged from 400 to 1,000 and includes about 75% of the female population. Thus, the controls approximate a random sample of the nonaffected population from which the cases arose. The controls were then selected by registration number closest to that of the patient since the registration is based on the time of first contact with a Mayo Clinic facility. Thus the controls are also matched on duration of prior medical history. Table 6 presents the age of the first registration and diagnosis of each of the 15 patients. Most of the reproductive periods of the patients and corresponding controls were covered by the Mayo Clinic records. In fact, the duration of medical history is slightly greater, for some of the patients and some controls were seen at other medical facilities that served the Olmsted County population at an earlier date.

The medical records of each patient and control were reviewed for any reference to the prescription or use of oral contraceptives. Infor-

TABLE 6.—PITUITARY ADENOMA
CASES CONFIRMED BY SURGERY
OR ANGIOGRAM, FEMALES 15–44

| FIRST MAYO CLINIC REGISTRATION | | DIAGNOSIS OF PITUITARY ADENOMA | |
|---|---|---|---|
| Age | Year | Age | Year |
| 0 | 1948 | 30 | 1979 |
| 0 | 1954 | 26 | 1980 |
| 0 | 1955 | 25 | 1980 |
| 3/12 | 1957 | 20 | 1977 |
| 10 | 1960 | 27 | 1977 |
| 9 | 1964 | 21 | 1976 |
| 15 | 1964 | 22 | 1971 |
| 17 | 1965 | 25 | 1973 |
| 23 | 1967 | 31 | 1975 |
| 19 | 1967 | 27 | 1975 |
| 16 | 1970 | 20 | 1974 |
| 26 | 1971 | 30 | 1975 |
| 18 | 1973 | 25 | 1980 |
| 39 | 1974 | 43 | 1978 |
| 21 | 1975 | 26 | 1979 |

mation on such exposure was sought at the Mayo Clinic, other medical facilities in Olmsted County, including the Olmsted Medical Group, and the County Family Planning Department. Data were also collected on gravidity, parity, smoking history, prior head trauma, and therapeutic radiation. Relative risks were estimated by the odds ratio with the correction factor of Fleiss.[18] Use of oral contraceptives prior to the date of diagnosis was indicated in seven of the 15 patients and 47 of the 58 controls on whom information was available. Two controls were dropped from the analysis, as there was a lack of information as to whether they had used oral contraceptives or not. The controls had a higher frequency of prior oral contraceptive use and the relative risk of only 0.2 is significantly less than unity (Table 7). When oral contraceptive use is restricted to durations of one, two, or three years, the relative risks are slightly higher but always far below one. In Table 8 the cases have been limited to the ten prolactin-secreting tumors. Again, the results are similar in that the relative risks are well below one. Therefore, prior oral contraceptive usage was not associated with pituitary adenomas in general or prolactin-secreting tumors specifically in Olmsted County.

A closer look at the temporal association between pituitary adenomas and oral contraceptives in our series does not support an etiologic relationship. Seven of the 15 patients in this study were between 20 and 25 years of age and would have had only five years or so of potential oral contraceptive exposure. If oral contraceptives were an etiologic factor in pituitary tumors with a short latency period, e.g., five years, one would have expected the upturn in incidence to have begun in the late 1960s rather than the late 1970s. If the association had been the result of a longer latent period, the recent increase would have been confined to women aged 30 and older rather than have occurred throughout the reproductive ages.

TABLE 7.—PITUITARY ADENOMAS AND ORAL
CONTRACEPTIVES (ALL TYPES) IN WOMEN 15–44

| ORAL CONTRACEPTIVE USE | USE | CONTROLS | RR | 95% C.I. |
|---|---|---|---|---|
| Any | 7/15 | 47/58* | 0.2 | 0.1–0.7 |
| 1 yr + | 6/15 | 36/56† | 0.4 | 0.1–1.2 |
| 2 yr + | 5/15 | 26/56 | 0.6 | 0.2–1.9 |
| 3 yr + | 3/15 | 21/56 | 0.5 | 0.1–1.2 |

*Two unknown.
†Two used oral contraceptives for unknown durations.

TABLE 8.—PROLACTIN-SECRETING PITUITARY
TUMORS

| ORAL CONTRACEPTIVE USE | USE | CONTROLS | RR | 95% C.I. |
|---|---|---|---|---|
| Any | 5/10 | 32/39* | 0.2 | 0.1–0.97 |
| 1 yr+ | 4/10 | 25/38† | 0.4 | 0.1–1.5 |
| 2 yr+ | 3/10 | 19/38 | 0.5 | 0.1–1.9 |
| 3 yr+ | 2/10 | 15/38 | 0.4 | 0.1–2.1 |

*One unknown
†Two used oral contraceptives for unknown durations.

## Other Risk Factors

Nulligravidity and nulliparity were more common in the patients than in the controls. Nine of 15 patients were nulliparous while 29 of the 59 controls were nulliparous at the time the adenoma was diagnosed. Other risk factors were not found to be present or were present in equal frequency in the cases and controls. These include a history of head trauma, therapeutic radiation to the head, seizures, smoking, central nervous system infections, thyroid disease and medications.

The patients and controls were reviewed by Dr. Coulam for evidence of prior chronic anovulation syndrome. This diagnosis was made in eight of the 15 patients and in two of the 55 controls for whom there was sufficient information. The resulting relative risk is high, 24.3 (95% confidence interval, 4.9–120.6). Thus, patients with chronic anovulation syndrome, which usually begins at menarche, are at considerable excess risk to having pituitary adenomas diagnosed. This association has also been investigated in a cohort study of all Mayo Clinic patients with a diagnosis of chronic anovulation syndrome between 1970 and 1979. In that study 508 patients have been followed 1,200 women-years after the diagnosis of chronic anovulation syndrome. The expected number of pituitary adenomas in this cohort, based on the Olmsted County incidence rates, is 0.09. Two patients with pituitary adenomas were observed, for a relative risk of 22.2 (2.7–80.2). Although the point estimate is weak the magnitude of increased risk is similar to that found in the case control study.

## Summary

Descriptive studies are needed in other populations to more fully evaluate the changing incidence rates of diagnosed pituitary tumors.

Additional case-control studies may detect possible causes. The restriction of the increased incidence to women of childbearing age is probably attributable to investigations that lead to the discovery of pituitary tumors that originate from complaints of galactorrhea, amenorrhea, and infertility.

## REFERENCES

1. Heshmat M.Y., Kovi J., Simpson C., et al.: Neoplasms of the central nervous system. *Cancer* 38:2135, 1976.
2. Brewis M., Poskanzer D.C., Rolland C., et al.: Neurological disease in an English city. *Acta Neurol. Scand.* (suppl 24):21, 1966.
3. Costello R.T.: Subclinical adenoma of the pituitary gland. *Am. J. Pathol.* 12:205, 1936.
4. Burrow G.N., Rewcastle N.B., Holgate R.C., et al.: Microadenomas of the pituitary and abnormal sellar tomograms in an unselected autopsy series. *N. Engl. J. Med.* 304:156, 1981.
5. Susman W.: Pituitary adenomas. *Br. Med. J.* Dec.:1215, 1933.
6. Close H.G., Lond M.D.: The incidence of adenoma of the pituitary body in some types of new growth. *Lancet* 1:732, 1934.
7. McCormick W.F., Halmi N.S.: Absence of chromophobe adenomas from a large series of pituitary tumors. *Arch. Pathol.* 92:231, 1971.
8. Chang R.J., Keye W.R., Young J.R., et al.: Detection, evaluation, and treatment of pituitary microadenomas in patients with galactorrhea and amenorrhea. *Am. J. Obstet. Gynecol.* 128:356, 1977.
9. Davajan V., Kletzky O., March C.M., et al.: The significance of galactorrhea in patients with normal menses, oligomenorrhea, and secondary amenorrhea. *Am. J. Obstet. Gynecol.* 130:849, 1978.
10. Annegers J.F., Coulam C.B., Abboud C.F., et al.: Pituitary adenoma in Olmsted County, Minnesota, 1935–1977. *Mayo Clin. Proc.* 53:641, 1978.
11. Friedman S., Goldfein A.: Amenorrhea and galactorrhea following oral contraceptive therapy. *J.A.M.A.* 210:1888, 1969.
12. Sherman B.M., Harris C.E., Schlechte J., et al.: Pathogenesis of prolactin-secreting pituitary adenomas. *Lancet* 2:1019, 1978.
13. Hardy J., Beauregard H., Robert F.: Prolactin-secreting pituitary adenomas: Transsphenoidal microsurgical treatment, progress, in Robyn C. et al. (eds): *Prolactin Physiology and Pathology.* New York: Elsevier-North Holland, 1978, pp 361–369.
14. Reichlin S.: The prolactinoma problem. *N. Engl. J. Med.* 300:313, 1979.
15. Thorner M.O., Besser G.M.: Bromocriptine treatment of hyperprolactinaemic hypogonadism. *Acta Endocrinol.* (suppl) 216:131, 1978.
16. Coulam C.B., Annegers J.F., Abboud C.F., et al.: Pituitary adenoma and oral contraceptives: A case-control study. *Fertil. Steril.* 31:25, 1979.
17. Schoenberg B.S., Christine B.W., Whisnant J.P.: The descriptive epidemiology of primary intracranial neoplasms: The Connecticut experience. *Am. J. Epidemiol.* 104:499, 1976.
18. Fleiss J.L.: *Statistical Methods for Rates and Proportions.* New York: John Wiley & Sons, 1973.

# Panel IV: Special Pituitary Problems

*Moderator:* RAYMOND RANDALL, M.D.
*Panelists:* JAMES T. ROBERTSON, M.D., ALLAN ROGOL, M.D., JOHN F. ANNEGERS, M.D.

RANDALL: The question has arisen with regard to thyroid and adrenal evaluation and replacement in patients prior to surgery, and I think everybody is going by their own experience. Dr. Emmanuel and I agree that severe hypothyroidism should be treated prior to surgery. I think most of us are in a somewhat different situation. Perhaps anesthesiologists are not quite as confident, and my own experience is colored by having had some problems even with diagnostic testing, but also anesthesiology, particularly as it relates to large tumors in people who are hypothyroid. So I just think replacement therapy is probably a reasonable approach, certainly in those who are severely hypothyroid, and maybe even the moderately hypothyroid patients and it makes it a bit easier on the anesthesiologist to manage fluid replacement, blood pressure, and so forth at the time of operation. Obviously, in mild hypothyroidism this is not critical, and that is the experience at Mayo Clinic. But I thought that for the rest of us who can wait, whose patients are likely to be closer to us for a period of time, it probably makes sense to go ahead and treat them and bring them in when they are euthyroid for surgery. This does not of course preclude following them postoperatively to see if they have normal thyroid and pituitary function.

Before we ask for questions from the audience, I would like to ask Dr. Rogol to tell us when and how he starts sex steroid replacement in children, because this is such a very important point if one is to provide maximum growth.

0-8151-3530-0/82/0006-0405-0410-$03.75

ROGOL: We start sex steroid therapy usually when the children tell us they want it. That is not as trite as it sounds. Many of the children, when the rest of the kids in their class are starting to go through puberty, start to talk about it. It does, of course, change their bone age relatively rapidly. If they are on growth hormone as well, we talk with them and ask them to wait as long as they possibly can. Some of these youngsters feel good about themselves and will go through high school without sex steroid replacement. When they get to the college age, they often would like to be treated and you cannot blame them for that. Usually it is around 16 or 17. When we replace the gonadal steroids in young men we use testosterone heptanoate, one of the long-acting esters, and begin with 50 mg a month. We do that for a few months and then escalate from 50 to 100 mg, and then to 150 and 200 mg (adult dose). Some adults may need 200 mg a month. Then we usually let them adjust the amount they receive. That means they need about 150 or 200 mg every three to five weeks, and what is enough for an adult has to do with their job and sexual function. That is pretty much how they know when they are "running out of gas" and they need to get steroid replacement. For girls it is a very simple choice: (1) conjugated estrogens (Premarin) and medroxyprogesterone acetate (Provera) and (2) birth control pills. We prefer to use the smallest amount of estrogen possible since these young ladies often will be receiving sex hormones for many years. The replacement dose of the conjugated estrogens is usually 0.625 mg (occasionally 1.25 mg), not the former doses of 1.25 or 2.5 mg per day. With the younger children, 5 mg of medroxyprogesterone acetate is usually enough to cause endometrial shedding but we often use 10 mg per day in the older children. The easiest course is for the children to receive the estrogen beginning on the first day of the month to the 25th day and to add the progestational agent on days 21 to 25 with no medication taken until the first of the next month before which vaginal bleeding has usually occurred. Sometimes, however, we will start them on estrogen alone for up to six months and then start the progestational agent as well. It is important to remember not to use estrogen alone for a prolonged duration. When to begin, again, is a difficult question but it is at the option of these patients after discussing the matter (e.g., ultimate height versus sexual development now).

RANDALL: Very good. It is often a battle or turmoil in the child's mind between desire for more height and desire for sexual maturity. This is usually where the difficulty comes in.

ROGOL: I certainly agree with that and that is why we talk with them and their families. Usually they are able to tell us, "Doctor, when you think I'm ready." But that is not very common.

RANDALL: Thank you. Now I will invite questions.

QUESTION FROM THE AUDIENCE: *Could I follow right up the question about boys in using a slightly less potent androgen such as oxandrolone (Anavar)? Might you get growth without maturation by judiciously using something like that?*

ROGOL: Oxandrolone or Anavar is a synthetic steroid made with the best ratio of anabolic to virilizing ability. Yes, we do use that. We use that in two to three different cases. We use it in some of the patients with constitutional delay, which we have much more experience with. We use it in some of the girls with Turner's syndrome. It is just that usually the boys, if they have hypopituitarism by the time they really feel they need the steroid, ought to go through puberty completely.

RANDALL: *Would you not follow liver functions? Some of these people may get liver function abnormalities.*

ROGOL: We follow liver function every six months to a year. We try to stay away from the oral 17-methyl derivatives because of cholestatic jaundice. Yes we do follow liver function, but we are a little bit different, and I'm sorry I did not say much about dose response, since I am a pharmacologist. If you look at Vincent Kelly's data (Dr. Kelly is from a clinic in Seattle), you will see that they use about 0.25 mg per kg per day, which turns out to be about 2 to 5 pills per day. We have far less difficulty with masculinization in the girls, which can be a problem in terms of hair and voice changes as well as liver function. As a matter of fact, during the six years that Drs. Ann Johanson, Bob Blizzard, and I have been at Charlottesville, we had no major and maybe no minor problems using 0.1 mg per kg of Anavar rather than the greater dosage.

QUESTION FROM THE AUDIENCE: *I would like to ask you and Dr. Robertson about the postoperative cortisol replacement in the Cushing's disease patient as well as, let's say, the prolactinoma patient. You suggested that you do not give any steroids for patients with prolactin-secreting adenoma after the operation, right? In other words, you measure plasma cortisone, and if it is normal, you give none?*

RANDALL: That's correct. If they are low or borderline, we do give replacement and reevaluate in three months.

QUESTION FROM THE AUDIENCE: *If the cortisol levels were low, what you would do?*

RANDALL: We hope they are low in Cushing's disease because that means the tumor has come out. Then they need replacement therapy.

If the values are absolutely normal (we have only had this happen a couple of times), we watch the patient, and follow him carefully. This means that the surgeon has not got out all of the tumor. Because they should not be normal, they should be depressed. I happen to remember one patient who had normal values and normal suppression. About nine months later, back came her Cushing's disease. So, she did not have a successful treatment. Dr. Robertson, would you like to take that?

ROBERTSON: Endocrinologists in our city manage the patient with Cushing's disease postoperatively in different ways. In an effort to regain function in the suppressed corticotropes around the tumor, one group will allow the patient to have very low cortisol levels in an effort to stimulate recovery of the ACTH-secreting mechanism. If patients do not have too many symptoms, the philosophy is to allow them to reestablish a normal pituitary-adrenal axis so that they will not require replacement therapy. This works surprisingly well for the young but not so well for the older individuals. It may take as long as 6–9 months to a year for them to recover full function of the ACTH-secreting mechanism after being suppressed by the autonomous tumor making ACTH. Other endocrinologists do not put the patient to this degree of discomfort and will give them replacement therapy immediately postoperatively and continue it. We do not routinely give cortisol coverage during surgery or cortisol replacement after surgery unless the patient demonstrates an impaired diurnal swing of cortisol in the preoperative study period. If they have a normal diurnal swing of cortisol preoperatively, we usually do not give them cortisol replacement. So far all of them have done very well on treatment based on these criteria.

RANDALL: Most of our patients with Cushing's disease do not live nearby, so we cannot watch them as carefully as you can.

QUESTION: *What is the incidence of severe headaches in patients with microadenomas?*

RANDALL: I can't tell you the incidence, but I can tell you that as we looked over our cases, we have found, much to our surprise, that some of the patients have had headaches that disappear when the microadenomas are removed. Now, whether or not this is a placebo effect, I don't know, but it has happened enough so that I am convinced that some patients who have microadenomas get headaches from them.

ROBERTSON: I agree. I am not sure exactly what the mechanism of the headache is. Whether it is placebo effect or not, it is a fact. Headaches certainly can be a major complaint. It seems to me to be more common in the acromegalic and prolactin tumors than it is in the Cushing's cases.

QUESTION: *In my experience the use of chlorothiazide or chlorpro-pamide has been very effective in the management of patients with diabetes insipidus. On a cost effective basis these pills were remark-ably cheaper. Is this a unique experience?*

RANDALL: No, mild diabetes insipidus can be readily treated as you mentioned. I have done it that way myself. I have purposely not used chlorpropamide because some reportedly have hypoglycemia from it. If one is dealing with severe diabetes insipidus that cannot be con-trolled with any combination of medication, DDAVP has it all over intramuscular Pitressin tannate in oil, as Dr. Rogol pointed out.

STATEMENT FROM THE AUDIENCE: There is a significant difference in price of these two, though. One costs like $100 per month and the other about $25 per month.

RANDALL: There are other things, though, to be taken into consid-eration. People with permanent DI, who get a lot of Pitressin tannate in oil in their muscles over a period of years, get granulomas and sometimes abscesses, and you are pretty hard put to find a site to put it in. DDAVP has been a godsend to them. I must say that I have yet to take a single person off Pitressin tannate in oil and start him on DDAVP who wanted to change back because of price or any other reason. It is just such a much better medication to take. Yes, it is more expensive. Yes, we do as you do. We tell them to adjust the minimum effective dose because it is expensive—$35 for 2.5 ml.

COMMENT FROM THE AUDIENCE: I had one patient on Pitressin tan-nate in oil. I offered her DDAVP. She tried it for one bottle and came back and asked for something else. She had been requiring a fairly sizable dose of the DDAVP, and we were able to control her nicely with a combination of chlorothiazide and chlorpropamide. I think there must be some patients who have enough residual func-tion to allow you to use the pills.

RANDALL: Yes. I imagine that a patient like yours whom you can control with a lesser medication probably was not using the DDAVP correctly. This is a very important point because if they let it dribble out the front of their nose, or more likely put that little tube inside the nose and blow so hard it goes down into the throat, they have lost it. So it is important that it be placed properly.

COMMENT FROM THE AUDIENCE: I would like to make a point about the proper use of DDAVP. We have had excellent success with pa-tients and its effects. But our biggest problem is when they come in the hospital, and for some reason as it sometimes happens, the nurse gives them the medication. We make our patients give it to themselves as soon as they are physically able to do so because the nurses are sort of unsteady in blowing something into someone's nose. This is the problem we have had when DDAVP "didn't work in the hospital."

# Index

411